Pilates Applications for
Health Conditions

of related interest

Fascia in Motion
Fascia-Focused Movement for Pilates
By Elizabeth Larkam
ISBN 978 1 90914 128 5
eISBN 978 1 91208 524 8

Centered, Second Edition
Organizing the Body through Kinesiology, Movement Theory and Pilates Techniques
Madeline Black
ISBN 978 1 91208 595 8
eISBN 978 1 91208 596 5

Pilates-Based Movement for Menopause A Guide for Teachers and Practitioners
Dinah Siman
Foreword by Elizabeth Larkam
ISBN 978 1 91342 667 5
eISBN 978 1 83997 647 6

A Movement Educator's Guide to Pregnancy and Childbirth
Jennifer Gianni
Forewords by Marie Jose Blom and Nora St John
ISBN 978 1 91342 653 8
eISBN 978 1 91342 654 5

Spinal Asymmetry and Scoliosis
Movement and Function Solutions for the Spine, Ribcage and Pelvis
Suzanne Clements Martin
ISBN 978 1 90914 172 8
eISBN 978 1 90914 173 5

Pilates Applications for Health Conditions

Volume 1

Multi-system conditions

Edited by

Madeline Black and Elizabeth Larkam

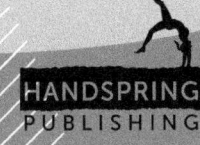

HANDSPRING
PUBLISHING

First published in Great Britain in 2025
by Handspring Publishing, an imprint of Jessica Kingsley Publishers
Part of John Murray Press

2

A CIP catalogue record for this title is available from the British Library and the Library of Congress

ISBN 978 1 91208 597 2
eISBN 978 1 91208 598 9

Printed and bound by CPI Group (UK) Ltd, Croydon, CR0 4YY

Jessica Kingsley Publishers' policy is to use papers that are natural, renewable and recyclable products and made from wood grown in sustainable forests. The logging and manufacturing processes are expected to conform to the environmental regulations of the country of origin.

Handspring Publishing
Carmelite House
50 Victoria Embankment
London EC4Y 0DZ

www.handspringpublishing.com

John Murray Press
Part of Hodder & Stoughton Limited
An Hachette UK Company

The authorised representative in the EEA is Hachette Ireland,
8 Castlecourt Centre, Dublin 15, D15 XTP3, Ireland (email: info@hbgi.ie)

Contents

Foreword

Diane Lee

It is an honour to write a foreword for the publication of two volumes on the application of Pilates to health conditions by editors Madeline Black and Elizabeth Larkam; two Pilates professionals well known not only in their discipline but throughout the world of musculoskeletal therapy.

I am not an expert in Pilates. I have trained extensively as a client with Pilates practitioners and witnessed the benefits for my own conditions. I am a physical therapist who practices/teaches a whole person/whole body model known as The Integrated Systems Model (ISM). In this approach, clients with complex stories and multiple impairments often have many things they cannot do well; walk/run, sit, sleep, lift etc. They also have many impairments due to multiple past traumas. Where to begin? In ISM, we begin by prioritizing the goal, or task, the individual would like to work on – this is called the meaningful task. From that point, everything (assessment, treatment, training) is focused towards that goal. When that task is improved, we pick the next one. I have not had this prioritized task experience in any Pilates program I have attended, to date.

There are several features and concepts in these two volumes on Pilates for health conditions that complement the principles of ISM and that I truly appreciate about this work.

- It is meaningful task, and individual, focused. We know from much research that strategies for movement are individual and *task specific*. Therefore, if assessment and treatment/training are not directed toward the task that is sub-optimal, then relevant deficits may not be appreciated, nor changed, and goals not met. The task chosen for every contributor to this work was gait. Every health condition including Multiple Sclerosis, (MS), Ehlers-Danlos Syndrome (EDS), Postural Orthostatic Tachycardial Syndrome (POTS), Mast Cell Activation Syndrome (MCAS), long COVID, Pelvic Girdle Pain (PGP) Diastatis Rectus Abdominis (DRA), Bone Health, Aging Well etc. impacts movement and this is reflected in one's gait. Two more volumes could potentially be written if the meaningful task was sitting; another highly meaningful task and I'm sure the programs in those two volumes would look very different! Programs must be task specific and individual. The only way to demonstrate the uniqueness of each program is to choose a task and show through a case report the specificity to an individual. The bulk of these two volumes is filled with individual case reports. If the chapters were *condition or body region focused*, and not client-centered, the detail required for individualization would be lost.

- Each chapter contributor was required to complete a standardized whole body/person assessment form that is incredibly thorough and the findings from this assessment led to an individualized program. There are no recipes for specific conditions and/or body regions in these two volumes because every assessment is unique to the individual *even though the task goal (gait) is the same*. While the focus is on improving gait and addressing mobility and control of the musculoskeletal system, the inclusion of cases that also have complex medical co-morbidities (such as those listed in #1 and more) allows us to see how the programs were adapted from the beginning, and on the fly, to accommodate the challenges these medical conditions present. Recovery, for most, is never linear and adding the self-report before every session allowed us to see how the program was paced/adapted.

- Many of the cases presented here would be excluded from a randomized controlled trial due to their multiple co-morbidities; yet, this is the practitioner's challenge. We see these individual's daily and it's extremely valuable for Pilates practitioners to now have these two volumes as a resource to provide guidance for assessment, treatment and training. While no two stories will ever be the same, there is enough convergence within the divergence presented here to find some help.

- Lastly, each chapter took us on a journey and revealed the progression of the program as well as the evolution of each individual's recovery. The concise theoretical information presented before each case and the clinical application of that knowledge in the Pilates program that followed reflects a high level of care – this work represents the state of the art/science of Pilates practice.

I'm sure these two volumes on Pilates Application for Health Conditions will be used by many for decades to come.

Diane Lee PT, South Surrey, BC, Canada

January 2025

Foreword

Kristi Cooper

Pilates is a practice that transforms lives. It extends beyond physical movement—it restores, strengthens, and empowers. Pilates Applications for Health Conditions represents a pivotal step in fulfilling Joseph H. Pilates' vision and establishing growing recognition of Pilates as a respected health and wellness practice.

I first met Madeline Black and Elizabeth Larkam about 15 years ago, at a pivotal time. I was in the early stages of launching Pilates Anytime, an online subscription platform dedicated to making Pilates accessible to all and preserving its oral history through the Pilates Legacy Project. They were established entities with prolific voices in preserving Pilates and sharing the application to individual health considerations.

I remember feeling nervous when I first approached each of them, hoping they would share my vision and contribute to what I was building. Thankfully, they both said yes! Thus began a longstanding personal and professional relationship with both. I have been in anatomical dissection courses with them at different times. You get to know a person in an anatomy lab! Through my business, I have also had the pleasure of working with and developing friendships with several of the contributors to this book.

I have witnessed Madeline and Elizabeth's unwavering individual commitment to honoring Pilates' legacy while continuously evolving its practice to meet the needs of diverse individuals and the industry. They never cease to inspire me and so many others. They constantly learn and always share the fruits of their efforts. I am a grateful recipient!

For those who have practiced Pilates, whether for fitness, rehabilitation, or as part of a journey to reclaim health, its impact is undeniable. Ask anyone with a regular practice—whether or not they have a diagnosed condition—and they will have their own story to tell. My journey with Pilates began over 40 years ago as a teenager. The reasons I practiced and became a teacher back then are vastly different from the reasons I returned after suffering a traumatic brain injury (TBI) in 2016. What I did know was that Pilates would be my path back to health, and I am forever grateful to those in this book—Elizabeth Larkam, Madeline Black, Dawn Marie-Ickes, Emilee Garfield, Rebekah Rotstein, and Jessie Lee—who supported me in my recovery.

This book is a treasure trove of expertise, offering practical applications and programs that give teachers confidence in their work. It is like having THE contact list of top professionals at your fingertips—what a gift!

This collection of wisdom, experience, and expertise will continue to shape the future of Pilates and its role in healthcare. It is an honor to witness this method's evolution and support the work of those who continue to use it.

The comprehensive scope of this book and meticulous attention to detail are a testament to the dedication of the co-editors and contributors. It is more than just a collection of knowledge—it is a guide, a resource, and an inspiration for those who seek to understand and apply Pilates in meaningful ways. Each exercise in every movement program is thoroughly documented in terms of its relationship to the vocabulary of JH Pilates, as recorded in the

NCPT Study Guide. Exercises attributed to teachers designated by Mr. Pilates trace their origins. In recognition of Pilates Legacy, this book also includes the contributions of Eve Gentry, Kathy Grant, Romana Kryzanowska, and Carola Trier.

Times have changed! Historically, Pilates teachers relied on apprenticeship to learn. Now, it is easy to be distracted by re-created shapes and performance-based Pilates often displayed on various social media channels. This book, however, contrasts those fleeting images with solid information from leading contributors in the industry. In short, this book is the ultimate resource for accompanying your in-person and online training and workshops to take your practice to the next level.

Whether you are a teacher, practitioner, or simply someone curious about the profound impact of movement on well-being, this book will offer valuable insights that stand the test of time. I wholeheartedly recommend this book and encourage you to immerse yourself in the generously shared wisdom.

Kristi Cooper, Co-founder of Pilates Anytime

Preface

Handspring Publishing invited us to co-edit a book based on Pilates research. During our initial meetings in the Spring of 2018, we reviewed the available research and found limited applicability to the studio environment. Research design does not provide the Pilates teacher with the pedagogical detail needed to customize results for each client.

The privilege of longevity in studying, teaching, and writing in the movement field through four decades contributes to our unique perspective on human movement and Pilates. Given that we work in a movement lab (the studio), not a research lab, we have the responsibility of designing a book that enhances the daily work of Pilates teachers. We bring our combined experience to serve Pilates practitioners and their clients with this book: *Pilates Applications for Health Conditions.*

Health may be considered from a variety of perspectives. According to Gabor Maté, MD, the root word of "healing" means "returning to wholeness" (Maté 2022). The World Health Organization Constitution (2020) defines health as "a state of complete physical, mental, and social well-being and not merely the absence of disease or infirmity."

> Health and illness are not random states in a particular body or body part. They are, in fact, an expression of an entire life lived, one that cannot, in turn, be understood in isolation: it is influenced by—or better yet, it arises from—a web of circumstances, relationships, events and experiences. (Maté 2022)

The perspective of this book considers health as a healing process, not an achievement of eliminating disease states. Diane Lee, BSR, FCAMPT, states: "Restoring health is about more than removing disease; creating optimal strategies for function and performance is about more than removing pain. What it means to be 'in health' is individually defined. It is linked to individual values and goals" (Lee 2011). As co-editors, we realize we are responsible for creating a book that addresses the complex health conditions facing Pilates teachers today. Many of these conditions were not prevalent when Joseph Pilates developed his system in the years from 1929 to 1967 (NPCE Study Guide 2021).

This book is distinct from all other Pilates resources. We value the uniqueness of the equipment designs and choreography of Joseph H. Pilates. We support a critical examination and application of the Pilates Method. We invited contributors with expertise grounded in years of experience and research studies to design, teach, and document Pilates movement programs. Our intent was to examine gait efficiency and its relationship to specific health conditions. Each contribution demonstrates how a customized Pilates program may fulfill movement potential, supporting the process of healing and living with a health condition.

For 40 years, Joseph Pilates taught his movement system of body conditioning (Contrology) in his New York gym (New York Times 1967).

> The period from the late nineteenth century until the beginning of World War I was characterized by optimism and new technology and medical discoveries. A cultural revolution in health and well-being developed during this period, especially in Germany. Joseph Pilates was one of many Europeans intertwining physical practice and discipline. (Larkam 2017)

He championed that the Pilates Method "corrects

and vitalizes the human body" (Larkam 2017). Mr. Pilates' perspective to "correct" the human body was derived from the culture of his time. "The back would be flat if the spine were kept as straight as a plumb line, and its flexibility would be comparable to that of the finest watch spring steel" (Pilates 1945). Mr. Pilates' publications describe movement practices that mold a body into his ideal alignment for the purpose of improved health. The cultural environment and lifestyle practices prevalent today have impacts on human health even Mr. Pilates did not predict. A postural strategy of sustained lumbar flexion contributes to a loss of torso reflexive activity. A study by Maaswinkel *et al.*, published in the *Journal of Biomechanics* in 2015, states that "the muscle pre-activation prior to the onset of perturbation was significantly lower in the flexed posture compared to neutral."

Appreciating and understanding how a person organizes themselves helps the movement teacher design effective movement sequences with a whole-person perspective. Evolving awareness of influences from past and present cultural biases impacts how we move and approach healing.

In contrast to the theory of biomechanics, current paradigms articulate new perspectives on human movement and its relationship to health. Both laboratory and clinical research publications have shown that static alignment and "straight spine" are not required for efficient movement or good health. Efficiency of movement requires an integrated neuromyofascial system to transfer forces through the tissues adapting to stimuli. The Integrated Model of Function developed by Diane Lee explains how form and force closure, together with motor control and emotional states, influence how loads are transferred through the lumbopelvic-hip complex (Lee 2011).

Stephen M. Levin, MD, conceived and defined the algorithm of biotensegrity in 1974 as a force vector model (Scarr 2018).

The language of Biotensegrity is the language of soft matter physics. It is tension and compression with continuity. The premise of Biotensegrity is non-linear continuous matter that is self-generated, self-organising, self-stressing, hierarchical, load distributing and low energy consuming. There are no shear moments, no bending moments, no levers, and no joints. (Sharkey 2015)

The compilation of movement programs in this book addresses the unique expression of gait as a human self-organizing and load distributing movement reflective of the healing process. This book contributes to the process of moving from the past belief systems and embracing new paradigms.

Madeline Black
Elizabeth Larkam

References

Larkam, E. (2017) *Fascia in Motion: Fascia-Focused Movement for Pilates.* Edinburgh: Handspring Publishing, p. 32, Figure 2.1; p. 31.

Lee, D. (2011) *The Pelvic Girdle: An Integration of Clinical Expertise and Research.* 4th Ed. Churchill Livingstone Elsevier, p. 52, Box 22; pp. 49–50, 164.

Maaswinkel, E., van Drunen, P., Veeger, D., van Dieën, J. (2015) "Effects of vision and lumbar posture on trunk neuromuscular control." *Journal of Biomechanics, 48,* 2, 298–303.

Maté, G., with D. Maté (2022) *The Myth of Normal: Trauma, Illness & Healing in a Toxic Culture.* New York City: Avery Publishing, Penguin Random House, pp. 9–11.

New York Times (1967) "Joseph H. Pilates, Body Builder, 86; Developer of 'Contrology' Operated 8th Ave. Gym." *New York Times,* October 10, 1967, p. 47. www.nytimes.com/1967/10/10/archives/joseph-h-pilates-body-builder-86-developer-of-contrology-operated.html. [Accessed August 1, 2023].

NPCE Study Guide (National Pilates Certification Exam Study Guide) (2021) Miami, FL: National Pilates Certification Program, Inc., pp. 94–97.

Pilates, J. H. (1945 [2010]) *Return to Life Through Contrology.* Miami, FL: Pilates Method Alliance, Inc., pp. 1–35.

Scarr, G. (2018) *Biotensegrity: The Structural Basis of Life.* 2nd Ed. Edinburgh: Handspring Publishing, p. xiii.

Sharkey, J. (2015) *Biotensegrity—the fallacy of biomechanics: Part 2.* December 23, 2015. www.johnsharkeyevents.com/research/2015/12/23/biotensegrity-the-fallacy-of-biomechanics-part-2. [Accessed August 1, 2023].

World Health Organization (2020) *WHO Director-General's opening remarks at the Empire Club of Canada.* November 20, 2020. www.who.int/director-general/speeches/detail/who-director-general-s-opening-remarks-at-the-empire-club-of-canada. [Accessed August 1, 2023].

Introduction

Madeline Black and Elizabeth Larkam

I only went out for a walk and...going out, I found, was really going in.

Hippocrates proclaimed that "walking is man's best medicine" (McCarthy 2023). Living day to day involves continuous adaptation and response. Individuals and social systems respond unconsciously and consciously to both internal states and external environments. This book focuses on human movement adaptations and responses influenced by health conditions. Specifically, gait is considered in relationship to health and the process of healing. Numerous studies indicate gait patterns are associated with early detection of health conditions, including Parkinson's disease (Gilat *et al.* 2017), cognitive decline (Bridenbaugh and Kressig 2015), and dementia (Kondragunta and Hirtz 2020). Each of the Pilates movement programs in this book documents the client's movement and gait adaptations. Each program reflects the client's experience of their healing process.

As co-editors we initially designed the methods and materials following the case report format. During the editing process we realized that the program documentation required for a cohesive, practical manuscript had evolved and no longer satisfied case report guidelines.

Each movement contributor followed the format of assessment, program design, teaching, and reassessment. Documents were provided to record the 12-session process (see Chapter 4). Each client program began with health history and an observational assessment of gait. Each contributor observed and documented their client's movement and gait strategies. Program design and pedagogy were developed based on the findings. During the home program and equipment practice, each client was guided to notice their self-organizing movement strategies. The teacher and client worked together as a team to consciously shift toward more efficient movement patterns. The final assessment documentation indicated a more efficient gait. Clients' self-reports expressed an improved attitude toward their healing process and health. The practice of skills acquisition promoted an uplifted sense of hope and self-efficacy.

We invited additional experts to provide perspectives on Pilates movement programs. Dr. Sherri Betz, DPT, details a history of Pilates research. Graham Scarr, DO, considers human movement within the paradigm of biotensegrity. Ken Endelman explains the variable resistance of springs. Variable spring resistance in the frame of Pilates equipment designs is distinct from other forms of resistance prevalent in exercise environments. The contributed movement programs reference J. H. Pilates' exercises and incorporate the pedagogy developed by Eve Gentry, Kathy Grant, Romana Kryzanowska, and Carola Trier. Sarita Allen wrote about working for Kathy Grant, her teacher and mentor. Alycea Ungaro contributes her perspective on her teacher, Romana Kryzanowska.

In this book you will find:

- Pilates movement programs of home exercise and studio equipment sequences for different health conditions
- An assessment observation guide you can use with your clients

- A glossary of terms and a list of abbreviations
- Photos
- Anatomical illustrations references
- A list of equipment and props for each movement program
- A delineation of the J. H. Pilates' movement vocabulary as documented in the *National Pilates Certification Exam Study Guide* (NPCE Study Guide 2021)
- Reference to teachers who studied with J. H. Pilates whose vocabulary is included in the contributed programs (Gentry, Grant, Kryzanowska, Trier)

Timeline of the book

The development of the book spans the years prior to and throughout the global pandemic. The book is shaped by the pandemic timeline and trends in health care. The global pandemic affected each book contributor and the program they designed, taught, and documented for their client. This book reflects how the global pandemic shaped the interactions of Pilates teachers and clients. Contributors started their programs prior to and during the pandemic. Some programs were conducted entirely in person prior to the pandemic. Some programs were hybrid, starting in person and completing on screen. Some programs were conducted entirely on screen.

How to use this book

This book is a thorough resource designed for in-depth study. It is a studio companion providing guidance and inspiration to Pilates teachers as they design, implement, teach, and document client programs. Become acquainted with the book, getting an overview by looking at the photos accompanying each of the programs. Become familiar with the anatomical illustrations in Appendix 1.

When you are ready to settle in and study:

- Focus on Chapter 4, assessment

- Complete the assessment documentation form included in Appendix 2 with yourself as the client
- Implement the assessment documentation; make video clips of your own gait
- Read the health condition program that is most interesting to you
- Prior to implementing any movement sequence during a client session, practice on yourself. Become familiar with the kinesthetic logic and cues
- Practice each suggested movement sequence noticing how your gait is influenced.
- With your client's permission, make video documentation of your client's gait. Both you and the client can observe changes in movement efficiency
- Repeat this process for each program included in the book
- Study the references for more detail and understanding
- Continue to study with references noted in this book

The truth you believe in and cling to makes you unavailable to hear anything new.

Pema Chödrön

Allow for the possibility that interacting with this book may upgrade your own practice and teaching skills and contribute to each client's healing process.

With gratitude
Madeline and Elizabeth

References

Bridenbaugh, S. A. and Kressig, R. W. (2015) "Motor cognitive dual tasking: Early detection of gait impairment, fall risk and cognitive decline." *Zeitschrift für Gerontologie und Geriatrie, 48,* 1, 15–21.

Chödrön, P. (2012) *The Wisdom of No Escape: How to Love Yourself and Your World.* HarperCollins.

Gilat, M., Bell, P. T., Ehgoetz Martens, K. A., Georgiades, M. J. *et al.* (2017) "Dopamine depletion impairs gait automaticity by altering cortico-striatal and cerebellar processing in Parkinson's disease." *Neuroimage, 152,* 207–220.

Kondragunta, J. and Hirtz, G. (2020) "Gait parameter estimation of elderly people using 3D human pose estimation in early detection of dementia." *Annual International Conference of the IEEE Engineering in Medicine & Biology Society. 2020,* 5798–5801.

McCarthy, A. (2023) "Whatever the problem, it's probably solved by walking." *New York Times,* March 25, 2023. www.nytimes.com/2023/03/25/opinion/walking-hiking-spring.html. [Accessed August 1, 2023].

NPCE Study Guide (National Pilates Certification Exam Study Guide) (2021) Miami, FL: National Pilates Certification Program, Inc.

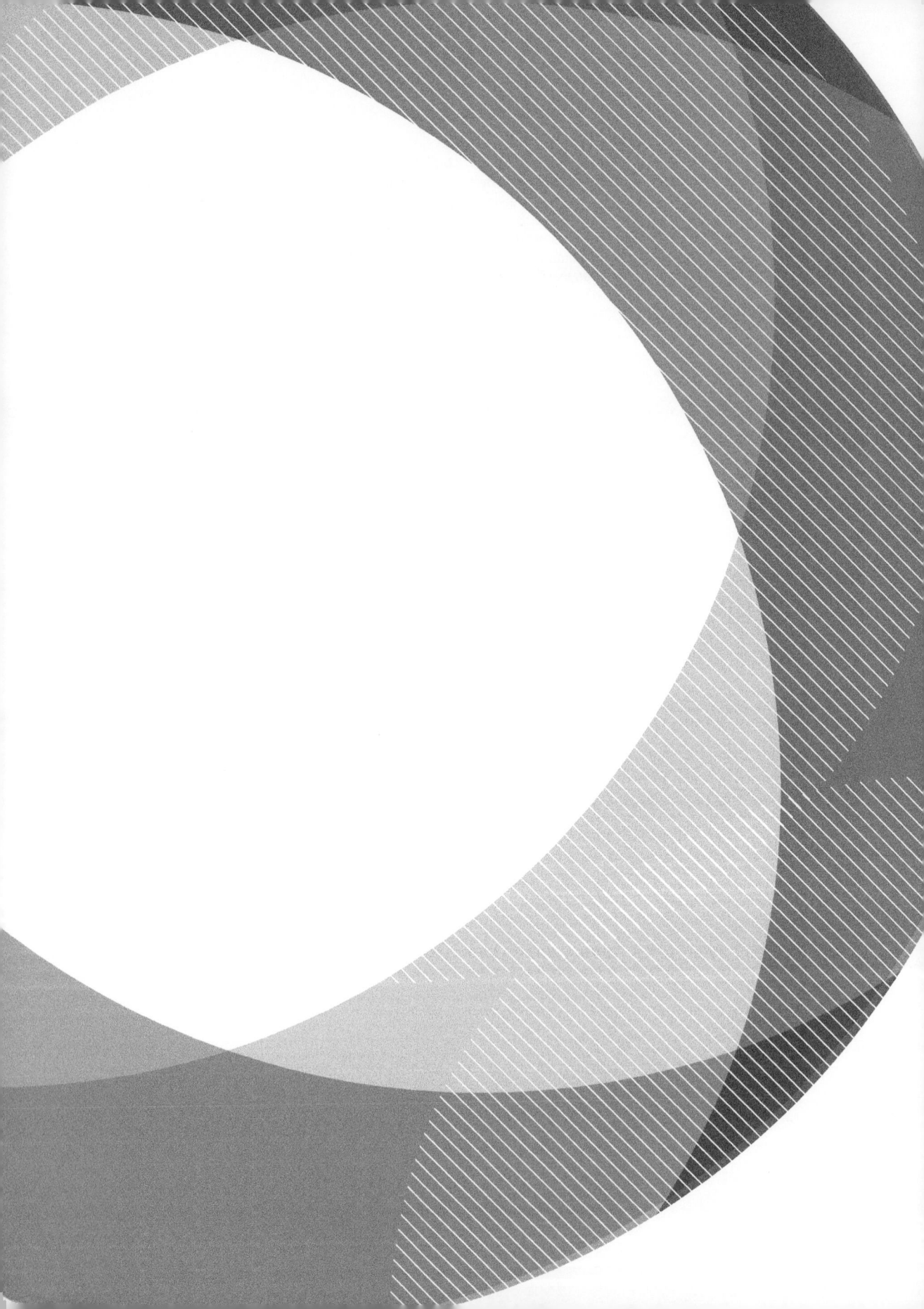

Contributor Biographies

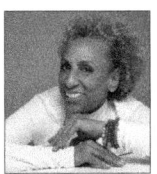

Sarita Allen

Sarita Allen is a classically trained dancer and was an original member of the Alvin Ailey Repertory Ensemble and Complexions Contemporary Ballet where she is currently an Artistic Advisor. Sarita has been a regular contributor to Pilates Anytime, Pilatesology, and Pilates Alliance. Her wellness and fitness work has been acknowledged in fitness publications including Self Magazine, Fit Life, and Very Well, the number one online fitness reference. She continues to be invited to teach Pilates workshops around the world in Brazil, Hawaii, Japan, France, and Italy.

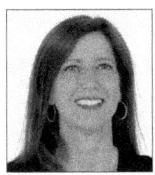

Sherri Betz

Sherri Betz, PT, DPT, is a physical therapist and director of Thera-Pilates® Physical Therapy Clinics in Louisiana and California, specializing in geriatrics and osteoporosis. She is devoted to improving awareness about geriatric exercise, bone health, and safe yoga- and Pilates-based exercise through professional and consumer education as well as through the promotion of low-cost, on-site, and virtual community exercise programs for fit and frail older adults. Dr. Betz is the recipient of both the PMA Deborah Lessen Award for her many years of dedicated service to PMA and the APTA Geriatrics Lynn Phillippi Advocacy for Older Adults Award. She continues to publish numerous articles, author book chapters, produce videos, and speak internationally about Pilates for special conditions and exercise for osteoporosis.

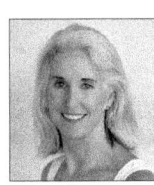

Madeline Black

A Nationally Certified Pilates Teacher, Madeline Black's life pursuit is the discovery of how the human body moves. Over 30 years in the field of movement, her curiosity has explored all aspects of movement in dance, Pilates, yoga, Gyrotonic®, fitness training, and, from studies of human biomechanics, applied biotensegrity, human cadaver dissection labs, and osteopathic and manual therapies. Madeline developed the Madeline Black Method™, a movement method that improves function and strength based on intelligent assessments, manual techniques, and exercise sequences that help people achieve their fullest movement potential. Her extensive study and widely respected accomplishments in the field of movement and fitness have fueled her rise as an international leader in movement and exercise education. She is the author of *Centered* (Handspring Publishing), now in its second edition.

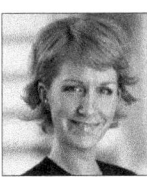

Jojo Bowman

Originally a professional ballet dancer with The Royal Danish Ballet, Jojo Bowman, NCPT, AMRSPH, is one of the pioneers of the Pilates Method Alliance initiative Heroes in Motion® and the director and co-founder of the medically endorsed Danish Wounded Warriors Project. She has received awards such as the Medal of the Danish Society of Military Medicine, the Anders Lassen award, and a special commendation by the Royal Society of Public Health amongst others. Jojo is a published author and lecturer, as well as a movement teacher for Paralympic athletes. Her most valued mentors are her wounded warriors, who continuously inspire her every day.

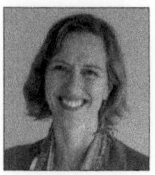

Marylee Bussard

Marylee Bussard, NCPT, ATSI, is an entrepreneur and educator dedicated to helping individuals experience freedom, comfort, and capacity in their bodies through a holistic, client-centered approach that draws on over 20 years' experience in movement and manual therapy. She has a passion for working with people who don't fit the mold of traditional fitness programs, such as those experiencing chronic pain, physical or emotional trauma, and "zebras" with invisible or difficult-to-diagnose conditions. Marylee is Founder of Chaturanga Holistic Fitness (est. 2010) and the Chicago School of Pilates and co-author of *Functional Anatomy of the Pilates Core* (North Atlantic). Marylee splits her time between Chicago and the Tampa Bay area.

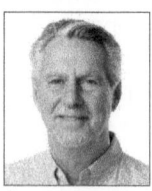

Ken Endelman

Ken Endelman, CEO, Balanced Body Inc., founded Balanced Body in 1976 after a Pilates instructor visited his furniture store in Hollywood, California and asked him to build an improved version of a Universal Reformer. After studying the Pilates methodology and original apparatus, Ken designed a modern Universal Reformer that was reliable, safe, and user-friendly. Under Endelman's leadership, Balanced Body has grown into the world's largest resource for Pilates equipment and education. He has collaborated with Pilates educators, studio owners, fitness club operators, physical therapists, athletic trainers, and home users to create equipment that combines Joseph Pilates' original designs with our modern understanding of human biomechanics. His innovations have been awarded over 43 patents in the United States and hundreds more worldwide.

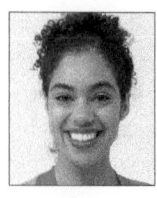

Rosa Marimba Gold-Watts

Rosa Marimba Gold-Watts, NCPT, RCST®, is currently an instructor on Apple Fitness+. Formerly a professional dancer, she began studying Pilates in 1997. She was certified at the Kane School of Core Integration in 2007. In 2012 she founded Articulating Body Inc. She has studied extensively with Christine Wright; Dr. Kate Klemer, DC, RCST; Marika Molnar, PT, LAC; Madeline Black; Jean-Claude West; and Kelly Kane. In 2018, Marimba won the Pilates Anytime Next Instructor competition. She has taught at Momentum Fest, the PMA, and IADMS conferences. She has taught Horton technique at the Ailey School since 2005, and throughout the US and Italy.

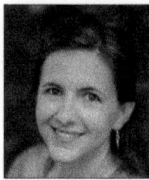

Amy Hershey

Amy Hershey, MS, is a graduate of the Pilates Center Advanced Teacher Training program in Boulder, CO. She has completed the Kathy Grant Heritage Training Program and holds a certificate as a Specialist in Pilates-Based Exercises for Neurological Conditions. In addition to her Pilates trainings, Amy has a master's degree in Applied Physiology and Kinesiology and is a certified corrective exercise specialist. Amy was first treated for Lyme disease in 2012 and in 2017 was subsequently treated for ehrlichiosis, which is one of the Lyme co-infections. In addition to her own medical journey, Amy began seeing a rise in clients over the years who were struggling with various symptoms associated with Lyme disease.

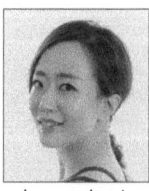

Ji Hyun Koo

Ji Hyun Koo, PMA-NCPT, ACSM-CPT, ACSM-CET, is a Balanced Body Master Instructor and Director of Korea Integrated Movement Academy, where she is also an anatomy instructor. She is CEO of Pilates the Balance Centum, co-author of *Pilates Bible*, instructor at Busan Student Culture and Arts Center and Busan School for the Blind, and Director of Haeundae Pilates Federation.

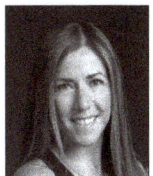

Meghann Koppele Duffy

Meghann Koppele Duffy, NCPT, MS, is an international Pilates educator, specializing in working with people with neurological conditions and a co-founder of The Neuro Studio. Meghann is a Kane School, Nationally Certified Pilates Teacher, as well as a Certified Strength & Condition Specialist since 2002. Meghann received a BS in exercise science from the University of Scranton and a master's degree in Applied Physiology from Columbia University. Along with her business partner Mariska Breland, Meghann created the first online movement education tool for people with Neurological Conditions, called The Neuro Studio. When Meghann is not working, she is spending time with her husband and their two dogs.

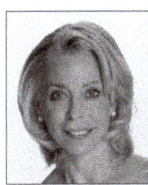

Elizabeth Larkam

Elizabeth Larkam, NCPT, is internationally recognized as an innovator of movement education. Elizabeth began her Pilates studies in 1985 while teaching dance at Stanford University, where she had received her bachelor's and master's education. A Gold Certified Pilates Method Alliance teacher, she was educated by the first-generation Pilates teachers. Elizabeth co-founded and co-owned Polestar Education. When Balanced Body Pilates Education was founded in 2004, she became a Master Teacher and Mentor, conducting courses throughout the world. Elizabeth is a Feldenkrais® practitioner, Franklin Method teacher, and Gyrotonic® and Gyrokinesis® instructor. She is qualified in Gyrotonic® II and Gyrotonic Specialized Equipment. She is the author of *Fascia in Motion: Fascia-Focused Movement for Pilates*, also published by Handspring.

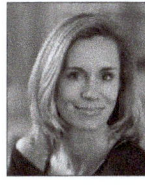

Jessie Lee

Jessie Lee is a Pilates, Gyrotonic®, and Gyrokinesis® instructor and has worked for more than 25 years in the field of movement rehabilitation. She is the founder and director of Copenhagen Pilates Studio and co-founder and director of the medically endorsed Danish Wounded Warriors Project (DWWP). She has received several awards for her humanitarian efforts, among others the Medal of the Danish Society of Military Medicine. Jessie is a lecturer within the field of movement strategies for trauma-related injuries. She is a published author and has presented her work at medical symposiums in Denmark and lectures and teaches workshops internationally.

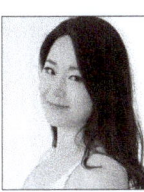

Eunju Lim

Eunju Lim, PhD, PMA-NCPT, ACSM-CPT, ACSM/ACS-CET, the headmaster of Return to Life & Health. She presented research at PMA (2018, 2019, 2021, 2022, 2023) and was invited as the lecture presenter of Korea at PMA 2022 in Las Vegas. Eunju accomplished special movement certifications and continue training for instructors such as Sissel Academy SPINEFITTER Senior Educator, EBFA(NABOSO), Oov Fitness/Group educator and Recovering Master. She is the translated author of Jillian Hessel's "Pilates Basics". Additionally, Eunju has been presenting at CKLZ (Best Fitness, Yoga, Pilates convention in Korea) since 2023 to deliver the post-rehabilitation approach of Pilates to many instructors.

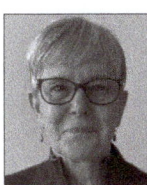

Julie Lyons

With master's degrees in both physical therapy and traditional Chinese medicine, I dedicated my career to integrative healing. My early work in hospitals and private clinics focused on osteopathic manual medicine and spinal rehabilitation. Later, I ran a private practice in Alameda, California, for nearly 20 years, combining acupuncture, herbal medicine, and osteopathic techniques to provide exceptional care. Diagnosed with multiple sclerosis in 2009, I've embraced movement as medicine, using Pilates, swimming, and cycling to stay active.

My lifelong passion for holistic health continues to shape my life, and I remain a dedicated advocate for people with disabilities.

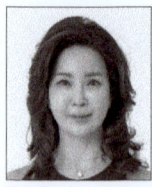

Su Yeon Roh

Su Yeon Roh, PhD, PMA-NCPT, ACSM-CPT, ACSM/ACS-CET, Lolita Disciples, Balanced Body Master Instructor, FMS, GFM, GRASTONE Technique, is a professor of Exercise Rehabilitation & Welfare at Gachon University. She is honorary president at the Korea Integrated Movement Academy. She studied, performed, and directed ballet, and started to teach Pilates in 2004. Su Yeon is certified with four main international Pilates instructor licenses: Polestar, Ellie Herman Studios, Balanced Body Master Instructor, and Lolita San Miguel as a Lolita disciple.

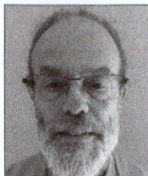

Graham Scarr

Graham Scarr, CBiol, FRSB, FLS, DO, has a particular interest in the morphology and mechanics of living structures and has been at the forefront of biotensegrity research for many years.

He is a Chartered Biologist, a graduate in microbiology, and a retired osteopath. He is a Fellow of the Royal Society of Biology and Fellow of the Linnean Society. His book, *Biotensegrity: The Structural Basis of Life* (Handspring), is now in its second edition, and with more than a dozen scientific publications, he presents at meetings and conferences in both the UK and internationally.

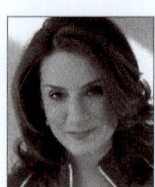

Alycea Ungaro

Alycea Ungaro, PT, MSACN, is the founder of the Real Pilates studios in New York City, and the author of five books including the best-selling *Pilates: Body in Motion* (DK). A student of Romana Kryzanowska, Alycea has been a voice for classical Pilates for decades. As the creator of the Real Pilates Teacher Training program, Alycea is committed to passing on her knowledge as a second-generation instructor. She lives in New York with her family. Visit her at realpilatesnyc.com and the teacher training site at realpilates.com.

Pilates Research: A Historical Perspective

Sherri Betz

PMA Research Committee

The PMA Research Committee was initiated by the Board of Directors of the Pilates Method Alliance in 2009 to validate the Pilates method of exercise. As a continuing education instructor for special populations, I began collecting and organizing Pilates research in 1999 to support the recommendations for modifications and precautions for osteoporosis, spinal and orthopedic conditions, pregnancy, postpartum, and neurological pathologies. This database of research provided evidence for the recommendations for special populations published in the PMA Study Guide for teachers who sought the third-party credential, now known as NCPT, National Certified Pilates Teacher. With the upsurge in the popularity of Pilates in the late 1990s, there was confusion about the definition, claims, and benefits of Pilates in both the fitness industry and in the consumer sectors. Expressing urgency for validation of the Pilates method to the PMA Board, they agreed to add a scientific symposium where authors of research would explain their reports to annual PMA conference attendees. In 2010, I began vetting and selecting oral research submissions to present at the conference each year. Selections were based on merit and rigor of scientific methodology with a variety of types of research placed on the agenda, from case reports to randomized controlled trials to systematic reviews. In the early years, almost every paper that was submitted was selected for the forum. Many Pilates teachers were eager to present their case reports but were unfamiliar with composing an organized report. I mentored them through the process of writing the abstract, creating their slide deck, and presenting the case in a professional manner at the forum. This mentoring process became one of the main functions of the committee, to nurture future research and let Pilates teachers know that they could present retrospective cases without having an academic affiliation with a university or institutional review board (IRB) approval if they had written permission from the client.

In 2015, the committee began to solicit research posters for submission to the 2016 PMA Annual Conference. The posters were displayed in the expo hall and each author was given a specific time to be at their poster so that interested attendees could come by to ask questions and discuss the author's research. These poster presentations became very popular and garnered more interest from Pilates teachers who were unfamiliar with this type of scientific publication. I mentored the authors by creating a template and providing feedback, editing, and guidance to those who wanted to present research in a poster format.

The evolving primary goal of the committee became education of Pilates teachers on the importance of research influencing knowledge translation of scientific outcomes on the practice of teaching Pilates. To fulfill this goal, there were two main functions of the committee: 1. collection, organization, and dissemination of relevant publications regarding the efficacy of Pilates exercise and 2. selection of authors of Pilates research to present their work at the annual conference.

In 2016, the Research Committee was expanded to garner the expertise of a prestigious group of university professors, research scientists, clinicians, and Pilates teachers.

The PMA Research Committee Members are:

Sherri Betz, PT, DPT, GCS, NCPT, Chair
Karyn Staples, PT, PhD, NCPT, Vice Chair
Anne Bishop, EdM, BS, NCPT, Secretary
Virginia Cowen, PhD, LMT, NCPTMB, NCPT
Rebecca Hess, PhD
Lise Stolze, MPT, DSc, NCPT
Craig Ruby, MPT, DEd, NCPT
Tom Welsh, MS, PhD, MA
Deborah Lessen, NCPT

The effectiveness and knowledge of this group catapulted the success of the research committee. A set of Standing Rules (below) was developed to establish the name, purpose, and objectives, as well as the leadership qualifications and responsibilities for each member.

Article I: Name and purpose

A. The name of the committee shall be the Pilates Method Alliance Research Committee. In these Standing Rules it will be referred to as the Research Committee.

B. The purpose of the Research Committee is the collection, evaluation, and selection of oral platform or poster research and special interest presentations for the PMA Annual Meeting and PMA publications as well as summarizing and updating current research on Pilates.

Article II: Objectives

A. Create an objective format for evaluating Pilates research

B. Build a robust team who can bring the importance of research to the forefront of the Pilates community

C. Keep the Pilates research reference list updated

D. Summarize current Pilates research for dissemination among the PMA community

E. Create an infrastructure that could eventually support the creation of a Pilates research journal

F. Establish and publish a Pilates research journal

Article III: Leadership qualifications and responsibilities

A. Committee member qualifications:

1. Baccalaureate degree from an accredited college or university
2. Knowledge and familiarity with current Pilates research
3. Understand research methodology and the levels of evidence in current research publications
4. Understand how to perform literature reviews
5. Understand how to read a peer-reviewed research paper and compose written commentary summarizing the paper

B. Committee member responsibilities:

1. Encourage excellence in Pilates-based research
2. Collect current Pilates-based research
3. Share current Pilates-based research
4. Evaluate Pilates-based research abstracts and posters for presentation at the PMA Annual Meeting
5. Summarize Pilates-based research for dissemination among PMA members
6. Attend the Research Forum at the PMA Annual Meeting
7. Attend one in-person meeting per year at the PMA Annual Meeting
8. Participate in three quarterly teleconferences calls per year

The Standing Rules could be changed with approval of the Executive Committee of the PMA. Where these Standing Rules were silent, the applicable PMA Bylaws would prevail.

By 2017, Pilates research publication numbers rose exponentially in the scientific literature, driving more and more authors to submit papers for the PMA Research Forum every year. Since there were now many committee members, a blinded selection was implemented to remove bias from the presentations. The committee aimed to present a sample of each type of research report representing varying levels of evidence (case report or case study, literature review, observational pre-post study, randomized controlled trial, and systematic review). To read, understand, and apply research, the following schematic and definitions are helpful.

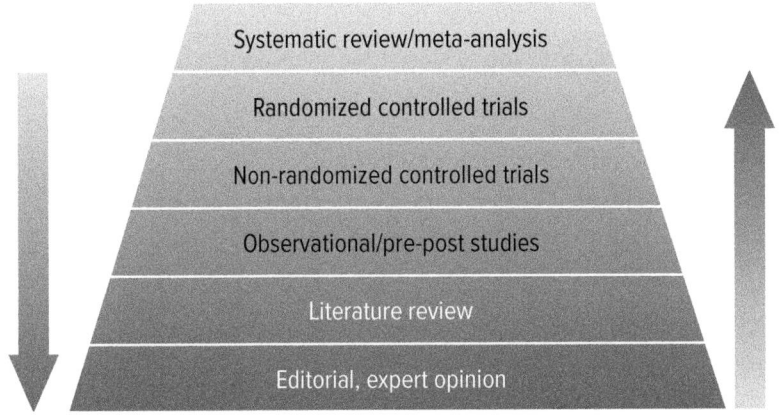

Figure 1.1
Research design: levels of evidence. Hierarchical format of research designs arranged by strength of levels of evidence
©2017 Dr. Sherri Betz

A systematic review is a summary of the medical literature that uses explicit methods to perform a comprehensive literature search and critical appraisal of individual studies, and that uses appropriate statistical techniques to combine these valid studies.

Meta-analysis is a particular type of systematic review that attempts to combine and *summarize quantitative data from multiple studies using sophisticated statistical methodology.*

A randomized controlled trial is an experimental, *prospective study* in which "participants are randomly allocated into an experimental group or a control group and followed over time for the variables/outcomes of interest" (Dang and Dearholt 2017).

An observational study or pre-post study is *a prospective or retrospective study.* The researcher is observing the effect of an exercise or intervention with no control group defined. Cohort studies and case control studies are two types of observational study.

A case study is *a prospective pre-planned intervention applied to a willing subject.* Case studies require institutional review board approval for research on human subjects to be published (Porcino 2016).

A case report is a *retrospective* detailed report of the management of an individual's single case or a group of subjects' unusual condition or a condition that is rare or poorly reported in the literature. Often a practitioner finds that a particular intervention worked quite well in achieving the desired goals or outcomes and would like to share that information formally with colleagues (Porcino 2016).

A literature review is an informative, critical synthesis known and unknown in a subject area. Literature reviews can be formatted as systematic reviews, theses, or dissertations aiming to evaluate and critically analyze relevant work in a particular field (Bolderston 2008).

Editorials and expert opinions: The clinical experience, expertise, and judgment of a respected health care professional do play important roles in evidence-based practice. Sometimes there will not be methodologically sound research to answer a clinical question, and expert opinion will be important in the decision-making process. When evidence has been insufficiently developed for a specific topic, a consensus opinion of experts can be valuable. There are two consensus methods for expert opinion: the nominal group technique and the Delphi method. The nominal group technique is a structured face-to-face meeting facilitating discussion and allows participants to voice their opinions. The key characteristics of the Delphi method are the use of panel experts to obtain data, no face-to-face discussions, the use of sequential questionnaires, and the systematic emergence of a concurrent opinion. The collective experience of our leading experts should not be dismissed in providing valuable guidance on best practices in teaching Pilates (Hohmann, Cote, and Brand 2018).

Keep in mind that both expert opinion and scientific research should be evaluated for selective use of evidence and other biases.

Published Pilates research papers

To date there are 259 papers published in peer-reviewed journals. Below are boxes listing the categories of research published with Pilates as a focus.

BOX 1.1
Categories of research

Systematic reviews or meta-analysis	36
Literature reviews	4
Randomized controlled trials	111
Non-randomized controlled trials	14
Descriptive or observational pre-post-design	70
Case reports	8
Expert opinion or editorials	16+
Total	259

The former PMA Research Committee kept a Pilates reference database updated yearly with categories of research, diseases, physical benefits, functional benefits, or specific muscle changes as outcomes.

BOX 1.2
Topics addressed in the published papers (there is overlap)

Physical or muscle benefit	80
Disease or disability (not including LBP)	66
Low back pain (LBP)	46
Older adults	34
Balance or fall prevention	27
Quality of life	26
Respiratory	15
Posture	13
Mental or cognitive	10
Sports or dance	9
Teaching	6
Adolescents	5
Rehabilitation	4
Cardiovascular	4
Pregnancy	3
Bone density	1

BOX 1.3
Papers focusing on the physical, functional, or specific muscle benefits of Pilates: 80

- Functional
- Fitness
- Flexibility
- Body composition
- Muscle strength, thickness, or activation
- Endurance
- Intra-abdominal pressure
- Motor control
- Pelvic floor

BOX 1.4
Papers focusing on disease or disability targeting through Pilates exercise: 111

- LBP (46 papers)
- Cancer
- Multiple sclerosis
- Osteoporosis
- Neck pain
- Obesity
- Total hip arthroplasty/total knee arthroplasty (THA/TKA)
- Ankylosing spondylitis
- Fibromyalgia
- Incontinence
- Scoliosis
- Menopause
- Diabetes
- Prostatectomy
- Arthritis
- Cardiovascular
- Cerebral palsy
- COPD
- Heart failure
- Hypertension
- Lateral epicondylosis
- Postpartum
- Spondylolisthesis
- Stroke
- Temporomandibular joint disorder (TMJD)
- Hypermobility (expert opinion)

Questionable-quality Pilates research

High-quality research helps us to validate Pilates and distinguish it from other forms of exercise. Pilates studies need improved methodological rigor and should be more clearly defined in scientific literature for measurable changes to actually be attributed to Pilates exercise. Often, Pilates gets muddled with physical therapy, massage therapy, or various forms of exercise in research papers. Results are then published, attributing Pilates exercise as the source of the benefits described in the study. If Pilates exercises get collapsed with balance devices, elastic bands, foam rollers, balls, or physical therapy, then the results cannot really be attributed to Pilates.

Most of the Pilates studies in the literature fall into one of three categories:

1. *Direct source* Pilates where most of the exercises are clearly described and recognizable as Pilates and are referenced directly from either Joseph Pilates' publications and videos or are from the NPCP (formerly PMA) Study Guide (NPCE Study Guide 2021; Pilates 1945).
2. *Hybrid* studies where Pilates is mixed with another modality, so that the results cannot be directly attributed to Pilates exercise.
3. *Inspired by* Pilates where there is no text or photographic description of the exercises included in the study and no recognizable Pilates exercise in the study. Hence, Pilates is noted in the title but is not included or described in the methodology of the study. The study is not repeatable; therefore, the results cannot be attributed to Pilates.

Development of the virtual forum

In 2021, the PMA Research Forum was shifted to a very successful and well-attended virtual format where eight presenters were selected from several countries to present in the usual 10-plus-5 format (10 minutes to present the abstract and 5 minutes for the Q&A).

The future of Pilates research

Pilates research publications should include *clearly defined* Pilates exercises within the methods section of the papers. Future Pilates research should continue to inspire and enhance the skills of Pilates teachers in critical thinking and improve the safety and benefits for clients of the Pilates method. Huge thanks to all of the former PMA Research Committee members, who contributed greatly to disseminating the evidence-based benefits of Pilates. I am so grateful to have embarked on this journey and am delighted to continue fostering higher quality Pilates research trials comparing Pilates head-to-head with other forms of exercise.

References

Bolderston, A. (2008) Writing an effective literature review. *Journal of Medical Imaging and Radiation Sciences, 39,* 2, 86–92.

Dang, D. and Dearholt, S. (2017) *Johns Hopkins Nursing Evidence-Based Practice: Model and Guidelines.* 3rd Ed. Indianapolis, IN: Sigma Theta Tau International.

Hohmann, E., Cote, M. P., and Brand, J. C. (2018) "Research pearls: Expert consensus based evidence using the Delphi method." *Arthroscopy, 34,* 12, 3278–3282.

NPCE Study Guide (National Pilates Certification Exam Study Guide) (2021) Miami, FL: National Pilates Certification Program, Inc.

Pilates, J. H. (1945 [2012]) *Return to Life Through Contrology.* 2nd Ed. Miami, FL: Pilates Method Alliance, Inc.

Porcino, A. (2016) "Not birds of a feather: Case reports, case studies, and single-subject research." *International Journal of Therapeutic Massage & Bodywork, 9,* 3, 1–2.

Pilates Movement and Apparatus in Health Care

Elizabeth Larkam

Contrology supported individual health and well-being during the life of inventor and teacher Joseph Hubertus Pilates (1883–1967). The movement system created by J. H. Pilates served the bedridden after World War I broke out in 1914, when he taught in a camp for enemy aliens in Lancaster, England. A photograph of Mr. Pilates on an early version of his Trapeze Table shows the metal frame of a hospital bed on casters to which he has attached a four-poster canopy and springs (Larkam 2017). Throughout four decades of work in his "Universal" Gymnasium, J. H. Pilates continued to develop his movement system, inventing over 20 items of exercise apparatus. The equipment frames provide eye bolts to which springs or straps may be attached, creating movement environments that support a variety of vectors (Larkam 2017; Steel 2020).

During the 50-plus years following his death, Pilates movement programs and equipment have been integrated into clinical and non-medical settings to address a variety of health conditions. The techniques and apparatus of J. H. Pilates have been incorporated into dance education programs, dance medicine centers, sports medicine practices, physical therapy clinics, chiropractic offices, and athletic training facilities. The Comprehensive Combat and Complex Casualty Care program of Naval Medical Center, San Diego, invested in Pilates equipment and movement techniques to develop gait and movement training for polytrauma patients including individuals with prosthetic limbs (Moore 2009). Medical practices specializing in treatment of a connective tissue disorder called hypermobile Ehlers–Danlos syndrome rely on the unique attributes of Pilates apparatus with variable spring resistance to provide supportive framing and scaffolding for movement training of individuals who lack connective tissue integrity (see Volume 1, Chapter 9). Research first published in 2022 in *Sports Health: A Multidisciplinary Approach* found that long COVID sufferers, who had been hospitalized with COVID-19 and had reported shortness of breath and fatigue since being discharged, saw their lung function increase by 34 percent following an eight-week Pilates mat program (Bagherzadeh-Rahmani *et al.* 2023) (see Chapters 12 and 13).

Documentation of customized movement programs in Pilates apparatus environments that improve gait efficiency may further develop appreciation of this underutilized movement system. Assessment of gait patterning is a dynamic approach to whole-body movement, an effective alternative to static posture. The writer Rebecca Solnit pointed out that walking "is how the body measures itself against the earth." And through such physical communion, walking offers up its crowning gift by bringing us emotionally, even spiritually, home to ourselves (McCarthy 2023).

Despite the growth of Pilates applications that address health conditions, the potential of Pilates has not yet been realized in health optimization practices. This may be attributed in part to the lack of published Pilates documentation perceived as relevant to health care. This deficit compromises professional communication among Pilates practitioners who are motivated to share best practices. Today, actualization of the potential of Pilates in health and wellness spheres requires specific spoken, written, and visual documentation that articulates assessment, design of movement sequences, pedagogy, and progress toward a client's short-term and long-term goals. The scarcity of Pilates client data that track measurable health markers hinders communication with health practitioners who are unfamiliar with Pilates.

Innovation may emerge from within a field, brought forth by recognized experts. Alternatively, innovation can be generated by influencers working outside of respected institutions. J. H. Pilates was self-taught through movement experience, observation, and reading (Larkam 2017). He did not have formal education from academic institutions. Mr. Pilates did not articulate his approach to therapeutic movement using vocabulary accepted by medical professionals. He created a unique repertoire for each of his equipment inventions and gave presentations to doctors, hoping to interest them in his method (Larkam 2017). In 1958, J. H. Pilates was awarded an Appointment of Merit in appreciation of his Valued Assistance in the Presentation of the Post Graduate Course of the Academy of Chiropractic, Inc. (Gallagher and Kryzanowska 2000).

Written documentation of client sessions designed and taught by J. H. Pilates and his associates are rare and not widely available to practitioners teaching today. The two books he published, *Return to Life Through Contrology* (1945) and *Your Health* (1934), champion the tenets of health and healthy behaviors espoused by Mr. Pilates. J. H. Pilates documented his mat and apparatus exercises with black-and-white photographs for which he modeled. The walls of his gym, approximately 15 ft (4.5 m) wide and 20 ft (6 m) long, were covered with black-and-white photographs of Mr. Pilates demonstrating exercises (Steel 2020).

Mr. Pilates made films to document his movement teaching. A film of Mr. Pilates instructing Eve Gentry on the Pilates Universal Reformer was made in 1956 following her radical mastectomy surgery, part of treatment for breast cancer. This film was intended to demonstrate to physicians the effectiveness of the Pilates Method in restoring motor control following surgery.

The education model demonstrated by J. H. Pilates was based on loyal apprenticeship prior to being granted permission to establish an independent business as a Pilates teacher (see Chapter 5). Mastery was obtained by observation of the teacher and supervised movement practice. Apprentices received coaching from their teacher or from advanced students. They practiced with peers. Those who apprenticed to J. H. Pilates established independent movement studios where they provided instruction to clients on apparatus he designed.

Each movement field has its own distinct physical, spoken, and written vocabulary. Practitioners and educators from Alexander Technique, Body Mind Centering®, Continuum Movement®, dance techniques, Feldenkrais Method®, Gyrotonic®, Pilates, and yoga learn the vocabulary used by their teachers and pass on these terms to their students. The descriptive names given by J. H. Pilates to his exercises do not translate to vocabulary used in professional communication by health care practitioners. Pilates mat exercise names include "Hundred," "Saw," and "Corkscrew" (Steel 2020). Pilates Contrology exercises on the Universal Reformer include "Swan Dive," "Horseback," "Stomach Massage," and "Russian-Stretch" (Larkam 2017).

Written documentation of Pilates movement sequences requires a vocabulary that can communicate effectively both with professionals within the Pilates field and with practitioners in other fields. Pilates practitioners have the responsibility to be conversant with the vocabulary physical therapists and other practitioners use to describe movement (see Abbreviations and Glossary at the end of this book). The contributed movement programs reference Pilates history, physical therapy, osteopathy, neurology, fascia research, and anatomy research. References are provided to position Pilates movement programs as practices that support the healing process and living with a health condition.

J. H. Pilates emphasized the value of whole-body

movement. The contributed programs reflect a whole-body perspective. This is congruent with fascial research on movement of connective tissue structure (Larkam 2017; Pilat 2022; Stecco 2015). The biomechanics of levers do not do justice to the complexities of Pilates movement. The principles of J. H. Pilates whole-body movement align with the algorithm of applied biotensegrity (Scarr 2018) (see Chapter 3).

Key contributors to Pilates in sports medicine, dance medicine, and health care

Rehabilitation of dancers provided the channel through which Pilates movement and apparatus entered clinical practice and medical organizations. Beginning in the 1980s, sports medicine centers in New York City and San Francisco integrated Pilates into patient care. Marika Molnar, Physical Therapist and Licensed Acupuncturist, a founder of Dance Medicine, and physical therapist for the New York City Ballet (1979–present), incorporated Pilates equipment into her treatment programs for dancers. In the mid 1970s Marika enrolled in New York University's master's degree in dance education where she studied ideokinesis with André Bernard. She took Pilates lessons from Kathy Grant (see Chapter 5). Upon graduation in 1979 with a degree in physical therapy Marika followed the advice of orthopedic surgeon Dr. Liebler and studied with Carola Trier (see Chapter 5). She established Eastside Dance Physical Therapy and Westside Dance Physical Therapy.

Saint Francis Memorial Hospital in San Francisco recruited orthopedist James G. Garrick, MD to establish and direct the Center for Sports Medicine. Dr. Garrick founded the Dancemedicine Pilates division in 1985. At this time there were no published studies validating the efficacy of Pilates. The inclusion of Pilates in a large hospital in a major US city was perceived as a medical "seal of approval." Dr. Garrick created a program for qualified dancers that prepared them to design and teach Pilates programs

to patients. The Dancemedicine Pilates specialists served as members of the Center's treatment team. Pilates apparatus and movement vocabulary were incorporated into a treatment model that included prescriptions from referring physicians, physical therapy evaluations, reevaluations, and chart documentation. Patient reports demonstrating progress toward short-term and long-term goals were submitted for insurance reimbursement.

Jean-Claude West, MS in Motor Learning, was the first to develop a private practice in New York City that integrated Pilates movement and customized apparatus with strength training and manual techniques learned from Rolfer author Louis Shultz (1996). Jean-Claude and Anna Schmitz developed close professional relationships with Pilates teachers Kathy Grant, Bruce King, and Eve Gentry (1983–1989). Professional dancers and noted artists flocked to their loft studio on Bleecker Street for individual sessions with Jean-Claude and Anna.

The evolution of Pilates equipment for therapeutic applications

Jean-Claude West was prolific in the engineering and construction of movement apparatus that evolved from and went beyond the original designs of Pilates equipment. In 1986 he built all the Pilates apparatus for his Bleecker Street studio using high-density foam upholstery to provide proprioceptive stimulation. Jean-Claude introduced Lazy Susan hardware for standing hip rotation in 1987. In 1988, he developed a prototype placing rotator discs on independent sliding platforms with spring resistance adjacent to a ballet barre. He used this training environment to refine dancer technique. Jean-Claude explored other inventions such as a plexiglass jump board to show foot loading and ground reaction forces (1990) and a Tee-Bar mounted on the Pilates Universal Reformer for leg biases (1991). Jean-Claude continued his innovations designing and engineering the JC5600 in 1990. This first four-in-one portable Pilates equipment combination could be assembled in 30 minutes. Jean-Claude developed the JC5600 for White Oak Project, founded by Mark Morris and Mikhail Baryshnikov, so he could provide sessions for the touring dancers (West 2023). Jean-Claude and Katy Keller, physical therapist, co-developed the Biomechanical Asymmetry Corrector (BAC). Their presentation of this comprehensive movement environment at the 1992 International Association for Dance Medicine & Science conference demonstrated a uniquely effective approach for managing scoliosis and spinal asymmetries. The modular design of BAC included the Functional Footprints (Keller and West 1995).

Ken Endelman, Founder and CEO of Balanced Body (formerly Current Concepts) (see Chapter 6), responded to requests from physical therapists and other practitioners teaching Pilates in clinical settings (Endelman 2023). The practitioners recommended altering Pilates equipment to improve client experiences in terms of safety, comfort, and ease of learning new patterns of motor control. Ken met Marika Molnar and Jean-Claude West in New York City in 1989 where Ken was introduced to their use of "Lazy Susan" technology for hip rotation. Marika suggested attaching rotator discs to the Universal Reformer jump board using Velcro®. This led to Balanced Body manufacturing rotator discs. Marika also suggested to Ken that he raise the height of the Universal Reformer and combine the Universal Reformer and Trapeze Table into one space-saving design (Molnar 2023).

Requests from Pilates practitioners working in clinical settings led to Ken separating the single pedal of the J. H. Pilates chair, creating the split-pedal chair. Marika used the split-pedal chair as a gait-training environment in the late 1990s. She and Madeline Black collaborated on a gait observation and assessment workshop for Pilates teachers sponsored by the Physicalmind Institute.

In 1992, Ken filed a patent application with the United States Patent Office for Universal Reformer innovations. The patent was awarded in 1994 (Endelman 1994). What became known as the "infinity footbar" was independently adjustable in vertical and horizontal dimensions. This accommodated client length as well as hip, knee, and ankle range of motion. A "proprioceptive T bar" provided an alternative to the footbar. It allowed the two legs to bear weight simultaneously yet independently, providing feedback for weight-bearing asymmetries. The headrest was independently adjustable in vertical and horizontal dimensions, respecting cervical integrity. The adjustable shoulder rests could also be removed, reducing pressure on the cervical and upper thoracic areas. This "clinical Universal Reformer" included 24 in. (61 cm) legs facilitating client transfer onto the carriage, as well as Velcro cuffs for thighs, ankles, elbows, and wrists. The jump board and standing platforms both had larger surface areas than those of previous Universal Reformers.

Movement practitioners teaching in Pilates environments benefit from interdisciplinary education that augments the curriculum focused on the repertoire of J. H. Pilates. Internationally respected physiotherapist, educator, and author Diane Lee incorporates Pilates into her clinical practice and courses. Her book, *The Thorax: An Integrated Approach*, includes a chapter on motor learning and movement training featuring sequences using the Balanced Body clinical Universal Reformer (Lee 2018). The gait-focused programs in this book continue the evolution of Pilates practice, documentation, and education in service of improving client quality of life and health.

References

Bagherzadeh-Rahmani, B., Kordi, N., Haghighi, A. H., Clark, C. C. T. *et al.* (2023) "Eight weeks of Pilates training improves respiratory measures in people with a history of COVID-19: A preliminary study." *Sports Health: A Multidisciplinary Approach,* *15,* 5, 710–717.

Endelman, K. (1994) United States Patent. Exercise Equipment. Patent number: US5338278A. Date of patent: August 16, 1994. https://patents.google.com/patent/US5338278A/en. [Accessed September 25, 2023].

Endelman, K. (2023) Personal correspondence with Ken Endelman, Founder and CEO of Balanced Body, April 6, 2023.

Gallagher, S. P. and Kryzanowska, R. (Eds.) (2000) *The Joseph H. Pilates Archive Collection: Photographs, Writings and Designs.* Philadelphia, PA: Bainbridge Books.

Keller, K. and West, J.-C. (1995) "Functional movement impairment in dancers: An assessment and treatment approach utilizing the Biomechanical Asymmetry Corrector (BAC) to restore normal mechanics of the spine and pelvis." *Journal of Back and Musculoskeletal Rehabilitation, 5,* 3, 219–233.

Larkam, E. (2017) *Fascia in Motion: Fascia-Focused Movement for Pilates.* Edinburgh: Handspring Publishing, pp. 18–19, 31, 34, 92–101, 148.

Lee, D. (2018) *The Thorax: An Integrated Approach.* Edinburgh: Handspring Publishing, pp. 275–276, 282–283, 286–290, 293–294, 296–298.

McCarthy, A. (2023) "Whatever the Problem, It's Probably Solved by Walking." *The New York Times,* March 25, 2023.

Molnar, M. (2023) Personal correspondence with Marika Molnar, founder of Dance Medicine, and physical therapist, New York City Ballet (1979–present), April 19, 2023.

Moore, J. (2009) Lower extremity amputation: Early management considerations. Workshop, July 28–30, Military Amputees Advanced Skills Training (MAAST) conference. Comprehensive Combat and Casualty Care Naval Medical Center, San Diego, CA.

Pilat, A. (2022) *Myofascial Induction: An Anatomical Approach to the Treatment of Fascial Dysfunction—Volume 1 The Upper Body.* Edinburgh: Handspring Publishing.

Pilates, J. H. (1934) *Your Health.* New York City: Printed by C. J. O'Brien, Inc.

Pilates, J. H. (1945) *Return to Life Through Contrology.* New York: J. J. Augustin Publisher.

Scarr, G. (2018) *Biotensegrity: The Structural Basis of Life.* 2nd Ed. Edinburgh: Handspring Publishing.

Shultz, R. L. (1996) *The Endless Web: Fascial Anatomy and Physical Reality.* Berkeley, CA: North Atlantic Books.

Stecco, C. (2015) *Functional Atlas of the Human Fascial System.* Edinburgh: Churchill Livingstone Elsevier.

Steel, J. H. (2020) *Caged Lion: Joseph Pilates & His Legacy.* Santa Barbara, CA: Last Leaf Press, pp. 11, 12, 15.

West, J.-C. (2023) Documents with inserts. Personal correspondence with Jean-Claude West, Kinesiologist in private practice, April 26, 2023.

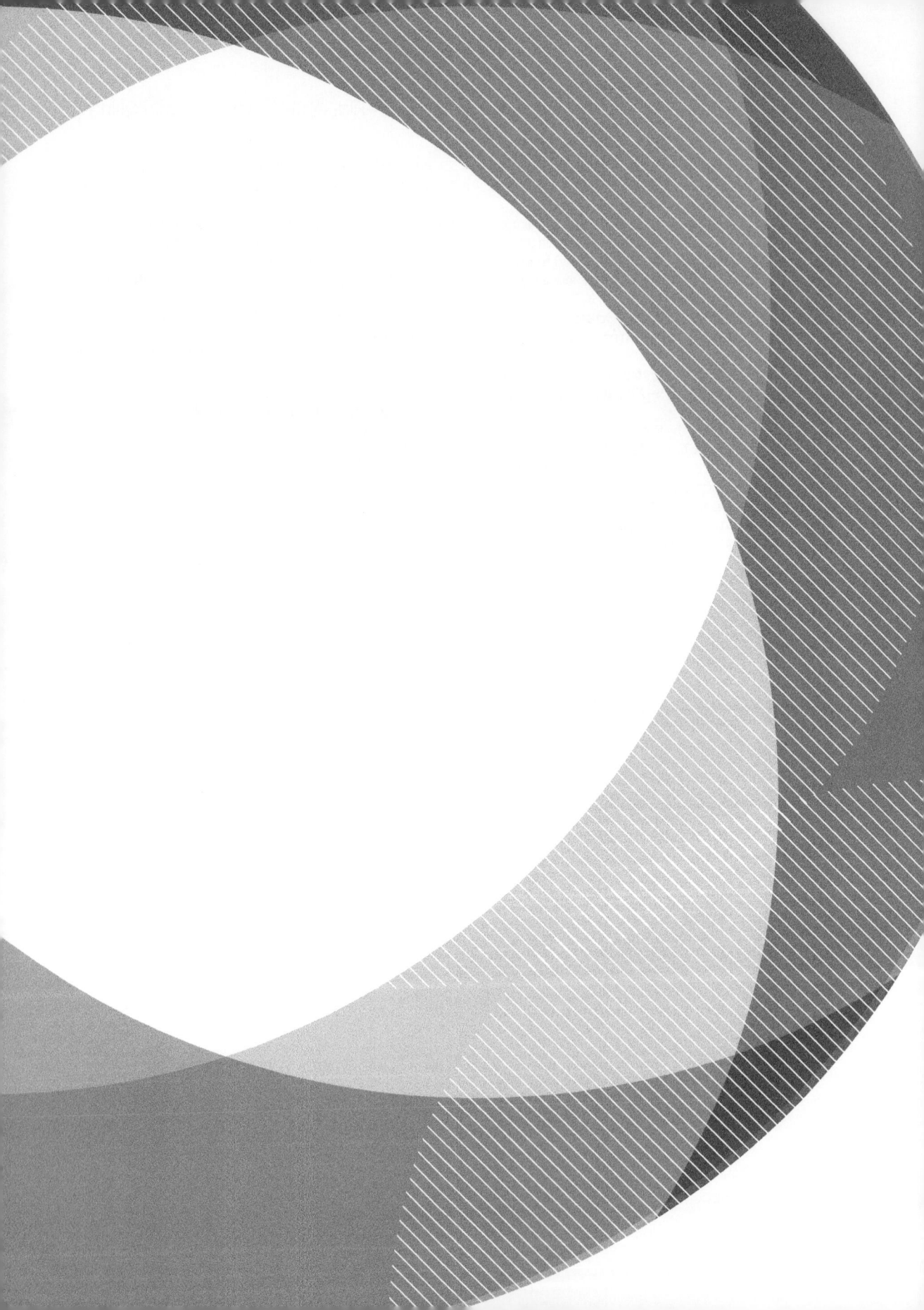

Movement is a Whole-Body Issue

Graham Scarr

Movement is the means that humans use to express life and must be carried out in a controlled way if it is to be meaningful. The way we walk, talk, eat, and meet are just as important to our health as contraction of the heart, peristalsis, and breathing because integrated motion represents the most efficient use of resources. It also produces useful information that feeds into every part of the body and enables us to live healthy and purposeful lives.

Unfortunately, we have all been taught that bones form the basic structural framework of the body and that muscles simply pull on the bones and cause movement, but this is far from the reality. Such a view derives from the workings of man-made machines from the 17th century, where bones and muscles operate as isolated lever systems and other tissues are relegated to mere supporting roles. It has thus given rise to the "musculoskeletal" duality and the notion that we can strengthen and stretch individual muscles during exercise, but the body is much more complicated than that (Scarr 2018).

Levers generate potentially damaging stress concentrations that would be likely to cause living tissues to collapse during development, and that would really be the end of them. As nature always does things in the most energy-efficient ways, and our bodies are relatively light, flexible, and capable of functioning much the same in any position, it probably uses a different system of mechanics altogether (Levin and Scarr 2022).

Biotensegrity

The biotensegrity concept recognizes that stability and ease of movement are not due to the strength of individual components but because of the way the system is configured to distribute mechanical forces: tension and compression. Here, the tissues are coupled in such a way that when one part moves, *everything* becomes involved. Tensegrity models consist of a set of compressed struts suspended within a tensioned network of cables, and are physical representations of the invisible forces that maintain their integrity. They are organized into continuous mechanical loops (closed kinematic chains) that enable every part of the system to move in a controlled way (Levin, Lowell de Solórzano, and Scarr 2017).

Closed kinematic chains

Kinematics is all about the "geometry of motion," and the simplest arrangement that enables the structure itself to control this is the "4-bar" mechanism, where the length and position of each bar (tension/compression element) determines the mechanical behavior of all the others in the system. Here, the triangular "3-bars" are relatively rigid and important because of their stability, while more complex configurations can have *any* number of bars oriented in *any* direction.

At first sight, these tensegrity configurations might just appear to be complicated lever systems, but this is not the case in a biological context where each part consists of a hierarchy of smaller structures organized according to the same principles. In simple terms, each anatomical "bar" ("cable/strut," bone, muscle, organ, tissue, cell, etc.) will be under tension *or* compression, and maintained in response to the forces flowing through it, and this system is far more complex than a machine.

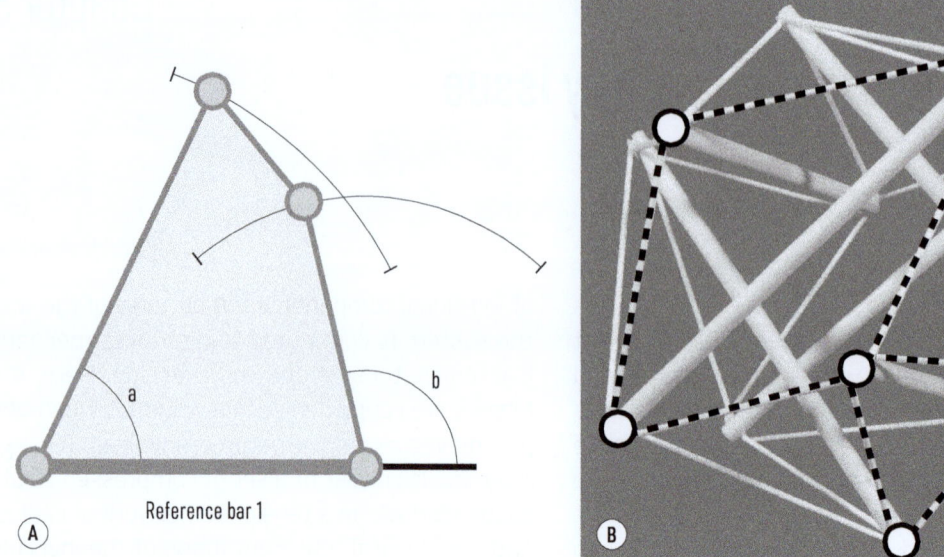

Figure 3.1
A A "4-bar" closed kinematic chain showing the motions of three bars in relation to a fourth (reference bar) with each one guided by the relative positions of all the others. **B** Tensegrity model highlighting some of the rigid "3-bar" triangles (white, 2-D) that allow the "4-bars" (dotted, 3-D) to change shape in a controlled way.
A: *Modified with permission from Levin, S. M., Lowell de Solórzano, S., and Scarr, G. (2017) "The significance of closed kinematic chains to biological movement and dynamic stability." Journal of Bodywork and Movement Therapies, 21, 664–672.*
B: *©Rory James, reproduced with permission from Scarr, G. (2018) Biotensegrity: The Structural Basis of Life. 2nd Ed. Edinburgh: Handspring Publishing.*

Such structural configurations would allow the body to respond *instantly* to rapidly changing conditions and regulate complex movements in ways that are beyond the sole capability of the nervous system (Cabe 2019), where the control of motion is embedded within the structure itself and efficiently reduces the amount of effort needed to coordinate changes. Like a drawing pantograph, they enable such systems to amplify (or attenuate) force, speed, and kinetic energy, with the structure itself guiding motion and acting in synergy with the nervous system.

Movement

The mechanics of biotensegrity thus applies equally well to the interactions within and between molecules, cells, tissues, joints—and everything else—with their responses intrinsically coupled through the multi-scale geometry. As the position of each bone is dependent on the interactions between many different tissues (fascial sheets, septa, aponeuroses, tendons, ligaments, etc.), so the effect of every muscle contraction becomes distributed over a much wider anatomical field than is often appreciated. Conversely, multiple muscles can transfer their power through these multi-scale couplings and enable movement patterns that might otherwise seem

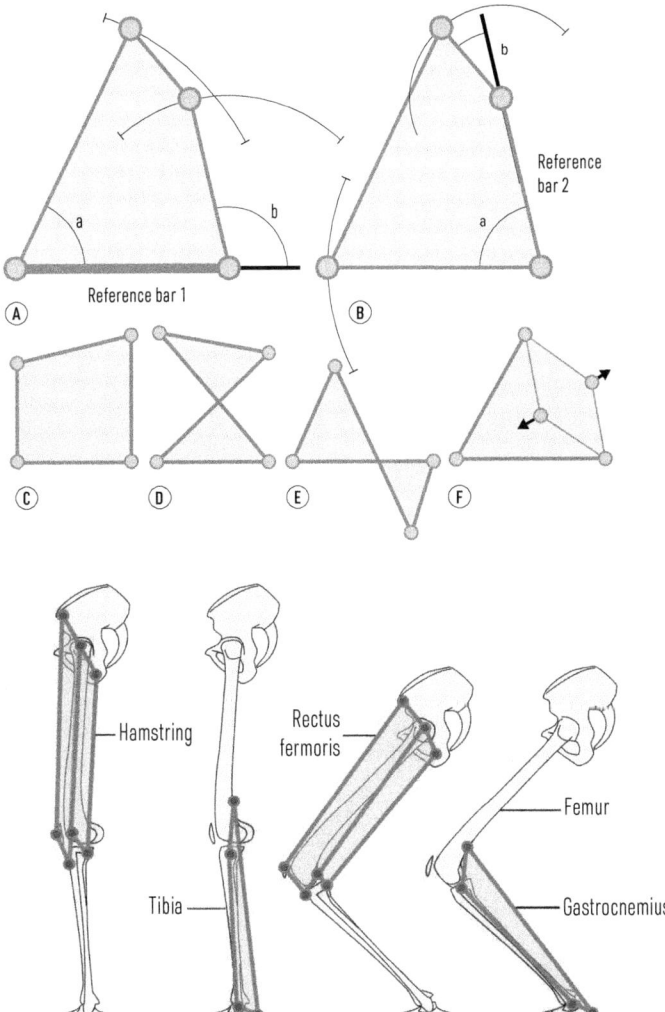

Figure 3.2
Closed kinematic chain showing how each part consists of similarly organized tensegrity structures at multiple-size scales.

Figure 3.3
Simplified schematic showing joint movements in the lower limb controlled by the closed kinematic chain geometry of bones and biarticular muscles.
Modified with permission from Levin, S. M., Lowell de Solórzano, S., and Scarr, G. (2017) "The significance of closed kinematic chains to biological movement and dynamic stability." Journal of Bodywork and Movement Therapies, 21, 664–672.

difficult to explain. For example, the biarticular muscles that cross the hip/knee and knee/ankle joints can be visualized as simple "4-bar" mechanisms that concentrate their combined power and enable us to jump much higher when starting from a crouched position than a standing one (Levin *et al.* 2017).

Of course, the effects of any "aberrant" movement pattern due to posture, injury, or pathology would also be transferred through the body in a similar way, and with the potential to cause problems, which is why an appreciation of this mechanical system is so relevant to modern therapeutic protocols.

Biotensegrity describes the *internal* mechanics of the body—the way it is organized and how it can function in the way it does—and it dismisses the contrived lever model and musculoskeletal duality because they are incomplete and out of date.

External movement patterns, of course, are the result of internal mechanics, and it is no coincidence that exercise regimes have developed that share obvious similarities with this kinematic system. Such routines clearly have therapeutic benefits, but it is important to note that some of the *labels* ascribed to them are often incorrect and misleading, and should be reconsidered before using them further (Di Fabio 1999).

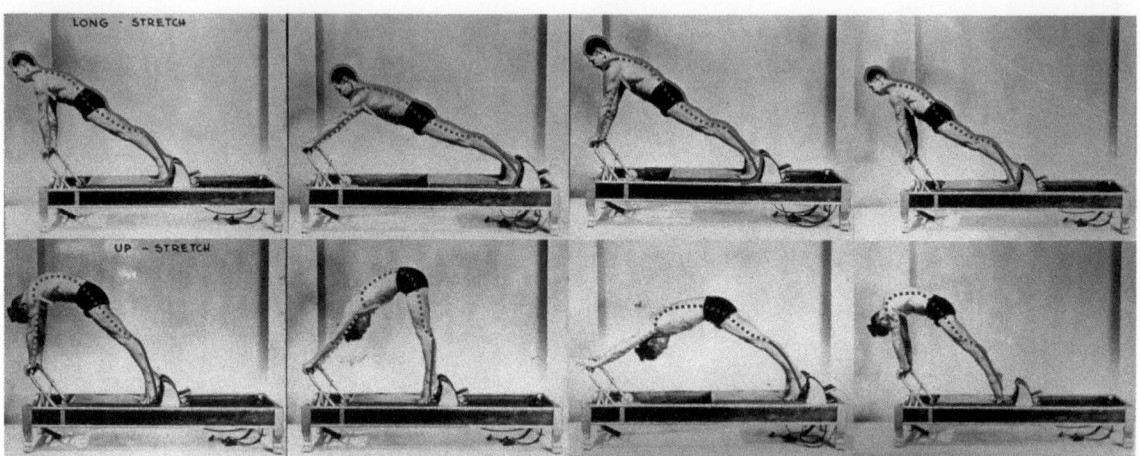

Figure 3.4
Joseph Pilates exercises illustrate how closed kinematic chains are able to control motion. Articulation of the Deep Front myofascial continuity in plank orientation. Top row: Long Stretch. Bottom row: Up Stretch.
Reproduced with kind permission from Balanced Body Inc. www.pilates.com.

Movement is a *whole-body* issue because everything is coupled together and nothing happens in isolation, and it is suggested that an appreciation of the body's internal mechanics (kinematic geometry) is at least as important as the behavior of individual bones and muscles. Our understanding of the human body comes from centuries of tradition, but we now have a new window into exploring its complexity and rethinking what we are doing as practitioners.

References

Cabe, P. A. (2019) "All perception engages the tensegrity-based haptic medium." *Ecological Psychology, 31*, 1–13.

Di Fabio, R. P. (1999) "Making jargon from kinetic and kinematic chains." *Journal of Orthopaedic & Sports Physical Therapy, 29*, 142–143.

Levin, S. M. and Scarr, G. (2022) "Biotensegrity and the mechanics of fascia." In: R. Schleip, C. Stecco, M. Driscoll, and P. A. Huijing (Eds.) *Fascia: The Tensional Network of the Human Body.* 2nd Ed. Elsevier, pp. 232–238.

Levin, S. M., Lowell de Solórzano, S., and Scarr, G. (2017) "The significance of closed kinematic chains to biological movement and dynamic stability." *Journal of Bodywork and Movement Therapies, 21*, 664–672.

Scarr, G. (2018) *Biotensegrity: The Structural Basis of Life.* 2nd Ed. Edinburgh: Handspring Publishing.

History of Assessment and Gait-Based Assessment Protocols

Madeline Black

"See that lady over there? She has her head at a tilt and that is because she takes a longer step with one foot which causes her to put that hip forward and that requires her to tilt her head to keep balanced" (Steele 2020). In Mr. Steele's memoir *Caged Lion* about his personal experience with Joseph H. Pilates, he describes a walk around Central Park in New York where Mr. Pilates points out various people's gait pattern. Mr. Pilates' keen eye observed how they are walking and identified potential physical issues that may result from gait strategies. Mr. Pilates had the ability to observe the human body, identify a person's movement strategy, and through his method create beneficial change.

Historically, assessment in Pilates teaching was not formal or structured. The teachers who worked with Mr. Pilates organically learned his pedagogy. They developed their own unique pedagogical approach to teaching Pilates from the synthesis of their dance education and other movement experiences. Eve Gentry (see Chapter 5) performed a thorough assessment during an initial appointment and wrote notes of the physical observations that were significant such as toe deviations, leg alignment, and spinal curvatures (Black 1992). Carola Trier (see Chapter 5) was known for her keen eye on evaluating posture using a mirror on wheels and specifically addressed alignment and posture. Kathy Grant (see Chapter 5) had extensive initial interview questions investigating one's history that included physical, life situations, and emotional aspects. Ms. Grant was known to have an intuitive sense for identifying the body's

history by observation. According to Brett Howard, Romana Kryzanowska (see Chapter 5) taught her teachers to "always teach the body in front of you." She educated by example, explaining how to assess the needs of the client (Pilates Anytime 2013). Today assessment, even as informal as Mr. Pilates', is the basis of a movement teacher's process.

Movement specialists are always observing and assessing movement for information to guide a client. It may be as simple as how a cue can change the client's focus, clarifying the movement function. A thorough analysis may determine an optimal starting intervention that progresses efficiently. Some physicians in New York City showed interest in the Pilates Method for its therapeutic potential. Mr. Pilates and Carola Trier developed a working relationship with Dr. Henry Jordan, Chief of Orthopedics at Lenox Hill Hospital in New York, who referred patients to them and invited Carola to observe surgeries (NPCE Study Guide 2021; Pilates Anytime 2013). The Saint Francis Memorial Hospital's Center for Sports Medicine's Dancemedicine division in San Francisco was the first clinical setting to incorporate Pilates as treatment modality. The center's director, orthopedic surgeon James G. Garrick, MD, hired Pilates teachers to be Dancemedicine Specialists, contributing to treatment teams. Physical therapists performed the thorough assessment of the patient. The Dancemedicine Specialists designed a Pilates program to meet short-term and long-term goals defined in the assessment. Dancemedicine Specialists documented patient progress in a SOAP (subjective, objective assessment, plan) note format. Physical therapists from sports medicine clinics around the world followed the example of James Garrick, MD and integrated Pilates into their treatment programs. This contributed to the inclusion of client assessment and client records in the Pilates practice.

As the evolution of a Pilates practice grew, assessment became part of the skill set for a Pilates teacher. The development of a national certification exam by the Pilates Method Alliance in 2005, now an autonomous certification program called the National Pilates Certification Program (NPCP), describes role delineations for Pilates teachers identifying three main domains that include assessment and evaluation (Domains I and II), and reassessment (Domain III) (NPCE Study Guide 2021). The assessment commonly used is a static posture-based analysis.

In this book, the co-editors introduce the use of gait as the basis for assessment rather than a static postural assessment. A unique assessment based on gait was customized for the movement programs (see Appendix 2). Gait highlights a person's structural patterns and movement strategies. It provides information about a person's physicality, nervous system responses, physiological states, and condition of health. Recent research indicates that assessing gait speed is significant for the measurement of health and measurement of decline (Rasmussen *et al.* 2019). Gait analysis is now being used as a determinant of quality of life in older age since it requires the integration of many physiological systems (Studenski *et al.* 2011). Health conditions involve physiological states that influence the neuromyofascial system, therefore affecting movement. The co-editors are interested in identifying the individual's unique gait pattern, to understand how the health condition impacts gait. Many of the movement programs in this book show that Pilates applications improve gait function, thereby lessening symptoms and enhancing a positive quality of life.

Gait analysis has been performed for decades in research studies using technology and visual observations. Phases of gait are well established strategies of how the person transfers weight from one foot to the other (Silva and Stergiou 2020). In these movement programs, the gait assessment is based on visual observations. Each author followed the movement program gait assessment in the Methods and Materials section.

The co-editors determined the important and easily observed movements of the body that are necessary for efficient gait. Starting at the ground, the feet adapt to the ground surfaces and forces. The ability of the foot to dorsiflex, plantar flex, supinate, and pronate are all required for adaptation and balance. In addition, the feet and ankles affect the distribution of forces through the body. The torso drives the motion of the pelvis and legs by its helical patterns of lateral flexion, rotations, and sagittal motions. The pelvifemoral motions for lateral shift of weight, abduction/adduction, and sagittal acetabular femoral joint movements were included in the movement program gait assessment. In lateral pelvic shift assessment, the pelvic listing, a slight inferior hemipelvis movement was observed with whole body response. Arm swing indicates how thoracic rotation contributes to the helical motion. Gait requires coordination and balance. The addition of simple timed tests of balance were integrated into the assessment.

The health conditions in this book range from joint limitations, neurological, autoimmune, and age-related health concerns. In some cases, additional assessment tests were required to address the specific condition. These are noted in the movement program chapter. During Session 12, the last session, the movement program gait assessment was repeated. The pre and post assessment findings are organized side by side so the reader can easily track the potential effects of the Pilates sequences.

Movement program gait assessment

The movement program gait assessment was followed by each contributing author. The contributing authors documented the findings of each assessment on the Movement Program Assessment Form (see Appendix 2). In context of this assessment, the terms *efficient* and *inefficient* are used to identify a client's movement strategies. Each assessment test is performed to the right and left directions. The notation of the findings is of the *inefficient movement* pattern. This allows the movement practitioner to design the appropriate program and to track the effectiveness of the movement sequences. For example, in the Hip Drop Test (see below), if the findings show the inability to lower the left hemipelvis, with limitations of thoracic translation and right pelvifemoral internal rotation, the notation will be left *inefficient movement.* Notes describing the efficient movement patterns are included on the form.

The following descriptions of the assessment tests prepare the reader to understand the logic and findings of the assessments.

1. General gait observation of subject's current state

a. Arm swing with thoracic rotation, relative pelvic motion, rear foot to forefoot adaptations
b. Torso's ability to react to the ground forces
c. Observe foot and ankle motion, noting the articulation from heel strike through propulsion

2. Standing full torso rotation

The end range of torso rotation is not the determinate of this assessment. The range may appear greater in one direction; however, notice the compensations such as flexing one knee to achieve the range.

a. Posterior view
  i. Sequential rotation from head to feet
  ii. Articulation of the thorax
  iii. Pelvic rotation on the femurs. This is pelvifemoral movement

  iv. Rear foot relative to forefoot adaptation of supination and pronation
b. Anterior view
  i. Pelvifemoral timing of pelvic rotation with a delay of acetabular femoral rotations
  ii. Noting acetabular femoral glide

3. Hip drop test

a. Pelvifemoral articulation
b. Lateral, translatory adaptation of the torso, specifically the lumbar and thorax
c. Posterior view
  i. Ability of inferior hemipelvis motion, pelvic list (see Glossary)
  ii. Lumbar lateral flexion and translation toward the lowering hemipelvis. This moves the convexity side toward the inferior hemipelvis
  iii. Thoracic translation toward higher hemipelvis
  iv. Pelvifemoral motion of higher hemipelvis with relative internal rotation/adduction of the acetabular femoral joint
  v. A pelvic list or inferior hemipelvis motion with thoracic translation occurs during swing phase transitioning from one foot to the other (Black 2022)

4. Hip hike test

a. Ability to elevate one hemipelvis and plantar flex the same side
b. Superior and inferior hemipelvis motions accompanied by pelvifemoral articulation
c. Posterior view
  i. Hemipelvis moves superiorly
  ii. Lumbar lateral flexion toward the rising hemipelvis
  iii. Thoracic translation toward elevating hemipelvis

5. Lateral pelvic shift

This transitional weight shift mirrors the moment when the body moves laterally, preparing to stand on one leg. A small shift of weight increases the load onto one leg without losing ground contact of the feet.

a. Posterior view
    i. The movement relationship of the thoraco-lumbar junction (TLJ) relative to S2
    ii. 5 degrees inferior hemipelvis motion of less weighted side
    iii. Lumbar lateral flexion with coupled movement of thoracic translation toward the more weighted side (Lee 2018)
    iv. Feet adaptation
        1. Side with increased weight supination maintaining 1st metatarsophalangeal (MTP) contact
        2. Side with less weight pronation with 5th MTP contact
b. Anterior view
    i. Acetabular femoral articulation
        1. Side with increased weight, internal rotation and adduction
        2. Side with less weight, external rotation and abduction

6. Seated tests

Sitting position locates the acetabular femoral joint 1 in. (2.5 cm) above the knee. In many cases, a person begins with the efficient side, placing more weight on one ischial tuberosity. It is important to note the organization in sitting prior to and throughout the movement task.

Each contributing author chose from the following:

a. Hip flexion without weight shift on ischial tuberosities or a posterior pelvic rotation and flexion
b. Knee flexion and dorsiflexion: slide the foot posteriorly, rear foot to forefoot in contact with the floor
c. Hip abduction and external rotation: slide plantar surface of the foot along opposite tibia
d. Ankle dorsiflexion: lift the mid-foot and forefoot while maintaining the calcaneus on the floor

e. Ankle plantar flexion: lift the calcaneus with the forefoot on floor

7. Seated torso rotation

This is an optional test as it was not performed in all the movement programs. Observing the torso rotation seated allows for a more specific view of the torso.

a. Sequential articulation of the thorax from the top down
b. Thoracic translatory movements
c. Weight shift on the ischial tuberosities

8. Sit and stand

Three times each view. There are three views: lateral, anterior, and posterior.

a. Hip and knee flexion and extension
b. Angle of torso
c. Rotating the TLJ and S2 vertical alignment
d. Ability to dorsiflex

9. Standing balance tests

One minute in length. The choice of appropriate balance test task for their subject was made by the authors.

a. Two-leg stance, eyes open
b. One-leg stance, eyes open
c. Two-leg stance, eyes closed
d. One-leg stance, eyes closed
e. Cervical rotation, two-leg stance

10. Final movement program gait assessment, Session 12

a. Detailed observation of the subject's gait pattern
b. Anterior and posterior views:
    i. Right step: weight transfer on to right foot
        1. Right ankle dorsiflexion and left foot push-off
        2. Pelvic rotation with oppositional thoracic rotation

3. Arm swing amplifying thoracic rotation
ii. Left step
   1. Left ankle dorsiflexion and right foot push-off
   2. Pelvic rotation with oppositional thoracic rotation
   3. Arm swing amplifying thoracic rotation

Each contributing author customized the Pilates program based on the subject's health condition and their observations during the movement program gait assessment. A post-assessment was conducted during Session 12.

References

Black, M. (1992) Notes from a private session with Eve Gentry gifted to her after Eve's death by Michelle Larsson, Eve Gentry Studio, Santa Fe, New Mexico.

Black, M. (2022) *Centered: Organizing the Body through Kinesiology, Movement Theory and Pilates Techniques*. Edinburgh: Handspring Publishing, p. 67.

Lee, D. (2018) *The Thorax: An Integrated Approach*. Edinburgh: Handspring Publishing, pp. 50–55.

NPCE Study Guide (National Pilates Certification Exam Study Guide) (2021) Miami, FL: National Pilates Certification Program, Inc., p. 11, pp. 95–96.

Pilates Anytime (2013) Documentary #1252. *In Honor of Carola*: 03:38–04:00, 06:35–07:25; Sarita Allen on Kathy Grant: 21:36–22:18; Cara Reeser on Kathy Grant: 11:28–12:20; Brett Howard on Romana Kryzanowska: 07:30–07:48.

Rasmussen, L. J. H., Caspi, A., Ambler, A., Broadbent, J. M. *et al.* (2019) "Association of neurocognitive and physical function with gait speed in midlife." *JAMA Network Open, 2,* 10. DOI:10.1001/jamanetworkopen.2019.13123.

Silva, L. M. and Stergiou, N. (2020) "The basics of gait analysis." In N. Stergiou (Ed.) *Biomechanics and Gait Analysis*. UK: Academic Press, pp. 225–250. www.sciencedirect.com/science/article/pii/B9780128133729000075. [Accessed July 31, 2023].

Steele, J. H. (2020) *Caged Lion*. Santa Barbara, CA: Last Leaf Press, p. 47.

Studenski, S., Perera, S., Patel, K., Rosano, C. *et al.* (2011) "Gait speed and survival in older adults." *JAMA, 305,* 1, 50–58.

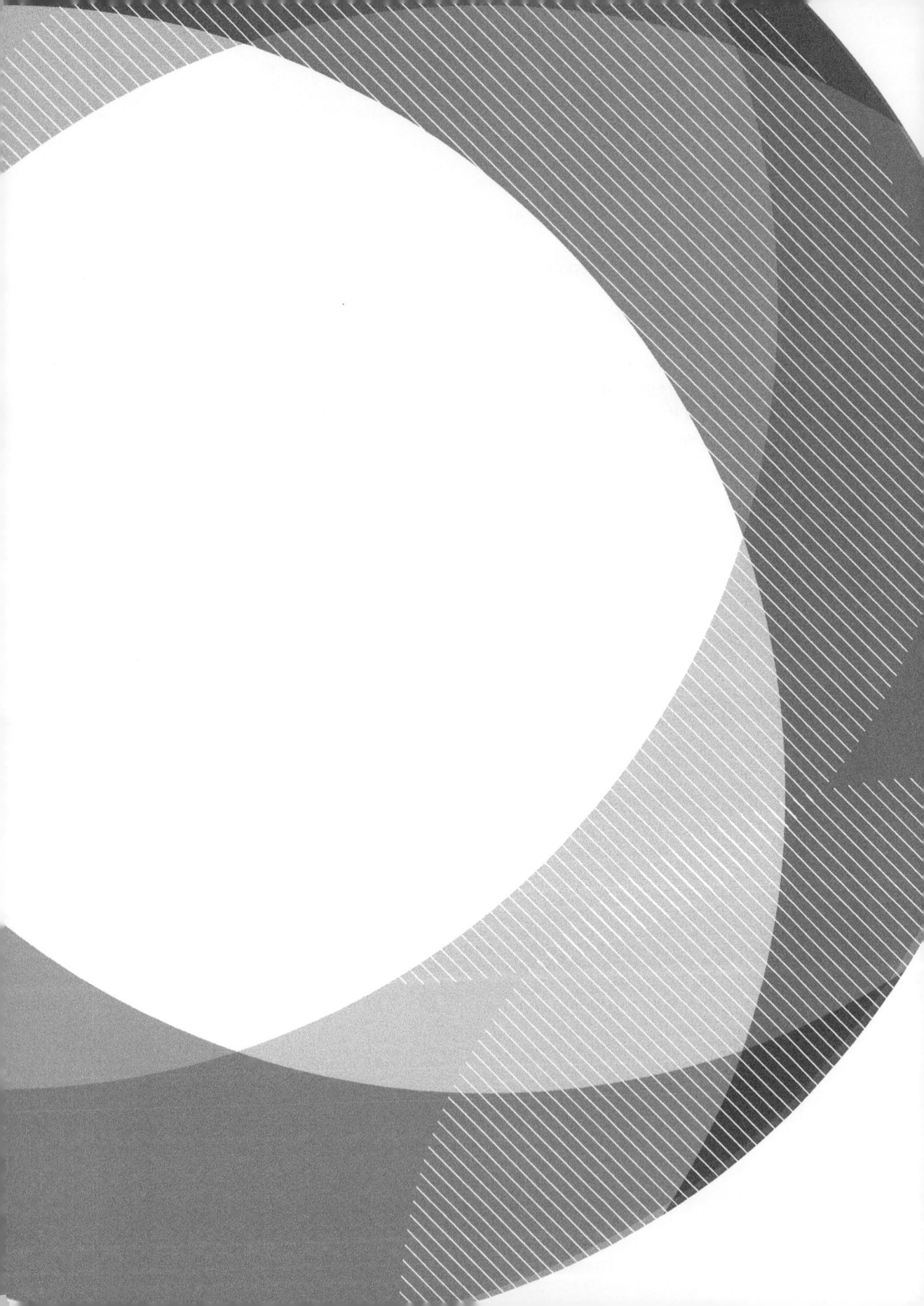

Movement Vocabulary Approaches

Contributions from Madeline Black, Sarita Allen, Alycea Ungaro, and Elizabeth Larkam

The majority of the movement vocabulary used in the case reports in this book is based on the movement sequences of J. H. Pilates that are documented in the NCPE Study Guide (2021). Each contributing author's unique expertise and experience influenced how they integrated the J. H. Pilates exercises. Many case reports included exercises developed by the teachers who studied with J. H. Pilates and worked as teachers at his studio. Eve Gentry, Carola Trier, Kathy Grant, and Romana Kryzanowska each evolved a pedagogical approach to the work of J. H. Pilates that is part of Pilates teachings today. This reference chapter is not an exhaustive list of all additional vocabulary—we focus on the vocabulary that appears in the case reports. Some contributors chose to include other variations of J. H. Pilates' vocabulary, integrating principles from contemporary theories for physical training. This chapter attributes the vocabulary to its source.

Eve Gentry approach
Madeline Black

Eve Gentry (Henrietta Greenhood) was born in 1909 in Los Angeles and began dancing at the age of five. She earned a scholarship to study a German form of modern dance influenced by Rudolf van Laban. In 1936, Eve joined the Hanya Holm Dance Company in New York City. A back injury brought her to J. H. Pilates' studio on 8th Avenue. She returned to dancing and assisted Mr. Pilates at his studio. In 1955, she was diagnosed with breast cancer and underwent a radical double mastectomy. Under Mr. Pilates' guidance, she restored her upper limbs to full function

and returned to performance. In 1968, she moved with her husband to Santa Fe, New Mexico, and established the Eve Gentry Studio. Later in her life, she contributed to the Physicalmind Institute previously known as the Institute for the Pilates Method. She continued to see clients with limited possibilities to move pain free after injury and illness at her studio until her death in 1994.

Eve Gentry studied with J. H. Pilates in New York City for over two decades. She developed a pedagogy of Pilates through her movement curiosity, explorations, and expression. She is known as an innovative movement specialist whose mission was to help an individual to move efficiently and cultivate their natural movement patterns. According to Michelle Larson (2007), Eve credited her Laban studies for her clarity of movement; Hanya Holm for movement concepts; and J. H. Pilates for her focus on breath and whole-body movement. Eve transitioned her life from the push of New York City to a calmer lifestyle in Santa Fe that allowed her to focus on developing her movement approach. Her sessions began with observing the client in movement to see the patterns, thereby understanding how to guide the session. Eve focused on moving from the bones with movements such as "imprinting" or "knee folds". She believed this focus of moving from the bones relieved excessive effort and freed the brain to choose more efficient patterns. Eve brought a somatic and movement correctives point of view to the Pilates method.

List of relevant exercises in case reports

- Knee folds to include unilateral, bilateral, and marching (Larsson 2007; Larsson and Kessel 2007)
- Eve's approach to encourage efficient hip flexion
  - Exhale, flex right hip with lower limb dangling for proximal activation to 90 degrees
  - Inhale at 90 degrees hip flexion
  - Exhale, moving lower right LE to the mat
  - Repeat for the left side
  - Alternate right to left
  - Bilateral flexion/extension
- Knee folds to leg slide
  - Slide right foot along the floor until leg is extended with femur in parallel
  - With extended right LE, externally rotate LE
  - In external rotation, flex/abduct the knee and hip, dragging the foot back into starting position
  - Perform the same movement again on each side by starting the hip in abduction/external rotation
  - Extend LE in external rotation with the foot in line with the ischial tuberosity
  - Internally rotate LE to parallel with extension
  - In parallel, flex knee and hip to return to starting position
- Knee stirs (Gentry and Gutterson 1982)
  - Exhale, flex one hip with lower limb dangling for proximal activation to 90 degrees
  - Place hand on top of ipsilateral knee
  - Place pressure into femur to facilitate posterior femoral glide
  - Circle the femur in the acetabulum
- Bellows breathing (Gentry and Gutterson 1982)
  - Inhale through the nose with lips closed
  - Exhale through the lips as if gently blowing out a candle
  - When seated place a towel or elastic band around the mid- to lower thoracic area, facilitating proprioception of the volume changes in the thorax. This is a bellows-like motion

- Nose circles (Gentry and Gutterson 1982)
  - Close your eyes, imagine a halo above your nose
  - Trace a circle with your nose, allowing the head to move along
  - Reverse direction
  - Let the circle grow as large as it feels good
- Spinal articulations/hip escalator (Gentry and Gutterson 1982)
  - Bridge movement with spine articulations
  - Variations: legs on spine corrector or wall
  - One-sided hip escalator
- Eve's Arm Swing Series (Gentry and Gutterson 1982)
  - Supine on mat
  - Windmill arms: bilateral or unilateral
- Puppet Arm Reaches (Gentry and Gutterson 1982)
  - Supine on mat with the arms at 90 degrees flexion, palms facing each other, elbows extended
  - Reach one arm to ceiling as if a puppeteer is pulling a string attached to fingers
  - Drop humeral head toward mat as if the string was released
  - Repeat with other arm
  - Repeat the above steps with both arms together
- Eve's Lunge (Larsson and Kessel 2007) is a safer alternative to standing on the Universal Reformer for J. H. Pilates Splits: Russian and Front (NPCE Study Guide 2021). It is performed standing beside the Universal Reformer with one foot on the carriage against the shoulder stop
- Wall: wall walks, straight-legged wall slide, pelvic tilts (Gentry and Gutterson 1982; Larsson and Kessel 2007)
  - Supine on mat with feet on wall
  - External rotation of hip joints, heels touching at midline/internal rotation of hip joints, 1st phalanges touching at midline
  - Walking feet on the wall, alternating external and internal rotation

- Legs extended on the wall, posterior pelvic tilt with pelvis lifted off floor, slide pelvis down the wall to floor
- Side Lying Imprinting (Larsson and Kessel 2007)
  - Segmental motion is a visualization of the bones moving into the mat and away from the mat in lateral motion
  - Begin at the pelvis, progressing to the head
- Propping with soft foam balls
  - Used in supine and lateral positions for re-organization of proprioception of the torso on the mat
  - Place soft foam balls underneath the areas of lightness or space
  - Breathe and rest for 1 minute or longer

We wish to acknowledge Debora Kowley and Kevin Bowen for their contribution of history and personal experiences of Eve Gentry for this reference.

Kathy Grant approach

Sarita Allen

Throughout her life, Kathleen Stanford Grant was a major influencer in the world of physical healing with her unique approach to the art of Pilates. While her contribution to Pilates was monumental, she made major contributions to the performing arts. Kathy had an illustrious dance career on Broadway and abroad. Two knee surgeries led her to Mr. Pilates. Kathy's interaction with Joseph Pilates was life-enhancing in terms of her physical well-being, her emotional confidence, and the support of her life purpose. Kathy began her apprenticeship with Mr. Pilates in 1964. She was the director of Mr. Pilates' studio at Bendel's in New York City. For over 20 years until her death, Kathy was on the faculty of the Tisch School of the Arts and ran her studio at NYU. She inspired a whole generation of Pilates teachers.

The combination of Kathy's work with Joseph Pilates and her love of dance compelled her to coach dancers. Her dance-focused clients ranged from the world's principal dancers to young dancers dreaming of having a career. Kathy's professional dance clients danced for prominent companies such as the Dance Theatre of Harlem, New York City Ballet, Paul Taylor Dance Company, Martha Graham Dance Company, Alvin Ailey American Dance Theater, and more. Kathy studied ballet, modern dance, and learned African dance in Africa. Her professional experience as a dance performance artist aided Kathy in her ability to serve this community. The combination of her insider knowledge of dance training and Mr. Pilates' method led her to create "Before the Hundred" practice, known today to teachers as "Pre-Pilates." These exercises were founded on the belief that people cannot come off the street and go straight into the Hundred. Kathy taught "Before the Hundred," helping her students move more efficiently, like when dancers prepare their bodies before class or rehearsal. She calmed the clients' mind to help them better connect to their bodies before engaging in dynamic and energetic Pilates exercises.

Kathy's breathing exercises

Kathy's breathing exercises and integration of sound are still used today to assist many in locating and activating their centers as well as relaxing their mind and body. Kathy would say, "Let your limbs be an extension of the breath!" While teaching at NYU, she developed what is called "Kathy's Song." Two key elements of this song include: ZIP (imagine you are zipping up a tight pair of jeans, which will cause you to pull your belly button to the lower part of your waist) and BUTTON YOUR VEST (imagine you are wearing a very elegant piece of cloth around your abdomen for awareness of rib connections to your center). Her breathwork also included accordion breathing, ball breathing, straw breathing, percussive breathing, hissing cat, and more. Humming, talking, singing, and breathwork were all key to Kathy's innovative approach to Pilates.

Kathy's insistence on finding movement from the inside out also proved essential to her method and practice. She never allowed her students to mimic a movement based on how it looked, but rather she asked them to understand the movement based on how it felt. She was emphatic that her clients find a grounded way of exploring their bodies in motion. Pulling from varied mediums, with influences from Mr. Pilates, Carola Trier, and Irene Dowd, Kathy Grant's creative and unapologetically distinct pedagogical approach to healing work, coupled with her undying curiosity to continuously expand her array of movement-based exercises, all added to her particular magic.

Exercises

- Ribcage Arms
  - Supine in hip and knee flexion with feet flat on mat, arms by sides
  - Raise arms to 90 degree shoulder flexion
  - Inhale, flex shoulder with extended elbows to a range of approximately 70–180 degrees
  - The range of shoulder flexion is in relation to the thoracolumbar junction contact with the mat
  - Exhale, extending the shoulders to 90 degree position
  - Option to hold a dowel, towel, or weighted bar
- Piston
  - Supine in hip and knee flexion with feet flat on mat, arms by sides
  - Wait until you have the sense of weight of the leg
  - With minimal effort, raise the foot a small amount off the mat
  - Feel the head of the femur as a piston moving deep into the socket
  - Place foot down

Romana Kryzanowska approach

Alycea Ungaro

I was a young dancer when I first met Romana Kryzanowska. In 1993, I came to study with her at the recommendation of her assistant, Steve Giordano.

She spoke few words in our meeting and charged me to return the next morning to teach a mat class according to an exercise list that she handed me. I was terrified.

Fast forward to a session several years later when I found myself subject to her prodding. "Bring this bone forward," she said, while simultaneously pressing her pointer finger against my sternum. She tapped that spot a few times for emphasis. I had little choice but to rearrange my skeleton accordingly and comply. She was right, of course, and the exercise suddenly went to work. I remembered our first meeting from long ago and how concisely she spoke and was reminded that too many words can be wasteful.

Romana taught Pilates with short simple cues. She shunned the use of anatomical terms and wasn't shy about saying so. She trained her teachers to speak in sound bites, actionable commands that would spark movement. Heavy imagery and lengthy explanations were best left to meditation and yoga—but not Pilates, as she explained. The breath was a final layer, she explained. "Get them moving" was the preferred approach.

In my time with Romana, I became aware of exercises that she had added to the Pilates repertoire including Side Kick exercises specifically for dancers or the jump board. For the most part she held to the work of her teacher, Joe Pilates. She reported checking her notes and shared her findings generously with her students and trainees. Above all she was expert at explaining everyday movements to her myriad clients to support their daily activities. Simple moves with simple words—this was her formula for success and the one she modeled and transmitted to the teachers she trained.

The Wall Series is a clear example of Romana's approach to the work using direct cueing and targeting simple movements. During final exams Romana could be heard asking soon-to-be graduates: "Who needs the Wall?" The entire gym would respond: "Everyone needs the Wall."

Read on to follow along.

The Wall Series

- Stand
  - Stand upright against a wall from heel to head
  - Work the base of your skull, the length of your spine, the backs of your legs into the wall
  - Draw the abdominals in and up
  - Breathe deeply as you work the back body into the wall
- Roll-Down
  - From your first exercise, walk the feet forward one step
  - Press the length of your spine into the wall from hips to head
  - Peel off the wall one bone at a time until you are about halfway down. Let your arms "dangle" (Romana's word)
  - Make tiny circles with the arms five times in one direction and then reverse
  - Roll back up the wall one vertebra at a time
  - Breathe naturally
  - Repeat 2–3 times

Editor note

An option is to hold light hand weights during the Roll-Down (see Volume 2, Chapter 4 Figure 4.4).

- Arm circles
  - From the end of the last Roll-Down stand upright
  - Raise the arms up to head height—pull the powerhouse in
  - Circle the arms down and around 5 times within the peripheral vision
  - Repeat 5 times in each direction
  - Breathe naturally

See Glossary: **powerhouse**

- Chair
  - From the end of the last Arm Circle, take the feet one large step away as you stay supported by the wall
  - Slide down the wall into a chair position. Ankles, knees, and hips are all at a sharp right angle. Raise the arms to shoulder height
  - Hold for 10 seconds. Build up to 1 minute. "Two minutes for Skiers," according to Romana
  - Breathe deeply

Editor note

For an example of how to use Wall Series: Chair in a home program, see Volume 1, Chapter 7, Session 3/12, exercise 4, Wall mini-squat.

Carola Trier approach

Elizabeth Larkam

Carola Trier was born Carola Beatrice Strauss in Germany in 1911. She died in 2000 in New York City at age 89. Mrs. Trier was trained in Laban and performed with the Joos Ballet. When a recital career was not economically viable in Germany, she became a hot rhythm tap dancer. In Paris she developed into a modern classic roller skating contortionist. She came to America with her act in 1942 to work in vaudeville and night clubs, spending 23 years in show business. Mrs. Trier was a staff member of the Marina Svetlova Ballet Academy and taught her specialty of preliminary exercises for acrobatics for actors and dancers at the Katherine Dunham School of Cultural Arts. She had a basic knowledge of anatomy and physiology of the musculoskeletal system acquired in part from her father (Ewing 2021) who was a research biochemist.

Mrs. Trier trained and worked with Joseph and Clara Pilates for ten years during the 1950s after his technique aided her in recovering from injuries resulting from a dance career. Mrs. Trier opened her own studio, the Carola Trier Studio—Body Conditioning and Correction in 1960 on 200 West 58th Street, New York, NY. The mechanical equipment and system of exercise used by Mrs. Trier were developed by Joseph H. Pilates.

Many clients were referred by doctors for rehabilitation. Self-referred dancers flocked to her practice. Dedicated students and teachers of the work of Joseph H. Pilates, including Romana Kryzanowska and Kathy Grant, worked as assistants in the Carola Trier Studio. Teachers working today who also taught in the Carola Trier Studio include Deborah Lessen (2013a; 2013b) and Roberta Kirschenbaum.

Dr. Henry H. Jordan, Chief of Orthopedic Surgery, Lenox Hill Hospital, referred patients to the Manhattan studio of Mrs. Carola Trier for a program of "heavy resistance" exercises designed to build up muscle strength and functional ability.

"When I am planning to refer a patient for exercises after surgery," said Dr. Jordan, "I often have Mrs. Trier in the operating room so she can watch the procedures and see the structures that are involved." He also provided her with information on the orthopedic condition and gave instructions on the particular muscle groups that required exercise. The programs customarily started with elementary training in deep diaphragmatic breathing and basic orientation by Mrs. Trier about the "totally integrated exercise system designed to train all muscles at the same time."

The Pilates programs in this book include movement sequences derived from the teaching of Carola Trier. These include:

- Universal Reformer
  - Stomach Massage with short box providing back support
  - Variations of the Knee Stretch Series
  - Variations of Long Spine Massage
- Trapeze Table
  - Leg Springs, fixed crossbar with central eye bolt
  - Breathing coordination
- Adjustable Ped-o-Pull arm springs

We wish to acknowledge Jillian Hessel and Roberta Kirschenbaum for their contribution of history and personal experiences with Carola Trier for this reference.

References

NPCE Study Guide (National Pilates Certification Exam Study Guide) (2021) Miami, FL: National Pilates Certification Program, Inc., p. 62.

Eve Gentry references

Gentry, E. and Gutterson, S. (1982) *The First Guide to your Daily Practice of Therapeutic and Corrective Exercise.* [Booklet]. Santa Fe, NM: Core Dynamics, pp. 2, 3, 8, 10, 12, 20.

Larsson, M. (2007) "All about Eve." Pilates Style Magazine, pp. 37–39.

Larsson, M. and Kessel, M. (2007) "Eve Gentry: The Power of Pilates DVD." Directed by Marion Kessel. Knee folds: 31:30–31:37; knee stirs: 28:17–28:20; hip escalator: 23:08–23:32; Eve's Lunge: 27:53–28:00; wall walks: 22:14–22:40; Side Lying Imprinting: 18:56–19:25.

Carola Trier references and further reading

Ewing, E. (2021) "Carola Trier." Archives of newspaper and magazine articles from Library for the Performing Arts. www.rhinebeckpilates.com/pilates-history-carola-trier. [Accessed August 3, 2023].

Lessen, D. (2013a) Tutorial #1202 Reformer Sequences. PilatesAnytime. October 09, 2013. [Video]. www.pilatesanytime.com/workshop-view/1202/video/Pilates-Reformer-Sequences-by-Deborah-Lessen. [Accessed August 3, 2023].

Lessen, D. (2013b) Tutorial #1319 Cadillac Methods. PilatesAnytime. November 18, 2013. [Video]. www.pilatesanytime.com/workshop-view/1319/video/Pilates-Cadillac-Methods-by-Deborah-Lessen. [Accessed August 3, 2023].

Variable Spring Resistance in Pilates

Ken Endelman

The unique characteristics of spring resistance differentiate the Pilates movement environment from all other exercise settings. Mr. Pilates' (1883–1967) insight was to choose springs for his equipment designs when most strength training equipment used metal weight plates. Throughout his four decades of work in the Pilates Universal Gymnasium (Gallagher and Kryzanowska 2000), J. H. Pilates continued to develop his movement system, inventing over 20 items of exercise apparatus that add assistance, resistance, and complexity to the organization and movement strategies required by the mat exercises. The equipment frames provide numerous places to which springs or straps may be attached, creating movement environments that support a variety of vectors (Larkam 2017). Springs support the Pilates principles of whole-body movement. These include Control, Breath, Concentration, Centering, Flowing Motion, and Precision (NPCE Study Guide 2021). Pilates teachers who understand the attributes of the variable spring resistance-assistance continuum of each apparatus can apply this knowledge when designing effective movement sequences for health conditions.

Spring manufacturing process

Springs can be made from metals, rubber, plastic, or other materials. The key characteristic is that, when the material is deformed, the spring returns to its original shape. This is called *memory*. Imagine molecular crystals interconnected in a very tight pattern. When you pull on a spring, the crystals begin to pull apart. Until the crystals reach their elastic limit, the crystals seek to return to their original formation (memory). Each spring is designed for an application that modifies the spring's performance. The behavior of a spring is a function of wire size, material composition, coil diameter, length, and manufacturing process. The manufacturing process involves several stages of pre-tensioning the spring followed by use of heat to reduce the tension. Each spring has unique properties resulting in up to 10 percent variability between springs.

Whether resistance is delivered by body weight, free weight, an elastic band, or a spring, it can be modified by friction, leverage, or trajectory. When lifting or pulling a weight the amount of resistance remains uniform throughout the stroke.

In contrast to the resistance delivered by weight(s), spring resistance predictably increases based on the design of the specific spring. For example, if 2 kg (4.41 lb) of force are required to extend a spring 10 cm (3.94 in.), extending the same spring to 20 cm (7.87 in.) will require 4 kg (8.82 lb) of force. Extending this spring to 30 cm (11.81 in.) requires 6 kg (13.23 lb) of force. The relationship between distance and resistance continues until the spring is pulled to its *elastic limit* when it deforms or breaks. This is known as Hooke's law.

Variable spring resistance in the J. H. Pilates Universal Reformer, Wunda Chair, and Trapeze Table

The application of the spring resistance within the frame of the apparatus influences the client's motor control response. Each Pilates equipment invention provides different challenges to motor control training.

If a client were to perform a leg press on a Universal Reformer custom-fitted with a 50 kg (110.23 lb) weight on a single pulley, the client would start by pushing 50 kg and continue with the same resistance until terminal leg press.

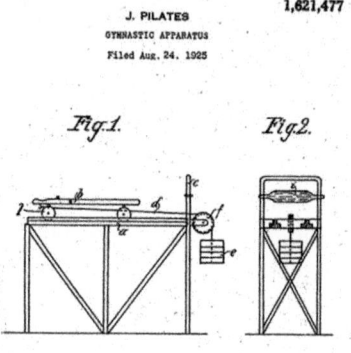

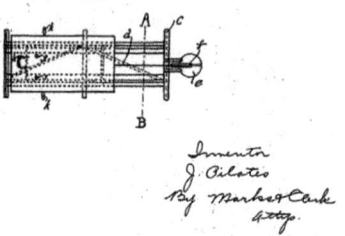

Figure 6.1
Pilates Universal Reformer patent drawing with weights
Reproduced with permission from Larkam, E. (2017) Fascia in Motion: Fascia-Focused Movement for Pilates. Edinburgh: Handspring Publishing, Figure 2.3, page 36

The linear progression of spring resistance means that a client can experience a wide range of resistances over a relatively small distance. With 4 medium (red) springs on a Universal Reformer the same client performing a leg press could experience a 12–92 kg (26.45–202.82 lb) variation (Singh 2022) in resistance from the beginning of the movement to terminal leg press.

Universal Reformer spring applications are complex. On the Universal Reformer, we start with a horizontal spring connected to a carriage. The carriage has its own mass and wheels that create friction. This friction is a result of rolling resistance caused by the type of wheel and the type of bearings used. This friction is compounded by the weight of the client. The amount of force (resistance) needed to move the carriage away from the spring attachment to the frame is a function of spring resistance, wheel friction, and inertia. Some Universal Reformers, like the Allegro 2, are designed to minimize wheel friction, and others, like the Balanced Body Contrology, capitalize on wheel friction.

On the Trapeze Table and Wunda Chair springs are used in conjunction with levers. The Trapeze Table push-through bar and the Wunda Chair foot pedal are examples of two different spring-lever systems. Levers distribute work (weight) by increasing and decreasing distance (travel).

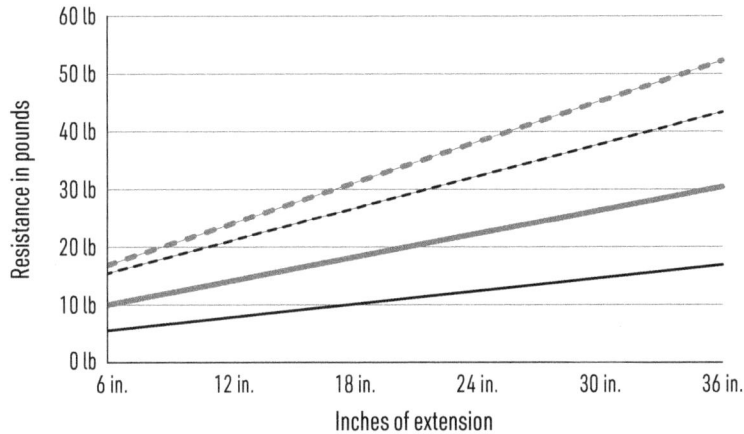

Figure 6.2
Springs on the Universal Reformer showing the length-resistance relationship

The mounting point of the spring is important to the pivot or fulcrum point of the lever. On the Trapeze Table push-through bar, the mounting point of the spring is directly over the pivot or fulcrum point when the push-through bar is sprung from the top. The resistance varies according to the arc of the push-through bar. For example, in the Cat (NPCE Study Guide 2021, p. 63) the client engages the spring moving the bar down, and the load increases until the bar begins to approach the point when the bar passes through bottom center, parallel to the vertical upright bars. The movement sequences of the spring-lever combination of the push-through bar sprung from above and sprung from below can be viewed in the video on the Cadillac Methods of Carola Trier narrated by Deborah Lessen (Lessen 2013).

The use of the lever in the Wunda Chair foot pedal is different from the Trapeze Table push-through bar. Here the pivot point is used more like a hinge. The forces are less linear and can be altered to take advantage of the client's strength profile.

Connective tissue response to spring resistance

An additional characteristic of spring resistance not commonly discussed is the vibration or oscillation that results as a spring expands and contracts. The amount and quality of the oscillation is determined by the type of spring and its application. This vibration creates additional variability and stimulation to the client's multi-sensory movement experience.

Editor note

The sensitivity of a Pilates client's response to variable spring vibration and oscillation may be attributed to fascia as a neurosensitive structure in which a complex functional network of interconnected and integrated body dynamics is assembled. In his book *Myofascial Induction: Volume 1—The Upper Body,* Andrzej Pilat cites studies that create a new vision of fascia different from the traditional view of the structure that envelops the muscle (Pilat 2022). The muscle is not considered as the exclusive protagonist of the movement. This role is extended to the myofascial unit, a group of highly specialized collagenous structures in a crossed-helical arrangement that are intimately linked to muscle fibers (Scarr 2018). The central nervous system and the autonomic nervous system receive most of their mechanosensitive information from the neurofascial system. The receptors, along with the peripheral nerves and the brain, constitute the somatosensory system which interacts with the autonomic nervous system.

In her book *Yoga, Fascia, Anatomy and Movement*, Joanne Avison writes:

> Fascia is known to conduct light through the body. It is suggested that the pre-stiffened tensegrity organization (which is the basic nature of the fibrils and fibers throughout the cells and the entire system) resonates with tissue-specific frequencies. That suggests fascia is highly sensitive to sound currents – as might be expected from a tension-compression structure. (Avison 2021)

For additional information on tension-compression structures see Chapter 3.

The variable resistance provided by the springs of the Pilates Universal Reformer, Wunda Chair, and Trapeze Table creates benefits supportive of a variety of health conditions.

References

Avison, J. S. (2021) *Yoga, Fascia, Anatomy and Movement.* 2nd Ed. Edinburgh: Handspring Publishing, pp. 170–171.

Gallagher, S. P. and Kryzanowska, R. (Eds.) (2000) *The Joseph H. Pilates Archive Collection: Photographs, Writings and Designs.* Philadelphia, PA: Bainbridge Books.

Larkam, E. (2017) *Fascia in Motion: Fascia-Focused Movement for Pilates.* Edinburgh: Handspring Publishing.

Lessen, D. (2013) Tutorial #1319 Cadillac Methods. PilatesAnytime. November 18, 2013. [Video]. www.pilatesanytime.com/workshop-view/1319/video/Pilates-Cadillac-Methods-by-Deborah-Lessen. [Accessed September 7, 2023].

NPCE Study Guide (National Pilates Certification Exam Study Guide) (2021) Miami, FL: National Pilates Certification Program, Inc.

Pilat, A. (2022) *Myofascial Induction: An Anatomical Approach to the Treatment of Fascial Dysfunction—Volume 1 The Upper Body.* Edinburgh: Handspring Publishing, pp. 155, 177.

Scarr, G. (2018) *Biotensegrity: The Structural Basis of Life.* 2nd Ed. Edinburgh: Handspring Publishing, p. 31.

Singh, H. (2022) Effect of springs on a Universal Reformer. Email correspondence with Harbir Singh, Engineering Manager, Balanced Body Inc., September 20, 2022.

Pilates and Multiple Sclerosis: Effect on Gait

Madeline Black

Multiple sclerosis (MS) is a disease of an immune-mediated process where an abnormal response of the body's own immune system is directed against the central nervous system (CNS), the brain, spinal cord, and optic nerves. The disease's name, multiple sclerosis, comes from the multiple areas of plaques that develop along the central nervous system creating multiple areas of hardening.

Multiple sclerosis occurs at any age from infancy to geriatric. MS is most diagnosed in one's 20s through 30s, making it the most diagnosed neurological disorder in young adults (National Multiple Sclerosis Society 2023a).

On average women are three times more likely to be diagnosed with MS than men. The cause of multiple sclerosis is unknown, and it may involve genetic, immune, and environmental sensitivities which in combination may result in a triggering of the disease. There is no cure for MS, nor can it be prevented. MS is not contagious. Currently numerous FDA-approved disease-modifying therapeutics (DMTs) are available to help reduce the severity of the disease in the hope of delaying progression.

In MS an abnormal response occurs within the body's immune system. This abnormal response incorrectly attacks healthy tissue of the CNS and causes inflammation that damages myelin, nerve fibers, and specialized cells that make up myelin. Myelin is the fatty substance that surrounds and insulates the CNS, providing the conductivity sheath for messages to travel from the CNS out to the peripheral nervous system (PNS). Myelin is the primary target of the immune system attack in MS.

When the myelin within the CNS is damaged, the messages from the brain, spinal cord, or optic nerve become patchy, slow, or incomplete. The result can be a conduction loss of motor and sensory information. The CNS dysfunction is not a peripheral motor loss. The PNS is still intact but cannot receive the message to complete the motor task of movement. This is the reason why the Bioness® transcutaneous neuromuscular system can work on some individuals with MS.

According to the National Multiple Sclerosis Society (2023b), common neurological MS symptoms are:

- MS hug (dysesthesia): the sensation of squeezing around the torso
- MS fatigue or lassitude commonly occurs in 80 percent of the MS population
  - General feeling of heaviness and moving slowly as if moving through concrete
  - Brain fatigue or brain fog
- The following may occur daily:
  - Poor sleep conditions
  - Nocturnal muscle spasms
  - Nocturnal bladder control problems
  - Depression
- Temperature intolerance increases in warmer external temperature conditions and when there is a warmer internal core temperature due to exercise or exertion
- Walking gait difficulties

- Spasticity or stiffness
- Numbness and tingling
- Vision changes or loss
- Vertigo and dizziness
- Weakness from damage to the nerve pathways
- Cognitive changes in 50 percent of the MS population may affect learning processes and the ability to recall new information, problem solving, focusing attention, and the ability to perceive the environment
- Pain is significant in 55 percent of people with MS, and almost 25 percent have a chronic pain condition
- Emotional changes from the daily stress of living with an unpredictable and chronic neurological disease and immune challenges

- Anxiety and depression

Not every person with MS has every neurological symptom, and each person has their individual presentation of multiple sclerosis.

Studies of people living with multiple sclerosis have shown that exercise can help with symptoms, improve strength, and result in increased participation in social activities. Exercise also slows down the progression of MS through the neurovascular system by improving smoother and faster communication between the brain and spinal cord (Ozkul *et al.* 2020).

Acknowledgment

The author would like to thank Julie Lyons P.T., L.Ac for providing the health condition description.

Client description: 55-year-old, identifies as female; physical therapist and licensed acupuncturist

Dates of case report: Session 1: December 27, 2019; Session 12: January 31, 2020

Studio apparatus and props
Pilates equipment

- Universal Reformer

Props used with equipment
- 4 heavy resistance bands, 6 ft (1.8 m), wrapping for proprioceptive input (see Chapter 7, Figure 7.2)
- Small, 1 in. (25 mm), pads, ¼ in. (6 mm) thick, for feet
- Ball, 9 in. (23 cm) in diameter, three-quarters inflated
- Konnector® attachment
- Air cushion disc
- Yoga strap

- Textured shoe inserts for proprioception stimulation
- Mat

> **Editor note**
> Konnector® was designed by Viktor Uygan. The four straps of Konnector® are attached through a series of pulleys to one rope. It is used in place of the Universal Reformer straps. The straps are connected to all four limbs to integrate the action of the limbs and torso. Konnector® creates an environment that stimulates the neuromyofascial system from the periphery to the torso, on the right and left sides, and in contralateral movement patterns (Uygan 2023).

Home program props

- Wall space
- 2 heavy resistance bands
- 4 dense half balls, 3 in. (76 mm) in diameter
- Yoga block
- Ball, 22 in. (55 cm) in diameter
- Ball, 9 in. (23 cm) in diameter, three-quarters inflated
- Rolled towel for head support
- Roller, 36 in. (90 cm) long, 6 in. (15 cm) in diameter
- Mat

Methods and materials

Session 1/12
1. Health history interview

- Subject initially diagnosed with relapsing-remitting MS; now after more than 25 years it has progressed to a secondary progressive form of MS
  - The change in diagnosis is based on yearly MRIs with contrast of the brain, thoracic, and lumbar regions showing no new lesions since approximately 2017
  - 2017: MRI showed a new lesion on the right optic nerve
  - Since 2017, no new lesions or new flare-ups but showing continued functional disability
- Early 1997: prior to diagnosis, client reports episodes of burning sensations and numbness on left side
- 2002–2003: after an episode of numbness of her face, doctor suggested possible MS
- February 2009: symptomatically diagnosed
  - MRI and blood tests showed thyroid insufficiency
- In 2010: client treated with radiation iodine for the thyroid condition
  - 1 year to find a balance of the thyroid medication
  - Infusion of Rituxan (immune suppressant) every 6 months
- December 19, 2019: most recent prescription
  - Prescribed Levothroid for the treatment of Graves' disease, an immune disorder affecting the thyroid

2. Symptoms

- General fatigue
- Left side
  - Foot drop
  - Loss of hip flexion and strength
  - Fine motor skills deficiency in the hand and numbness in hand
- Stress increases symptoms
  - Currently transitioning out of career
  - Sale of acupuncture and physical therapy (PT) practice

3. Movement aids

- 2 canes to walk
- Daily task of climbing stairs to bedroom
  - Belt attached on banister to pull and pauses one step at a time
  - Maneuvers one step at a time seated
- Bioness device in use for ankle dorsiflexion during gait

Final result of case report

Client was able to walk with a faster pace due to improved thoracic rotation and lumbopelvic femoral motions. She was able to climb her home stairs without pulling herself up with a belt or banister. Client is standing with improved bilateral weight distribution and feels more balanced.

Session 2/12: Initial assessment

1. General observations of gait

◆ Bioness activated, wore sneakers, used 2 canes

◆ No apparent thoracic rotation, excessive lateral motion

◆ Excessive right rib translation and left hemi-pelvis superior motion for left leg swing

◆ Cane usage inhibits thoracic rotation by pressing right cane into ground for left leg stability

◆ Cane powered by shoulder motion

◆ Heel strike sufficient on both sides

● Left heel strike possible with Bioness device activated

◆ Propulsion phase: plantar flexion was minimal on both sides

2. Standing tests

◆ Full torso rotation

● Observations of inefficient side: left
  ■ Left rotation
  ■ Minimal sequential thoracic rotation
  ■ Initiates from thoracolumbar junction (TLJ)
  ■ Minimal pelvis rotation on femurs
  ■ Right foot supinated, left did not adapt

◆ Hemipelvis inferior motion

● Observations of inefficient side: left
  ■ Inability to lower the left innominate

Session 12/12: Post-assessment

1. General observations of gait

◆ Bioness activated, wore sneakers, used 2 canes

◆ Improved thoracic rotation, less lateral shift and thoracic translation

◆ Pelvis motion balanced, less left hip hiking

◆ Improved sagittal plane hip and knee swing

◆ Cane usage facilitated better thoracic rotation and arm swing

◆ Heel strike sufficient on both sides

● Left heel strike possible with Bioness activated

◆ Propulsion phase: plantar flexion on right, not left

2. Standing tests

◆ Full torso rotation

● Observations of inefficient side: left
  ■ Left rotation
    ○ Visible sequential thoracic rotation with a differentiation of thorax to pelvis
    ○ Improved pelvis on femur rotation
  ■ Right foot pronated, left did not adapt

◆ Hemipelvis inferior motion

● Observations of inefficient side: left
  ■ Left hemipelvis inferior motion

- ■ Thorax translates right

- ◆ Hemipelvis superior motion

- ● Observations of inefficient side: both
  - ■ Right hemipelvis superior motion
  - ■ Inability to transfer pelvis over left leg
  - ■ Lack of left ankle plantar flexion
  - ■ Left hemipelvis superior motion
  - ■ Left innominate already elevated

- ◆ Lateral pelvic shift

- ● Observations of inefficient side: left
  - ■ Left shift
  - ■ Excessive right thoracic translation
  - ■ Feet not adapting
  - ■ Limited right femoral abduction and left femoral adduction

3. Seated tests

- ◆ Thoracic rotation

- ● Observations of inefficient side: right
  - ■ Seated heavily on right sitz bone
  - ■ Thorax held in a right translation inhibiting right thoracic rotation
  - ■ Thoracic flexion with right scapula retraction

- ◆ Hip joint and knee flexion

- ● Observations of inefficient side: both
  - ■ Seated heavily on right ischial tuberosity
  - ■ Thorax held in a right translation inhibiting right thoracic rotation

improved a small degree due to the right hip joint's ability to adduct

- ◆ Hemipelvis superior motion

- ● Observations of inefficient side: both
  - ■ Right hemipelvis superior motion
    - O Thorax orientated toward midline
    - O Plantar flexion on right foot improvement
  - ■ Left hemipelvis superior motion
    - O No excessive translation of thorax to right
    - O Left unable to plantar flex

- ◆ Lateral pelvic shift

- ● Observations of inefficient side: left
  - ■ Left shift
    - O Right innominate: slight degree of inferior motion
    - O Less thoracic right translation
    - O Feet not adapting, left foot unable to supinate

3. Seated tests

- ◆ Thoracic rotation

- ● Observations of inefficient side: right
  - ■ Seated evenly on ischial tuberosities
  - ■ Increased right rotation with transferring weight on left ischial tuberosity
  - ■ Torso in midline
  - ■ Scapula balanced

- ◆ Hip joint and knee flexion

- ● Observations of inefficient side: both
  - ■ Weight distributed evenly on ischial tuberosities
  - ■ Decreased right thoracic translation
  - ■ Able to maintain midline

■ Thoracic flexion with right scapula retraction

Author note

Included dorsiflexion and knee flexion test. Neither were efficient. On the right client was able to flex knee and dorsiflex ankle. Increased right thoracic translation and torso flexion required to perform the task. On the left side, she was unable to perform the task. Included hip abduction with external rotation. Neither were efficient. Right side was able to perform the task with increased right thoracic translation and torso flexion. Left side was unable to perform the task.

4. Sit and stand

◆ Lateral view

● Good bilateral pelvifemoral motion in flexion and extension
● Maintaining torso sagittal curves
● Seems cautious, moves slowly

◆ Anterior view

● Knees adduct, more on left than right

5. Standing balance

◆ Two-leg stance, eyes open

● No canes, Bioness on but not activated: 60 seconds

◆ One-leg stance, eyes open

● Using 2 canes
  ■ Left leg: 5 seconds
  ■ Right leg: 22 seconds

Author note

Included dorsiflexion and knee flexion test. Left was inefficient. Improved right dorsiflexion. Left side was unable to perform the task. Included hip abduction with external rotation. Left was inefficient. Left side was unable to perform the task.

4. Sit and stand

◆ Lateral view

● Good form, practices this movement on a daily basis, appears to have more confidence
● Transitions faster between stand and sit

◆ Anterior view

● Right knee aligned in flexion
● Left femur adducts slightly in flexion, less than in pre-assessment

5. Standing balance

◆ Two-leg stance, eyes open (with Bioness deactivated)

● No canes: 60 seconds

◆ One-leg stance, eyes open

● Using 2 canes
  ■ Left leg: 45 seconds
  ■ Right leg: 60 seconds

Session 3/12: Home program

Fatigue scale 5

Pain scale 1

Client self-report ● Anxious, excited

Key changes observed by author at end of Session 3/12
● No discomfort
● Accurate physical response to verbal cues
● Able to adjust normal compensations to a more optimal movement

Reason behind choice of sequencing
● Facilitate proprioception and sensory feedback with standing on unstable surface
● Balancing finding midline
● Thoracic articulation
● Addressing sagittal curves of thorax and lumbar region
● Challenge in variable positions: side, prone, and quadruped
● Hip activating through closed kinematic chain environment

Session movement sequence

1. Standing on half rubber balls (Black 2022)

Intent
● Challenge balance
● Sensory input to feet

Gait reasoning
● Proprioception of foot contact
● Sensory input to adapt to ground surfaces

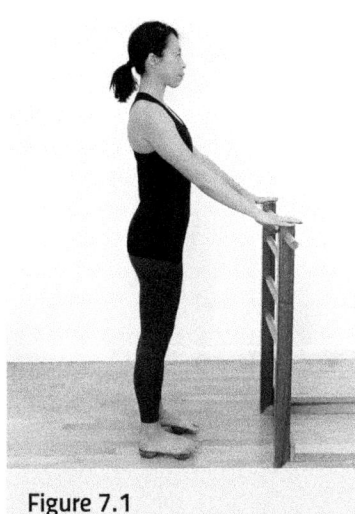

Figure 7.1

Starting position ● Standing on half rubber balls, all flat side up
  ■ Rear foot half ball placed with cuboid contact
  ■ Forefoot half ball placed with metatarsal arch supported
● Holding a bar for balance

Movement description ● Feet parallel, balance for 1 minute
● Shift weight to medial edge of feet tipping balls
● Shift weight to lateral edge of feet tipping balls
● Repeat alternating for 15 seconds' duration
● Pause
● Shift weight toward toes tipping balls
● Shift weight toward heels tipping balls
● Alternate in a rocking motion
● Allow body to adjust naturally with the weight shifts
● 20 seconds' duration
● Pause
● Shift feet around in same direction in small circle
● Circle 5 times then reverse the circle
● Circle in opposite directions
● Circle 5 times then reverse the circle
● Pause
● Figure 8 pattern with oppositional dorsiflexion and plantar flexion

2. Wall horizontal torso press

Intent ● Closed kinematic chain extension of torso
● Thoracic and lumbar articulation orientating to midline
● Posterior femoral head positioning

Gait reasoning ● Verticality of torso for improved three-dimensional motions
● Hip joint centration for hip swing

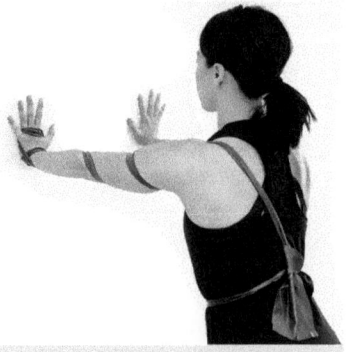

Figure 7.2

Starting position	• Stand facing the wall
	• 2 resistance bands wrapped around upper extremity (UE)
	• Place hands on wall with elbows extended
Movement description	• Flex at hip so that torso is parallel to floor
	• Flex knees if necessary
	• Using hands, press away from wall
	• Reach right ischial tuberosity away from wall and send the breath into left ribs
	• Maintain this position
	• Shift thorax laterally emphasizing motion to left
	• Circle the ribs 3 times in each direction emphasizing the motions of left translation and thoracic extension
	• Walk feet toward wall
	• Flex and articulate torso to upright position

Author note

A long theraband was used to wrap the hand along the UE to the torso for sensory feedback of UE activation. The subject had difficulty sustaining hand pressure on the wall and elbow extension.

3. Wall squat using a 22 in. (55 cm) ball

Intent	• Sustain torso vertical orientation while flexing and extending hips
	• Increase dorsiflexion
Gait reasoning	• Verticality of torso for improved three-dimensional motions
	• Hip joint articulation for swing phase
	• Increase lower extremity (LE) load
Starting position	• Place ball against wall
	• Lean torso on ball at TLJ
	• Feet parallel, placed forward for 90 degrees hip and knee flexion
Movement description	• Lean into ball
	• Squat, rolling ball up and down wall
	• Hip and knee flexion rolling ball up
	• Hip and knee extension rolling ball down
	• 10 repetitions

4. Wall: mini-squat Derivative of Wall Series (see Chapter 5, Kryzanowska)

Intent
- Activate LE to torso focus on femoral joint position
- Activate torso through UE shoulder girdle
- Flexion and extension articulation of the torso from top down

Gait reasoning
- Stimulate activation of torso distally from UE and LE in closed kinematic chain
- Limbs to torso coordination

Starting position
- Back against the wall, with contact points occiput, thorax, lower ribs, sacrum
- Small squat position with 9 in. (23 cm) diameter ball three-quarters inflated placed between LE at mid-femur
- Arms reaching at 45 degree angle forward without shoulder blade protraction

Movement description
- On an inhale, slide the occiput up the wall nodding the chin down
- Exhale, thorax slides up wall which moves head off wall
- Engage ball continually to stimulate flexor response
- Hold for 2 breath cycles
- Inhale, sequentially move from thorax to head to upright position against wall
- Repeat 3–5 times

5. Side lying articulation Derivative of Side Lying Imprinting (see Chapter 5, Gentry)

Intent
- Side lying position allows gravity to assist in lateral motion
- Sequential articulation of torso from bottom up
- Gliding of surrounding connective tissues
- Activation of torso
- Improve lateral translation for rotation

Gait reasoning
- Orientate the torso toward midline orientation
- Improve thoracic rotation and lumbar lateral flexion

Starting position
- Lying on left side on mat
- Support head with small bolster or rolled towel
- Lie orientating torso to midline
- Hip flexion 70 degrees
- Place roller vertically from knees to ankles
- Lower limb resting on roller

Movement description
- Segmental motion is a visualization of the bones moving into the floor and away from the floor in lateral motion
- Begin at the pelvis
  - Feel left upper innominate move into mat as coccyx arcs toward ceiling in a small right hemipelvis superior motion
  - Feel inferior left greater trochanter into the mat as coccyx arcs toward mat in a small right hemipelvis inferior motion
  - Repeat this lateral pelvis motion 10–15 times
- Thoracic movement
  - Feel left inferior ribcage move into mat
  - Feel superior left ribcage into mat as left inferior ribcage moves away from mat
  - Repeat this 10–15 times
- Head movement
  - Gently rock head in side arc
  - Feel top of ear into mat
  - Feel bottom of ear into mat
  - Repeat arc 10 times

6. Side lying with roller

Intent
- Side lying position allows gravity to assist in lateral motion
- Sequential articulation of torso
- Gliding of surrounding connective tissues
- Activation of torso
- Improve rotation

Gait reasoning
- Orientate torso toward midline orientation
- Improve lateral translation for thoracic rotation

Starting position
- Lying on left side on mat with extended left LE
- Place roller in front and parallel to mid-torso and LE
- Right lower limb rests on roller in 70 degrees hip flexion with knee in comfortable flexion
- Rest right hand on roller with elbow flexed

Movement description
- Roll roller forward rotating pelvis toward floor, left pelvic rotation
- Pause before thorax moves
- Return to starting position sequentially, feel head of femur move into acetabulum posteriorly initiating right pelvic rotation
- Repeat this 3–4 times

- Add right thoracic rotation as pelvis rotates left
- Lean left lateral thorax into mat as it rotates right
- Return thorax and pelvis at the same time to side lying position
- Lie on right side
  - Place a triple-folded towel under the thorax at the mid-point of the curve
- Place left hand behind head and reach left elbow toward ceiling for left thoracic translation
- Roll roller forward rotating pelvis toward floor, right pelvic rotation
- Pause before thorax moves
- Return to starting position sequentially, feel head of femur move into hip joint posteriorly initiating left pelvic rotation
- Repeat this 3–4 times

Author note

On the left side the emphasis is the left thoracic translation allowing gravity to assist by leaning into the floor. On the right side, the triple-folded towel supports the excessive right thoracic translation bringing the thorax toward midline. The left upper extremity position facilitates the expansion of the left ribs to counter the tendency to approximate the ribs on the left.

7. Side kick on the ball Derivative of J. H. Pilates Side Kick (NPCE Study Guide 2021, p. 49)

Intent
- Sagittal plane articulation of hip joint
- Activation of hip flexion, extension, abduction, adduction
- Sustained activation of torso during active leg movement

Gait reasoning
- Stance leg balance
- Maintain torso verticality during LE movement

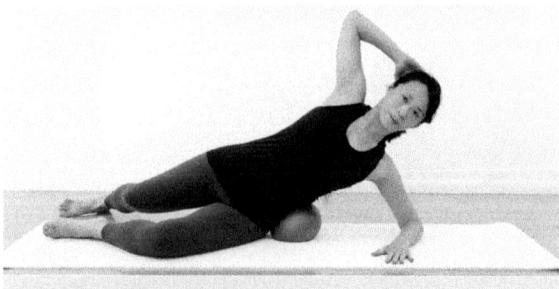

Figure 7.3

Starting position	• Lying on left side on mat
	• Place a 9 in. (23 cm) diameter inflated ball under waist at superior innominate
	• Place upper part of bottom leg with elbow in flexion on mat
	• Hips and knees in flexion to 70 degrees
Movement description	• Slide right foot along mat posteriorly to extend hip while maintaining knee flexion
	• Slide foot anteriorly flexing hip to 70 degrees
	• Maintain foot on mat throughout the arc of the leg
	• Repeat 5 times
	• Change to other side

8. Quadruped

Intent	• Torso adapting to various weight distributions
	• Loading torso distally from 4 limbs to 2
Gait reasoning	• Adapt to changes of ground forces
	• Practice torso strategy of midline orientation during limb changes of support
	• Alternate UE activation for improved thoracic rotation and arm swing
Starting position	• Kneel in quadruped position on mat with torso in optimal position for the task
Movement description	• Unweight right hand and left knee without changing torso orientation
	• 5 repetitions, alternating sides

9. Prone torso rotation

Derivative of J. H. Pilates Swan Dive (NPCE Study Guide 2021, p. 48)
(Black 2022, "Tom Swan")

Intent	• Activate torso extensors through torso articulation focused on thoracic rotation
	• Posterior LE activation
	• Activation of posterior hip to opposite side shoulder girdle
Gait reasoning	• Contralateral patterning
	• Extensor activation for push-off
	• Improve thoracic orientation to pelvis and feet for improved rotation
	• Challenge torso against gravity

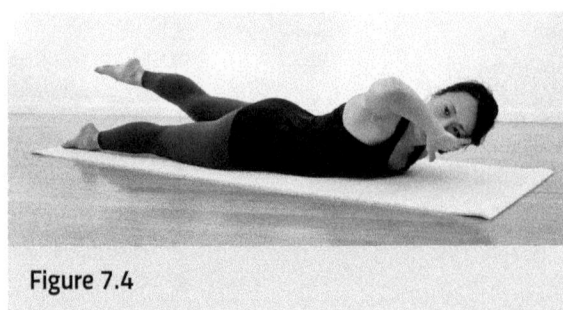

Figure 7.4

Starting position	● Prone on mat
	● Head rotated to the right with right dorsum side of hand on left zygoma bone
	● Eyes directed to right elbow
	● Left arm extended by side
Movement description	● Begin with eyes looking in the direction of the right shoulder
	● Upper thorax extends and rotates right lifting UE and head together
	● Extend left LE
	● Repeat 3 times on each side

10. Rotating hips (Black 2022)

Intent	● Pelvifemoral rotation initiating from foot in closed kinematic chain
	● Improve torso rotation
Gait reasoning	● Improve stance leg support through awareness of LE to torso movement strategy
	● Oppositional thoracic rotation to pelvis

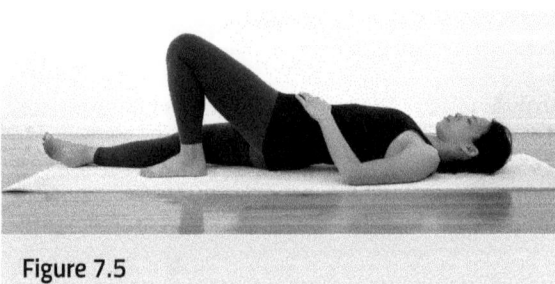

Figure 7.5

Starting position	● Supine with right hip and knee flexion, foot placed on mat
	● Extend left LE
	● Use non-skid rubberized mat under right foot
Movement description	● Right knee moves over the 3rd toe increasing dorsiflexion
	● Pelvis rotates to left
	● Look over right shoulder for right thoracic rotation
	● Left lateral side of ribcage remains in contact with mat
	● Right LE maintains its starting position during pelvic rotation
	● Do not adduct the right femur
	● Repeat 5 times on each side

11. Bridge

Intent	● Femoral glide from flexion to extension
	● Activate posterior-lateral hip and torso extensors
	● Load LE for weight-bearing capacity
	● Torso orientation to midline
Gait reasoning	● Activate pelvifemoral motion for stance and swing phases
	● Improve LE weight bearing for stance phase
	● Torso midline orientation for improved rotation and extension
Starting position	● Supine with knees flexed, feet in line with ischial tuberosities
	● Place 9 in. (23 cm) diameter inflated ball in between mid-femurs
Movement description	● Shift weight on feet from rear foot toward midfoot increasing ankle dorsiflexion
	● Hip joint extends and pelvis lifts off mat
	● Focus on right femur pressing into ball
	● Articulate through torso to rest on scapulae
	● Press firmly into mat with feet
	● Articulate in flexion from scapulae to pelvis, returning to starting position
	● Repeat 5 times

Author note

Subject was challenged with sustaining the right femur centration. The sensory feedback of the ball between the femurs assisted in activating the right femoral head into the acetabulum for improved centration.

12. Standing calf raises

Intent
- Improve ankle joint articulations of dorsiflexion and plantar flexion
- Torso orientation with elevation and lowering of rear foot
- Proprioception in standing organization in gravity

Gait reasoning
- LE function for push-off and landing
- Improve functional LE movement from feet
- Torso adapting in standing with ankle movements

Starting position
- Stand holding on to a bar
- LE in parallel stance
- Hips and knees extended

Movement description
- Shift torso forward as weight moves toward forefoot
- Rear foot elevates into plantar flexion
- Slowly dorsiflex to standing starting position
- 10 repetitions

Session 11/12: Studio session

Fatigue scale 3–4

Pain scale 1–2

Client self-report
- Pain scale based on knee discomfort from biking
- After least session, less fatigue and more energy
- Due to feeling less fatigue biked 15 minutes longer than usual on Saturday
- On Sunday was exhausted from extra time bike riding

Key changes observed by author at end of Session 11/12
- Improved thoracic rotation with arm swing and use of canes
- Fluid integration of leg swing with lumbopelvic rhythm
- In hip flexion bringing the knee and foot forward to heel strike without a lateral shift
- Lower kinematic chain coordination facilitated ankle plantar flexion in push-off phase
- Sacrum, TLJ, and occiput organized to midline in all three planes resulting in improved rotation

Reason behind choice of sequencing
- In final movement session performed all exercises in sequence
- Sense of completion of a program
- Client recognizes achievement in coordination, endurance, concentration, and awareness

Session movement sequence

1. Supine femur circles on Universal Reformer (See Chapter 5, Gentry: knee stirs)

Intent
- Motor control of hip joints
- Spring resistance for support of LE

Gait reasoning
- Improve ability to flex and extend hip
- Medial and lateral hip glide and coordination
- Torso organization toward midline during hip joint movement

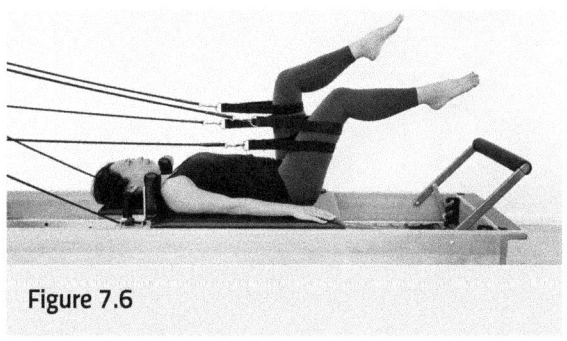

Figure 7.6

Set-up
- 2 medium springs
- Konnector® with Tri Loops attachment

Starting position
- Supine on carriage, feet on footbar
- Place Konnector® straps around mid-femurs one at a time
- Begin in 90 degrees hip flexion with lower limb hanging

Movement description
- Bilateral hip flexion and extension
  - 5 repetitions
- Abduction and adduction
  - Unilateral: one LE holds as opposite LE abducts and adducts
  - Bilateral abduction and adduction
  - 5 repetitions

CUES
- Right hip abduction: cue to anchor the posterior left thorax prior to right hip abduction
- Right hip adduction: cue left thoracic translation, roll the pelvis left, prior to adduction
- Left hip movement had better control through the torso, no specific cueing needed

Author note

This client has significant deficit of hip control. Specific cues for her right hip were to bring attention to the thorax sensation on the carriage of the Universal Reformer prior to right hip movement. This attention activated the torso and dynamically stabilized the torso to move the unilateral LE. The Konnector attachment provided the individuation of leg movement through its single-rope pulley system challenging the client's motor control. A less effective variation of this exercise can be practiced using the Universal Reformer cords. See Editor note on Konnector at the beginning of the chapter.

2. Footwork on Universal Reformer

Derivative of J. H. Pilates Footwork on Universal Reformer (NPCE Study Guide 2021, p. 52)

Intent
- Establish foot contact and ground force reactions
- Stimulate intrinsic aspects of the feet
- Movement rhythm of ankle, knee, and hip joint in flexion and extension

Gait reasoning
- Coordination between forefoot, mid-foot, and rear foot
- Enhance sensory feedback of feet
- Increase proprioception by novel stimulation using textured insoles and bands
- Stimulate better control of hips

Author note

Studies have shown that sensory and motor function in MS responds well to novel stimulation to improve gait by enhancing sensory information at the feet (Hatton *et al.* 2016).

The band wrapping began at the feet to internally rotate the forefoot so that the metatarsals meet the footbar. The interaction of the forefoot with a support surface (footbar and band) may increase rear foot eversion during mid- to late stance phase and may cause proximal changes throughout the lower extremity closed kinematic chain (Souza *et al.* 2009). The intention was to stimulate the forefoot through the LE to activate better control of the hip. The continuation of the band around the LE to the pelvis is for proprioceptive feedback.

Set-up
- Springs: 2 medium and 1 light
- Footbar placed for 75 degrees hip flexion
- Placed textured insole inside socks to stimulate feet
- Wrapped a band for a heel cuff to enhance forefoot internal rotation and ankle dorsiflexion

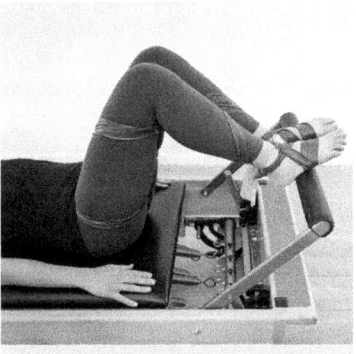

Figure 7.7

- Band wrap continued following the inward spiral of LE to hip

Starting position
- Supine on carriage with feet on footbar

Movement description
- Doming parallel feet
  - Feet placed at the front of the heel with cuboid contact
  - 5 repetitions
- Prehensile parallel feet
  - Move apart
  - Move together
  - 5 repetitions
- One leg on the front of the heel
  - 2 medium springs
  - 5 repetitions
- 30 degrees external rotation
  - 5 repetitions
- Ankle dorsiflexion and plantar flexion
  - Maintain knee flexion
  - Universal Reformer carriage remains at home
  - 10 repetitions
- Hip and knee extension
  - Heel lowers (dorsiflexion and plantar flexion)
  - 5 repetitions

3. Knee Stretch on Universal Reformer

Derivative of J. H. Pilates Knee Stretch Series on Universal Reformer (NPCE Study Guide 2021, p. 60)

Intent
- Torso dynamically stabilizing during articulation and activation during hip joint flexion and extension
- UE and shoulder girdle supported torso organization to midline
- Motor control of flexion and extension

Gait reasoning
- Increase ability to coordinate hip joint flexion and extension
- Torso organization toward midline during LE movement
- Organize transfer of force through torso from LE rhythmic movement and hands on footbar

Set-up
- Springs: 1 medium and 1 light
- Footbar in high position

Starting position
- Kneeling on carriage in quadruped position
- Feet against shoulder stops
- Hands on footbar
- Elbows extended
- Torso in client's optimal sagittal plane organization

Movement description	<ul><li>Inhale, press feet into shoulder stops</li><li>Hip extension moves carriage away</li><li>Exhale, eccentric control of hip flexion controls carriage return</li><li>5 repetitions in a rhythmic timing</li></ul>

CUE
- Breathe into the left side of ribs for left thoracic translation maintaining midline orientation throughout the movement

4. Down Stretch on Universal Reformer

(NPCE Study Guide 2021, p. 55)

Intent	<ul><li>Closed kinetic chain shoulder flexion and extension</li><li>Sustain activation of extensors throughout the movement</li></ul>
Gait reasoning	<ul><li>Increase ability to sustain spinal midline orientation</li><li>Arm-supported torso organization to midline</li><li>Shoulder flexion and extension for arm swing amplifying thoracic rotation</li></ul>
Set-up	<ul><li>Springs: 1 medium and 1 light</li><li>Footbar in high position</li></ul>
Starting position	<ul><li>Kneeling on the carriage</li><li>Hands on footbar</li><li>Elbows extended</li><li>Torso upright, slight extension</li><li>Hips extended</li><li>Feet against shoulder stops</li></ul>

CUE
- Maintain midline orientation throughout the movement

Movement description	<ul><li>Shoulder flexion presses carriage out maintaining midline orientation</li><li>Extension of upper thorax and then shoulder extension controls carriage return</li><li>3 repetitions</li></ul>

CUE
- Cue for carriage return: extend upper thorax by bringing the sternum forward and up

5. Breaststroke on Universal Reformer	Derivative of J. H. Pilates Long Box: Breaststroke on Universal Reformer (NPCE Study Guide 2021, p. 55)

Intent
- Stimulate the extensors by pressing into belt
- Sustain torso extension from a prone position

Gait reasoning
- Increase ability to sustain torso in extended position
- Posterior extensor activation for push-off phase

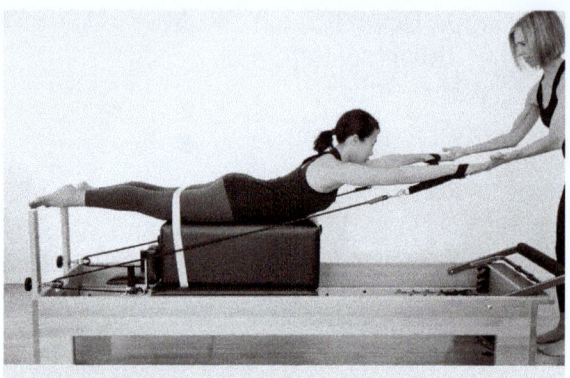

Figure 7.8

Set-up
- Light spring with carabiner (yellow recommended)
- Risers in high position
- Box in long position
- Footbar down
- Yoga belt around the box to anchor legs to the box

Author note

The strap around the box anchors the legs enabling the client to press the legs against it to stimulate the posterior extensors. A light trainer assist was necessary to guide the client's UE orientation and assist extension.

Starting position
- Prone on long box head facing footbar
- Hold straps with elbows flexed, forearms pronated
- Straps from underneath the axilla to hands

Movement description
- Press legs into the strap
- Pull straps superiorly (trainer assisted)
- Extend the torso
- Return to starting position

6. Rowing Back variation on Universal Reformer

Derivative of J. H. Pilates Rowing Back: Flat Back on Universal Reformer (NPCE Study Guide 2021, p. 53)

Intent
- Improve inefficient thoracic rotation with oppositional motion of pelvis

Gait reasoning
- Align TLJ with S2 in three planes
- Left thoracic translation coupled with right thoracic rotation
- Simultaneous oppositional pelvic rotation left

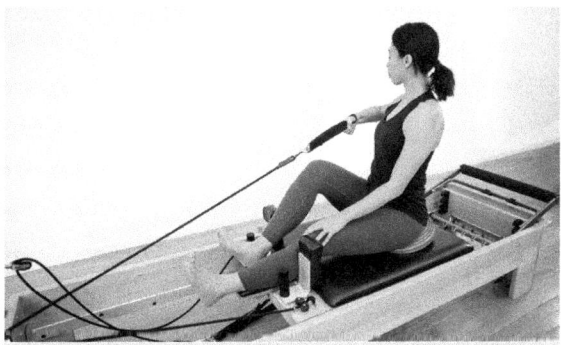

Figure 7.9

Set-up
- Light spring
- Air cushion disc on carriage, apex of disc slightly left of center of carriage
- Risers at high setting
- Loop for handle

Author note

The height of the riser and the line of the strap will change the force vector from the UE into the thorax. Using the loop versus handle facilitates proximal thoracic rotation by minimizing the initiation from the hand. The grip of a handle encourages distal initiation. In addition, the loop contact on the palm and wrist facilitates glenohumeral rotation.

Editor note

The air cushion disc is an air-filled soft, pliable PVC disc that allows each person to adapt to weight shifts during a variety of movements. The air cushion disc provides sensory feedback to the client allowing the righting reflex response to organize to midline. In this exercise, the client is seated in a placement where her left ischial tuberosity is slightly left of the apex. This stimulates the client to distribute the weight toward the left ischial tuberosity, reorganizing the thorax to midline. This reduces right thoracic translation.

Starting position
- Seated with feet toward straps
- Seated on air cushion disc, left ischial tuberosity slightly left of the apex
- Left knee flexion, left ankle dorsiflexion, foot on headrest
- Right knee extended, dorsiflexed ankle, posterior calcaneus on headrest
- Right hand holds strap from left riser, elbow extended, left thoracic rotation
- Right hand through the loop, around wrist, grasping from palm

Movement description
- Activate left pelvic rotation by sliding right heel away from pelvis
- Simultaneously, left heel presses into the headrest anchoring left ischial tuberosity
- Breathe into left lateral ribs initiating proximal thoracic rotation to right
- Pull strap with right elbow flexion

- Return to starting position
- Repetitions are based on the integrity of the thoracic organization
- Right side only

CUES
- Sink right ischial tuberosity into cushion
- Breathe into left ribs for left translation as thorax rotates right
- During thoracic rotation, imagine a light shining from the sternum up and to the right
- Observe rotation from the thorax and not scapula retraction

7. Mermaid on Universal Reformer Derivative of J. H. Pilates Mermaid on Universal Reformer (NPCE Study Guide 2021, p. 58)

Intent
- Activate lateral flexion
- Midline orientation of thorax

Gait reasoning
- Balance thoracic movement
- Improve inefficient left thoracic translation
- Lateral motion

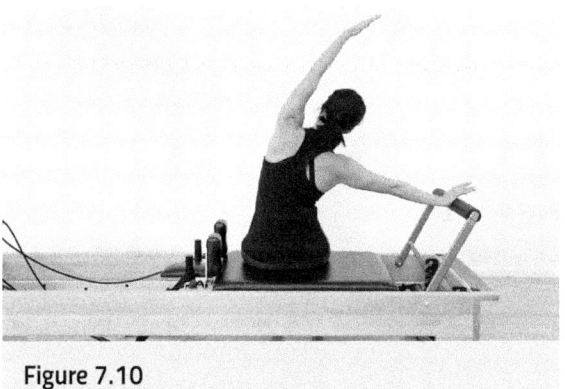

Figure 7.10

Set-up
- Medium spring
- Footbar in low position

Starting position
- Side seated, no air cushion
- Right hand on footbar, elbow extended
- Left arm abducted 90 degrees

Movement description
- Right arm abduction and thoracic translation left presses carriage away from footbar
- Reach left hand toward ceiling amplifying translation of thorax to left
- Slight lateral flexion of thorax with emphasis on translation and left rib expansion
- Return to starting position
- Left side only

CUE
- Breathing into the left ribs assists thoracic translation

Author note
All previous sessions used an air cushion disc to sit upon allowing the subject to sit level and sink the left ischial tuberosity into the disc for equal weight on the ischial tuberosities. No air cushion was used in this session.

Practiced gait patterning with cane usage

Intent
- Practice new organization of body in gait pattern
- Reinforce changes of client's organization
- Novel skills of thoracic rotation
- Leg swing in more sagittal plane
- Push-off phase

Gait reasoning
- Gait practice

Movement description
- Walking

Author note
At the end of each session, gait was practiced integrating the experience of the sessions to reinforce improved gait patterning and build endurance.

The journey to Session 11

Session 4/12
Client self-report

- Felt soreness on right to left anterior oblique line of torso
- Fatigue scale 3
- Pain scale 0

Key changes observed

- Sensing feet in contact with footbar
- Coordinating oppositional hip joint motions
- Ability to move torso toward midline for improved rotation

Reasoning behind choice of movements

- Begin session with feet to increase sensory feedback and proprioception
- Establish foot contact bilaterally
- Facilitate torso movement necessary for gait

Session movement sequence
1. Wall horizontal torso press

- Added a resistance band in wall plank for proprioceptive feedback of UE extension and closed kinematic chain of UE to contralateral hip (see Figure 7.2)

2. Side lying roller added extending hip/knee, ankle circles

3. Prone torso rotation

4. Fine-tuned quadruped to activate torso

5. Universal Reformer

- Supine femur circles
- Footwork focusing on doming and prehensile
- Knee Stretch
- Down Stretch
- Mermaid using air cushion disc

6. Additional movement

- Gait integration with right foot forward and left thoracic translation

Session 5/12
Client self-report

- Felt soreness of right side, internal oblique area
- Fatigue 4–5
- Pain 4–5

Key changes observed

- Right translation and right hemipelvis superior motion were more pronounced, reported had not done home program prior to session
- As the session progressed, torso organization moved toward midline

Reasoning behind choice of movements

- Sensory input to posterior torso and limbs for vertical axis
- Activate extensors for propulsion
- Practice motor control of thoracic translation and rotation

Session movement sequence
1. Universal Reformer

- Supine femur circles
- Footwork focusing on doming and prehensile
- Knee Stretch
- Down Stretch
- Mermaid
  - With air cushion disc
- Breaststroke

- ▪ Yoga belt
- Short box preparation

2. Additional movement

- Gait integration with right foot forward and left thoracic translation

Session 6/12
Client self-report

- Fatigue scale 5
- Pain scale 0
- Back to work this week

Key changes observed

- Short box preparation: no ability to lean back (see Author note below)
- Sustained vertical torso in seated Mermaid prior to lateral flexion
  - ▪ Prop not necessary

Reasoning behind choice of movements

- Practicing torso verticality to increase thoracic rotation
- Thoracic/rib translation to left to improve thoracic rotation
- Continue activation and proprioception of feet

Session movement sequence
Universal Reformer

- Supine femur circles
- Footwork focusing on doming and prehensile
- Knee Stretch
- Down Stretch
- Mermaid
- Breaststroke
- Short box preparation

Author note
The client attempted a modified version of Short Box Series. She was unable to lean back due to lack of control of eccentric torso activation and unable to maintain vertical axis. She discontinued this exercise.

Session 7/12
Client self-report

- Fatigue scale 4
- Pain scale 1
- Feels stiff and tight
- Possibly coming down with a cold

Key changes observed

- Execution of familiar exercises smoother and well performed
- Difficulty in extension of torso and UE in Rowing Back
- Cueing to press legs improved extension
- Improved proprioception of whole-body integration
- Ability to feel thorax translate toward midline while walking

Reasoning behind choice of movements

- Building feeling sense of helical motion
- Awareness of rotation of thorax in both directions
- Develop more confidence overall

Session movement sequence
Universal Reformer

- Supine femur circles
- Footwork focusing on doming and prehensile
- Knee Stretch
- Down Stretch
- Rowing Back (new exercise)
- Mermaid (no prop)
- Short box preparation

Session 8/12
Client self-report

- Trying to recover from work transition and not giving self enough time to rest
- PT session confirmed improved strength and rotation of thorax
- Fatigue scale 5
- Pain scale 0

Key changes observed

- Challenging session due to fatigue
- Inability to control torso
- Down Stretch
  - Not able to sustain torso position
- Rowing Back
  - Finding the position, no pulling of straps
  - Unable to support torso in leaning back

Reasoning behind choice of movements

- Continue to develop the program
- Address setback due to fatigue and personal stress positively
- Encouragement to continue to move in the capacity possible

Session movement sequence
Universal Reformer

- Supine femur circles
- Footwork focusing on doming and prehensile
- Knee Stretch

- Down Stretch
- Breaststroke
- Rowing Back (lean back with straps only)
- Mermaid (no prop)

Session 9/12
Client self-report

- Having difficulty getting through home program
- Stressed about work transition
- Right rib discomfort
- Fatigue scale 4
- Pain scale 2

Key changes observed

- Increased ability to rotate thorax to right with left rib translation and right hemipelvis inferior motion

Reasoning behind choice of movements

- Continue developing support of new available movement in torso
- Integrate new organization in gait and use of canes

Session movement sequence
1. Universal Reformer

- Supine femur circles
- Footwork focusing on doming and prehensile
- Knee Stretch

- Down Stretch
- Breaststroke
- Rowing Back (lean back with straps only)
- Mermaid (no prop)

2. Gait integration with right foot forward and left thoracic translation

Session 10/12
Client self-report

- Increased stress
- Working with the lessons every day
- Walking up stairs without a belt or banister
- Discomfort of right posterior ribs at T5
- Fatigue scale 4
- Pain scale 2

Key changes observed

- Gait is the best yet
- Developed awareness and ability to move in economical way that feels good to her
- In Footwork unable to feel contact of right foot

Reasoning behind choice of movements

- Chose new position of feet on footbar: abduction and adduction of legs to facilitate proprioception of right foot into footbar
- Right foot was placed in center of bar and left foot left of center noting maintaining pelvic position in order for hips to be in an adducted and abducted position
- Seated, she was able to transfer weight onto left ischial tuberosity and translate thorax to left

Session movement sequence
1. Universal Reformer

- Supine femur circles
- Footwork focusing on doming and prehensile

- Knee Stretch
- Down Stretch
- Rowing Back with rotation (new)
- Mermaid

2. Gait integration

- Practice

References

Black, M. (2022) *Centered: Organizing the Body through Kinesiology, Movement Theory and Pilates Techniques.* Edinburgh: Handspring Publishing, pp. 26–28, 127–131.

Hatton, A. L., Dixon, J., Rome, K., Brauer, S. G., Williams, K., and Kerr, G. (2016) "The effects of prolonged wear of textured shoe insoles on gait, foot sensation and proprioception in people with multiple sclerosis: Study protocol for a randomised controlled trial." *Trials, 17,* 208 (2016). DOI: 10.1186/s13063-016-1337-x.

National Multiple Sclerosis Society (2023a) Who gets multiple sclerosis? Epidemiology of MS. www.nationalmssociety.org/What-is-MS/Who-Gets-MS. [Accessed September 24, 2023].

National Multiple Sclerosis Society (2023b) Pathways to wellness in MS. www.nationalmssociety.org/Resources-Support/Library-Education-Programs/PathwaystoWellness. [Accessed September 24, 2023].

NPCE Study Guide (National Pilates Certification Exam Study Guide) (2021) Miami, FL: National Pilates Certification Program, Inc.

Ozkul, C., Guclu-Gunduz, A., Eldemir, K., Apaydin, Y., Yazici, G., and Irkec, C. (2020) "Combined exercise training improves cognitive functions in multiple sclerosis patients with cognitive impairment: A single-blinded randomized controlled trial." *Multiple Sclerosis and Related Disorders, 45.* DOI: 10.1016/j.msard.2020.102419.

Souza, T. R., Pinto, R. Z., Trede, R. G., Kirkwood, R. N., Pertence, A. E., and Fonseca, S. T. (2009) Late rearfoot eversion and lower-limb internal rotation caused by changes in the interaction between forefoot and support surface. *Journal of the American Podiatric Medical Association, 99,* 6, 503–511.

Uygan, V. (2023) Why Konnect? Konnect® Method. www.konnectmethod.com. [Accessed September 24, 2023].

Pilates and Parkinson's Disease: Effect on Gait

Meghann Koppele Duffy

Parkinson's disease (PD), the second most common neurological disorder in the US, is a progressive neurodegenerative disease caused by the loss of dopamine neurons. It affects roughly 7.5 million people worldwide. While primarily people are diagnosed with idiopathic PD, Secondary Parkinson's can be caused by pesticides and environmental toxins, a virus, concussion, lesions from a stroke or tumor, drugs, or long-term use of antipsychotics. Despite an increased understanding of PD, there is no definitive diagnostic test, and the diagnosis is based on clinical criteria. Diagnosis requires the presence and specific presentation of the following cardinal signs: distal resting tremor of 3 to 6 Hz, rigidity, bradykinesia, and asymmetrical onset to rule out another related disorder. PD patients can experience non-verbal communication issues due to rigidity in the facial muscles, kyphosis, shuffle gait, fine motor skill issues, small or cramped handwriting, dystonia, and loss of sense of smell. People with PD can also experience emotional symptoms such as flat affect, nervousness, and anxiety.

Editor note

Facial alterations incite functional deficits in expressions and can influence the social and emotional aspects of a person's life (Pilat 2022).

Without dopamine, the neurotransmitter that is significantly decreased in PD, smooth movement at the basal ganglia loop is compromised leading to the disordered movement you see in PD. Decreased dopamine will affect speeding up, slowing down, changing directions, or transitioning to different body positions. Evidence shows exercise to increase dopamine needs to be more intense than the person's normal activity. Combining exercise with techniques to increase neuroplasticity such as using repetition, task-specific movement, and adding both sensory and auditory feedback (music, a beat, tapping, cadence of voice) to boost dopamine are also helpful for Parkinsonism symptoms.

Important considerations when working with PD is understanding that non-verbal communication will be affected, and facial expression often does not match what the person is feeling. Posture and balance can also be affected due to decreased proprioception especially in the cervical region, sacroiliac joints (SIJs), and feet. Unlike when working with other conditions, it is important to help the client with PD to relax into effort with mindful movement without over-complicating the movements. Due to the lack of dopamine, performing multiple complex movements at once can cause rigidity and freezing. Beginning sessions with big, less complex movements that increase blood flow followed by more specific and precise movements has a better effect than over-concentrating. Creating better movement patterns is crucial for clients with PD, to address not only the symptoms of PD. Diagnosis is often around the age of 60 years old, so there will also be musculoskeletal issues that will need to be addressed while remembering that a PD diagnosis is just a part of the person's story. Each individual body tells a different story based on previous injuries and life experience, so exercise selection should be based on those factors, not just PD. Major contraindications will be based on previous injuries and experiences. If a client has a brain implant, which is used to help decrease tremors, make sure you understand the location of the device and position the client in ways that do not increase tremors or discomfort.

Client description: 68-year-old biologic male, identifies as male; social worker specializing in mental health and addiction

Dates of case report: Session 1: August 27, 2020; Session 12: October 6, 2020

Studio apparatus and props
Pilates equipment

- Universal Reformer-Trapeze Table combination
- Trapeze Table
- Wunda Chair with split pedal

Props used with equipment

- Heavy resistance band, 10 ft (3 m)
- Proprioceptive mat
- 3 lb (1.3 kg) hand weights
- Yoga block, 3 in. (7.62 cm)

Home program props

- Heavy resistance band, 10 ft (3 m)
- Yoga block, 3 in. (7.62 cm)
- Hand towel

Methods and materials

Session 1/12
1. Health history interview

- Client was diagnosed with PD in 2018 after noticing tremors in right hand
- Heart disease, with multiple stents implanted in 2017
- Sleep apnea for 8 years
- Diverticulitis for 10 years
- Arthritis in left knee and left elbow
- Prostatitis and bladder issues
- Fractured both elbows 50 years ago, which never healed correctly. Joint capsule is locked, and client cannot straighten both arms and radial mobility is very limited
- Torn ACL 20 years ago and has had knee pain since playing high school soccer
- Medication includes: Sinemet (carbidopa/levodopa) and Azilect for PD, Flomax, Proscar, BRILINTA, Lipitor, aspirin

2. Symptoms

- Resting tremor in left upper extremity (UE)
- Masked face
- Knee pain on left side
- Lack of sensation in both hands, especially when walking
- Fatigue
- Shallow voice

3. Movement aids

- No movement aids

Final result of case report
Client had a significant decrease in left knee pain, increased joint mobility, and less rigidity overall. He is still experiencing tremors and numbness in his hands when walking. He has learned strategies to manage symptoms. He is experiencing a decrease in frequency of urination at night.

Session 2/12: Initial assessment

1. General observations of gait

◆ Shuffle gait with limited foot and ankle movement

◆ Limited knee flexion

◆ Limited hip joint extension

◆ Minimal push-off bilaterally

◆ Tends to lean back to initiate leg swing

◆ Excessive toe extension when walking barefoot

◆ Limited thoracic rotation coupled with excessive lumbar rotation

◆ Limited arm swing

◆ Limited pelvic motion

◆ Head forward/kyphosis due to looking down

Editor note

The shuffle gait, known as Parkinson's gait, refers to quick-stepping and a short stride. The push-off phase of gait is non-existent or limited. In normal gait, the push-off is generated by the forefoot, especially the 1st phalange pushing off the ground with extension to propel the body forward. Without the push-off, a shuffling, flat-footed gait occurs.

2. Standing tests

◆ Full torso rotation

● Observations of inefficient side: right
  ■ Limited head-cervical rotation
  ■ Poor sequential rotation, rotation only occurring from approximately T10 to L3
  ■ No pelvic movement on femurs on either side

Session 12/12: Post-assessment

1. General observations of gait

◆ Shuffle gait improved

◆ Inability to push off limits forward momentum

◆ No longer leaning back

◆ Improved heel strike and articulation through foot

◆ Arm swing and thoracic rotation present

◆ Upper extremities are no longer hanging and pulling on his neck

2. Standing tests

◆ Full torso rotation

● Observations of inefficient side: right
  ■ Rotation improved on both sides
  ■ Increased pelvifemoral motion bilaterally
  ■ No excessive supination and pronation

◆ Hemipelvis inferior motion

- Tibial torsion on both sides
- Right rotation: excessive supination in right foot and pronation in left foot
- Left rotation: excessive supination in left foot and pronation in right foot

◆ Hemipelvis inferior motion

● Observations of inefficient side: both
  - Unable to coordinate the task
  - Increases pelvic translation to the right

◆ Hemipelvis superior motion

● Observations of inefficient side: both
  - Lacked coordination
  - Strategy was to elevate shoulders

Editor note

The ability to plantar flex is necessary for the hemipelvis to move superiorly. In addition, the pelvifemoral motion of abduction and adduction and lumbar region lateral flexion needs to be available for the coordination of hip hiking.

◆ Lateral pelvic shift

● Observations of inefficient side: both
  - No lateral shift of pelvis in either direction
  - Limited pelvifemoral glide and lumbar lateral flexion
  - Compensated in mid-thorax
  - Excessive movement of subtalar joints

3. Seated tests

◆ Thoracic rotation

● Observations of inefficient side: both
  - No rotation of thorax
  - Rotation at thoracolumbar junction and upper lumbar regions

◆ Hip joint and knee flexion

● Observations of inefficient side: right

● Observations of inefficient side: right
  - Coordination difficult
  - Able to maintain thorax position

◆ Hemipelvis superior motion

● Observations of inefficient side: left
  - Able to coordinate movement bilaterally; however, movement is limited
  - Limited plantar flexion of both feet

◆ Lateral pelvic shift

● Observations of inefficient side: right
  - Limited right pelvifemoral glide
  - Able to coordinate the movement
  - Improved pelvifemoral glide to left

3. Seated tests

◆ Thoracic rotation

● Observations of inefficient side: both
  - Limited thoracic rotation
  - Adjusted movement to let arms hang and swing to find more rotation bilaterally

◆ Hip joint and knee flexion

- Significant range of hip joint flexion bilaterally, left more than right
- Compensation of flexion in lumbar region
- Knee flexion limited, compensated with tibial rotation and foot eversion

Author note

Included dorsiflexion and knee flexion test. Dorsiflexion limited bilaterally with excessive toe extension. Plantar flexion limited with loss of toe position on the floor. Excessive flexion in metatarsophalangeal joint when attempting to plantar flex bilaterally. Included hip abduction with external rotation. Right hip joint external rotation: shifted weight to the left ischial tuberosity.

4. Sit and stand

◆ Lateral view

- Excellent range of bilateral hip joint flexion
- Hip joint extension limited bilaterally
- Excessive flexion in C7 caused by looking down

◆ Anterior view

- In sit to standing shifts weight left at the thorax
- Shifts left to avoid right knee pain
- Extends phalanges of toes to stand

5. Standing balance

◆ Two-leg stance, eyes open

- 60 seconds

◆ One-leg stance, eyes open

- Left leg: 10 seconds
- Right leg: 20 seconds

- Observations of inefficient side: right
  - Significant range of hip joint flexion bilaterally, left more than right
  - Improved weight distribution on ischial tuberosities

Author note

Included dorsiflexion and knee flexion test. Improved dorsiflexion with toes extended at proximal interphalangeal, distal interphalangeal, and metatarsophalangeal joints. Included hip abduction with external rotation. Improved weight distribution on ischial tuberosities.

4. Sit and stand

◆ Lateral view

- Excellent range of bilateral hip joint flexion with slight shift to left
- Improved hip joint extension bilaterally
- Gaze is no longer down

◆ Anterior view

- Decreased shift to left side
- No knee pain during knee extension
- Left phalanges flexion, gripping floor

5. Standing balance

◆ Two-leg stance, eyes open

- 60 seconds

◆ Two-leg stance, eyes closed

- 60 seconds

◆ One-leg stance, eyes open

- Right leg: 35 seconds
- Left leg: 20 seconds

Session 3/12: Home program

Fatigue scale	2
Pain scale	1

Client self-report
- Expressed he would like to feel less stiff
- Seems tired and serious although reported a low level of fatigue

Key changes observed by author at end of Session 3/12
- Facially expressive and more talkative at the end of the session
- Increased energy moving with ease and smoothness
- Tendency to force movement
- Responded well to hands on and simple cues

Reason behind choice of sequencing
- To work on shoulder girdle and pelvifemoral organization to create a better framework for improving torso movement
- Avoided supine exercises due to a strain on his voice (see Author note below)
- Enjoys movement but tends to do very linear movements, so program includes many planes of movement
- Due to extreme workload, needs a clear, concise program that could be completed in under 20 minutes

Author note

Kyphosis is a very common presentation in Parkinson's disease, combined with forward head and eyes looking down (Breland 2018). If this presentation is observed, avoid starting with supine exercises. Supine facilitates poor sensory mapping of the shoulder girdle, torso, and eye position. The disruption of proprioception from poor sensory input will affect changing movement patterns. Support the cervical region, SIJs, or scapulae to increase proprioception when performing supine exercises. Beginning with eye movement helps facilitate increased torso movement.

Session movement sequence

1. Push-off standing drill with hemipelvis superior motion/inferior motion

Intent
- Encourage foot articulations
- Challenge coordination of the hip joint, knee, and ankle while standing
- Increase proprioception of the feet
- Introduce the idea of the foot influencing the hip joint
- Explore pelvifemoral movements

Gait reasoning
- Improve push-off
- Increase proprioception of the feet
- Improve pelvic motions: pelvifemoral glide and lumbar lateral flexion

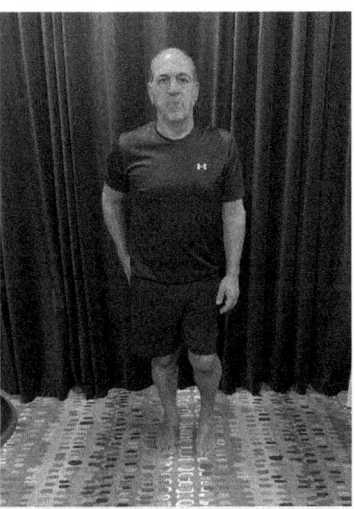

Figure 8.1

Starting position
- Standing on proprioceptive mat with knees extended and feet hip-joint-distance apart
- Hands against wall with elbow flexion

Movement description	● Flex right knee and hip joint as right heel lifts
	● Left hip joint and knee extended
	● Extend right knee and hip joint, place heel down
	● Repeat on right side 5–8 times
	● Hold the last repetition of right side
	● Press right hand gently into side of right pelvis at greater trochanter (GT) and right pelvis presses back into right hand
	● Maintain right lower extremity (LE) in flexion with heel up
	● Maintain left LE extended
	● Arc pubic bone toward left LE (right hemipelvis superior motion/left hemipelvis inferior motion)
	● Arc pubic bone to right LE (left hemipelvis superior motion/ right hemipelvis inferior motion)
	● Focus on swinging the pelvis left and right without movement of LE
	● Return to starting position
	● Repeat on left side

2. Quadruped flexion and extension

Intent	● Challenge pelvifemoral and shoulder loading while articulating the torso
Gait reasoning	● Torso articulation for improved motion in all planes
	● UE swing amplifying thoracic rotation
	● Organization and relative motions of limbs and torso in gait pattern
Starting position	● Quadruped position
	● Hands placed under shoulders, elbows extended
	● Hip joints centration
Movement description	● Articulate torso in flexion and extension 3–5 times
	● Focus on moving pelvifemoral and glenoid fossa-humeral head motions
	● Eyes look down toward the feet during flexion
	● Eyes look up the wall in front during extension

3. Seated rotation with eye tracking

Intent	● Encourage full torso rotation
	● Facilitate rotation through eye motion
Gait reasoning	● To facilitate thoracic rotation

Editor note

It has been shown that the effect of gaze direction may facilitate improved range of motion (ROM). The cerebellum's role of coordination coherence in the sensorimotor system includes ensuring the precision and accuracy of ocular movements regardless of changes in head or body positions (Beh, Frohman, and Frohman 2017). The interrelationship between the neuromyofascial continuity of the cervical region and the eyes has shown increases in cervical rotation (Bexander, Mellor, and Hodges 2005; Goffart, Hafed, and Krauzlis 2012). Moshe Feldenkrais was innovative with the use of eye gaze to facilitate efficient movement (Kresge and Elgelid 2021).

Starting position
- Sitting in chair with feet flat on floor
- Flex right UE with right thumb up
- Thumb in line with nose

Movement description
- Look at thumb
- Maintain the UE position
- Rotate head to left maintaining focus on thumb
- Repeat 3 times without taking eyes off thumb
- Abduct UE to the right as eyes follow thumb without moving head or torso
- Return to start
- Repeat 3 times
- Continue to move the arm and eyes, adding head and torso rotation
- Return to start
- Repeat on other side

4. Standing Saw   Derivative of J. H. Pilates mat exercise Saw (NPCE Study Guide 2021, p. 48)

Intent
- Standing balance
- Standing rotation
- Challenge motor control of rotation from UE in standing

Gait reasoning
- Standing balance
- Torso rotation with shoulder girdle glide
- Proprioception of hands and feet
- Sensory input of ground forces from feet

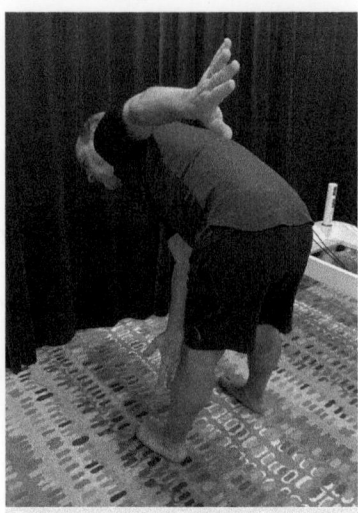

Figure 8.2

Starting position
- Stand with feet hip-joint-distance apart
- Abduct UE
- Elbows extended

Movement description
- Reach right UE across midline toward left LE
- Left torso rotation and flexion sliding hand inferiorly along left LE
- Allow left LE adduction and right LE abduction slightly
- Return to starting position
- Repeat on other side

5. Side lying abduction/adduction with resistance band

(See Figure 8.3A)

Author note

The resistance band is for sensory feedback, not for resistance. It is not to increase the challenge or resistance. The intention is to improve sensory awareness of the hip joint and its relationship to the opposite shoulder girdle (Koppele Duffy 2018). The band set-up is on the non-moving side to stimulate the reflexive stability of that side.

Intent
- Increase proprioception
- Improve femoral joint glide

Gait reasoning
- Improve femoral joint articulation
- Increase proprioception
- Foot to pelvis activation

Starting position
- Tie one end of band in a loop
- Place loop around right superior femur
- Place other end of the band posteriorly on torso to left shoulder
- Hold band over shoulder with left hand
- Lie on left side with head support
- Bilateral hip and knee joints in 90 degrees flexion

Movement description
- Rock pelvis anteriorly and posteriorly to sense the GT of bottom hemipelvis
- Press bottom femur into mat
- Extend right hip and knee joint maintaining position of bottom LE
- Abduct and adduct hip without torso lateral flexion
- Change band set-up to right side
- Repeat on other side

6. Side lying pelvifemoral circles with resistance band

Intent
- Improve femoral joint proprioception
- Shoulder girdle reflexive stability
- Torso reflexive stability

Gait reasoning
- Rhythm of pelvifemoral motion
- Posterior-lateral pelvifemoral to shoulder girdle neuromyo-fascia communication (Black 2022)
- Improve femoral joint articulation to enhance proprioception
- Foot to pelvifemoral activation

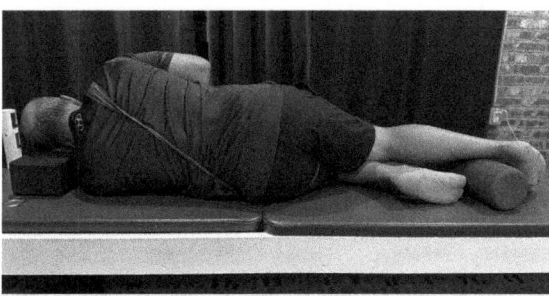

Figure 8.3A

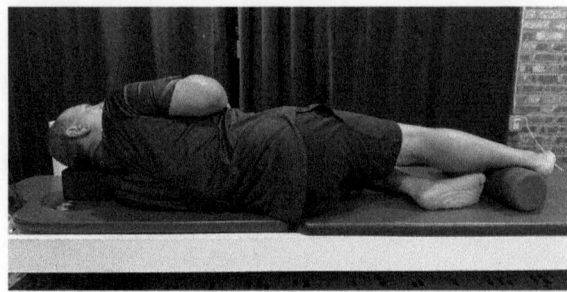

Figure 8.3B

Starting position	● Note which leg loop is on and why
	● Tie one end of band in a loop
	● Place loop around right superior femur at inguinal fold
	● Place other end of band posteriorly on torso to left shoulder
	● Hold band over shoulder with left hand
	● Lie on right side with head support
	● Bilateral hip and knee joints in flexion
Movement description	● Move pelvis to sense bottom GT
	● Press right femur into mat
	● Extend left hip and knee joint maintaining position of bottom LE
	● Left foot is on mat
	● Use a roller or yoga block to support the left foot if necessary
	● Rotate pelvis on right femur in diagonal direction, transverse-sagittal plane
	● Repeat 3 times
	● Settle pelvis on top of right femur
	● Perform 5 small circles of left pelvis in both directions
	● Change band to left side
	● Repeat on other side

7. Side lying leg kick with rotation   Derivative of J. H. Pilates Side Kick (NPCE Study Guide 2021, p. 49)

Intent	● Improve pelvifemoral motion
	● Torso rotation with leg swing
Gait reasoning	● Coordination of motions of thorax and pelvis
	● Proprioception of hip joint
	● Improve torso rotation

Starting position	(See Figure 8.3A) ● Tie one end of band in a loop ● Place loop around right superior femur at inguinal fold ● Place the other end of the band posteriorly on torso to left shoulder ● Hold the band over shoulder with left hand ● Lie on right side with head support ● Left hip and knee joint extended ● Right hip and knee joint flexed
Movement description	● Rock pelvis anteriorly and posteriorly to sense GT of bottom hemipelvis ● Press bottom femur into mat ● Kick left LE into extension with right torso rotation ● Kick left LE into flexion with right torso rotation ● Right LE remains in position ● The intention is to move the pelvis around the bottom femur

Author note

Side lying work is a preferred position integrating lateral stimulation unilaterally, awareness of asymmetries, and sensory input from the floor. This helps facilitate activation that is necessary for the lateral shift during gait. Side lying reduces gravitational force providing the accessibility of limb motion on the torso in combination with eye movements. This may improve the motor control of limb motions during gait. Side lying may also eliminate the potential bracing pattern that restricts the gait motions in all three planes (Koppele Duffy 2022).

8. Half high kneeling with torso rotation

Intent	● Challenge torso rotation in a split-stance position ● Improve balance ● Improve supination and pronation ● Increase grip strength ● Improve shoulder girdle strength and mobility
Gait reasoning	● Torso rotation while coordinating reciprocal movement of the LE ● Increase proprioception of hands to help hand to shoulder girdle connection

Starting position	● Kneel in half high kneeling
	● Right LE forward, hip and knee joint flexion, external rotation, foot planted on floor
	● Left hip joint extended kneeling
	● Hold towel with hands shoulder-distance apart
	● Elbows flexed
	● Right upper limb in supination
	● Left upper limb in pronation
Movement description	● Press down through right foot
	● Right rotation of torso
	● Extend elbows, hands to shoulder height
	● Cue to bring humeral head posteriorly in opposition to elbows extending
	● Flex elbows, left rotation of torso toward kneeling left LE
	● Repeat 8 times
	● Repeat on other side

9. Dual task training: modified Swan with counting

Derivative of J. H. Pilates Swan Dive (NPCE Study Guide 2021, p. 48)

Editor note

The ability to perform simultaneous tasks may be impaired for those with PD. For example, walking and talking requires different brain processes. Dual task training (DTT) consists of a primary task and an additional secondary task. The primary task in this exercise is torso extension. The secondary task is counting to 10. DTT can improve the automatization of the primary task, that is, the primary task will need less cognitive capacity. DTT may result in faster information processing. DTT is a promising approach for improving gait and balance (Feng *et al.* 2020; Hofheinz, Mibs, and Elsner 2016).

Intent	● Improve extension
	● Dual task training
Gait reasoning	● Improve upright orientation
Starting position	● Prone with head supported
	● Forearms and hands on mat, elbows flexed
	● Elbows close to torso

Movement description
- Looking up to lift head
- Maintain gaze on a point
- Slowly lower head and lower eyes
- Repeat 3 times
- On 4th repetition maintain gaze
- Extend torso
- Extend elbows articulating torso into increased extension
- Count to 10
- Slowly lower torso articulating sequentially to starting position
- Count backwards from 10
- Repeat 3 times

10. Dual task training: contralateral balance from quadruped with memory vocalization

(See Editor note above in exercise 9)

Intent
- Coordination of thorax and pelvis
- Reciprocal UE and LE movements
- Challenge dynamic stability

Gait reasoning
- Improve contralateral motion of UE and LE

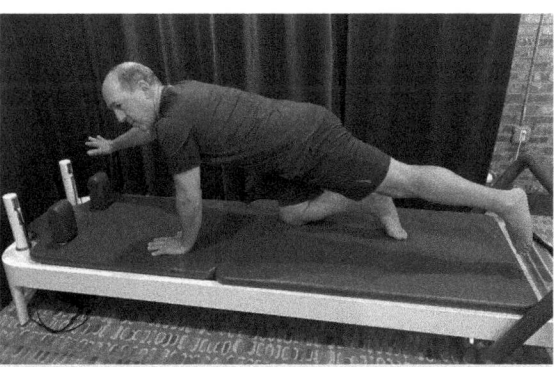

Figure 8.4

Starting position
- Quadruped position
- Find a position with lumbar and cervical extension pain free
- Medial borders of scapulae lined up with SIJs

Movement description	● Flex right shoulder and extend left hip joint
	● Return to start
	● Repeat on other side
	● Continue movement until naming 10 countries
	● Increase difficulty by saying the first letter of the country

11. Dual task training: quadruped push-up with memory vocalization

(See Editor note in exercise 9 above)

Intent	● Coordination of thorax and pelvis
	● Reciprocal UE and LE movements
	● Challenge dynamic stability

| Gait reasoning | ● Improve contralateral motion of UE and LE |

Starting position	● Quadruped position
	● Find a position with lumbar and cervical extension pain free
	● Medial borders of scapulae lined up with SIJs

Movement description	● Flex elbows toward knees
	● Extend left LE posteriorly
	● Extend elbows, flexing left knee and hip joint
	● Flex elbows
	● Extend right LE posteriorly
	● Extend elbows, flexing right knee and hip joint
	● Continue to alternate LE
	● During the movement name 10 foods
	● Other options are foods starting with a certain letter, foods that grow on trees, foods that are unhealthy, etc.

12. Standing push-off in tandem stance

Intent	● Encourage feet adaptation
	● Challenge pelvifemoral, knee, and ankle coordination in standing position
	● Increase proprioception of feet and response to the hip joints

Gait reasoning	● Improve push-off
	● Encourage multiple joint coordination for diminishing shuffle gait
	● Improve proprioception at the feet to stimulate hip joints

Starting position	<ul><li>Standing with knees extended</li><li>Feet hip-joint-distance apart with left foot slightly in front of right</li><li>Weight evenly distributed on both feet</li></ul>
Movement description	<ul><li>Tandem stance</li><li>Plantar flex right ankle, flex right hip and knee joints simultaneously</li><li>Return to starting position</li><li>Repeat 4 times</li><li>On 5th repetition shift weight forward into left foot</li><li>Maintain left hip and knee joint extension</li><li>Return to starting position</li><li>Repeat 5 times</li></ul>

Session 11/12: Studio session

Fatigue scale	1
Pain scale	0
Client self-report	<ul><li>First time without knee pain in 10 years, is now able to turn his head to look back when riding his bike and plans on adding Pilates to his routine</li></ul>
Key changes observed by author at end of Session 11/12	<ul><li>Improved flow and ease of movement</li><li>Able to coordinate multiple joint movements and self-correct with pain or rigidity as a factor for adjustments</li><li>Holds head higher with confidence</li></ul>
Reason behind choice of sequencing	<ul><li>Began on Universal Reformer to challenge his vestibular and proprioceptive system</li><li>Coordinated UE and LE movement with unilateral movement</li><li>Facilitated torso movements with limb</li><li>Flowing sequence on chair was to help with smoothness of movement</li><li>Standing roll-up combined with push-off drill to help coordination and balance throughout gait cycle</li></ul>

Session movement sequence

1. Single Leg Footwork on Universal Reformer

Derivative of J. H. Pilates Footwork on Universal Reformer (NPCE Study Guide 2021, p. 52)

Intent
- Use Magic Circle as tool for centration of femoral head and reflexive stability of unsupported LE during the movement
- Coordination challenge
- Feeling success at beginning of session increases dopamine and increases blood flow
- Establish awareness of foot through torso
- Ground through the feet with optimal LE organization

Gait reasoning
- Improve coordination and reciprocal LE movements
- Introduces LE opposition in a position of less body weight to build on success
- Optimal distribution of ground force reactions

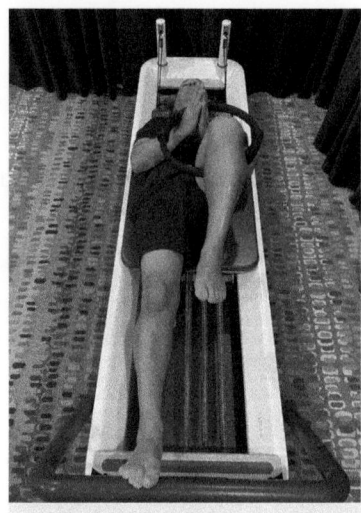

Figure 8.5

Set-up
- 2 medium springs

Starting position	● Supine on carriage with left foot on footbar
	● Right leg at 90 degrees hip and knee joint flexion inside Magic Circle
	● Posterior femur presses lightly on circle
	● Alternative foot positions
	■ On metatarsals, plantar flexion focusing on phalangeal extension
	■ On arch of foot
	■ On heels, dorsiflexion without over-extension of phalanges

Movement description	● Unilateral right hip and knee joint flexion and extension
	● 5 repetitions
	● Added left hip and knee extension during right hip and knee joint flexion
	● 5 repetitions
	● Repeat on other side

CUES

◆ Press the LE in the Magic Circle at a level of 2 for consistent sensory feedback of the non-working LE

◆ A helpful cue for the client is to not increase or decrease the pressure into the circle

Author note

Playing music or snapping fingers to a beat helps the client move smoothly. Rhythmic auditory cues bypass the basal ganglia loop, the area of the brain that is affected by Parkinson's (see Health condition description). Research suggests that rhythmic auditory stimulation (RAS) might provide an external rhythm that can compensate for the defective internal rhythm of the basal ganglia (Muthukrishnan *et al.* 2019).

2. Single Leg Circles on Universal Reformer	Derivative of J. H. Pilates Footwork on Universal Reformer (NPCE Study Guide 2021, p. 52) and Single Leg Circle (NPCE Study Guide 2021, p. 46)
Intent	● Improve hip joint glide
	● Activate non-moving LE
Gait reasoning	● Improve reciprocal leg movements: stance LE and swing LE
	● Establish subconscious motor control of stance and swing
	● Increase awareness of hip joint ROM with torso reflexive organization

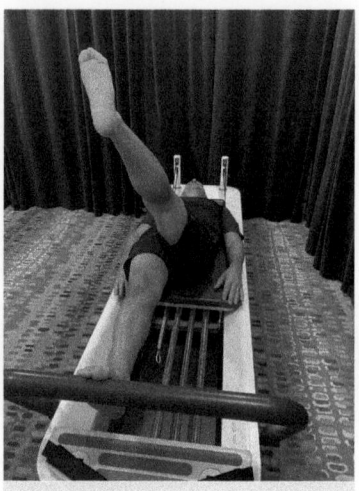

Figure 8.6

Set-up	● 2 medium springs
Starting position	● Supine on carriage
	● Right foot on footbar
	● Right hip and knee joint flexion, carriage at the stoppers
	● Left 90 degrees hip and knee joint flexion
Movement description	● Press carriage away extending right knee
	● Maintain right knee extension
	● Extend left knee with hip flexion
	● Perform circles with left LE 5 times in each direction
	● Take a break between directions
	● Repeat on other side

CUES

◆ Remain focused on the footbar extended LE
◆ Maintain foot pressure on the footbar
◆ ROM of the circles depends on the control and sustained activation of the footbar LE

Author note

The ROM of the circling leg is less important than maintaining the position of the standing leg. Prior to the movement, cue the client to place the hands (palm) down under the sacrum. Ask the client to notice how the pelvis moves side to side when the standing leg is not activated. This hands-on option was very helpful for increasing proprioception of hip joint motion and reflexive stability.

3. Supine single arm on Trapeze Table
Derivative of J. H. Pilates Arm Springs: Circles Supine on Trapeze Table (NPCE Study Guide 2021, p. 69)

Intent
- Establish reciprocal UE swing with thoracic rotation
- Unilateral UE to focus on the differences of usage
- Activating UE and LE continuity

Gait reasoning
- Encourage reciprocal UE movements with reflexive stability from ground forces

Set-up
- Light spring
- Strap

Starting position
- Supine on table
- Hip and knee joint to 90 degrees flexion
- Right UE to 90 degrees flexion, elbow extended
- Left UE by side palm down, palm up or thumb up
- Each UE position was challenged by a few deep breaths
- Choose UE position where the deepest breath has ease
- Once arm position is established hold strap with right hand with elbow extended

Movement description
- Shoulder flexion and extension 5 times
- Elbow flexion and extension 8 times
- Shoulder flexion, abduction, extension, adduction, flexion
- Perform 5 times in each direction

CUES
- Purposely varying the UE directions ensures attention
- Pulling the strap unilaterally while the hip and knee joints are in 90 degrees flexion challenges the strategy of torso adaptation
- Combined cueing of humeral head congruency relative to the thorax and shoulder girdle organization enables improved unilateral UE movement

Author note
The client enjoyed this series and reported he felt his body "working together." Bringing attention to LE activation allowed for freer movement of the UE. The change in the ability to take a deep breath by changing his arm position was empowering to him. At first, he was confused about varying the three UE movements. Once he understood the goal, he was able to complete a full set of 8–12 movements with optimal movement patterning.

4. Modified Coordination on Universal Reformer

Derivative of J. H. Pilates Coordination on Universal Reformer (NPCE Study Guide 2021, p. 53)

Intent
- Challenge concentration while coordinating different limb movements
- Introduce torso flexion while moving limbs

Gait reasoning
- Facilitate a smoothness in gait rhythm
- Improve coordination of the complex, reciprocal movements
- Establish the need for the eyes to converge throughout gait cycle

Editor note

Smoothness in the gait cycle is lost with decreased levels of dopamine (Gilat *et al.* 2017). (See Health Description paragraphs on dopamine and neuroplasticity.)

Editor note

Vestibulo-ocular reflex (VOR) maintains a stable perception of the world during normal movements such as walking. The eye structures create an eye movement opposite to the head movement at the exact same speed to readjust the visual world. This stabilizes the retinal image by keeping the eyes still in space, focusing on an object despite head movement (Somisetty and Das 2022).

Set-up
- Medium spring
- Footbar up if necessary for a break

Starting position
- Supine on carriage
- Hold straps, right forearm supination and left forearm pronation
- Elbows to 90 degrees flexion
- Hip and knee joint to 90 degrees flexion

Movement description
- Extend both elbows
- Abduct and adduct with elbows extended
- Return to starting position
- Repeat 5 times increasing the number of abduction/adduction movements by 1 for each repetition
- 5 repetitions
- Offer a break, feet on footbar
- Return to starting position
- Repeat entire series adding torso flexion and knee extension
- Add abduction/adduction of hip joints with knees extended
- 5 repetitions

CUES

- Over-cueing can lead to more confusion and an increase in a tremor response (Breland 2018). A good rule of thumb is say less, and focus on positional and/or sensory cueing (Koppele Duffy 2022). Offer one option at a time to maintain focus throughout the ROM and facilitate success. Cerebellum-based cueing bypasses the basal ganglia loop decreasing potential confusion and tremor response (see Author note below). For example, establish cueing to move around a specific part, such as pelvis on femur or a pressure point for sensory input.
- Add verbally counting during the abduction and adduction of arms and legs
- Use a yoga block above client's umbilicus at an angle that can be seen in torso flexion. Cue to continue to look at yoga block throughout the exercise

Author note

Counting out loud helps with low speech volume, a symptom of PD. If speech volume is reduced during torso flexion, it is a sign that the torso flexion is restricting the breath and of forced positioning. If the voice is shaky or volume is reduced, take a break. Reestablish the humeral-thoracic-shoulder organization.

Increase the challenge to unilateral LE after the client executes bilateral LE movement with precision. This increases the intensity and heart rate and boosts dopamine and BDNF (brain-derived neurotropic factor) which is necessary for neuroplasticity.

Author note

The cerebellum is responsible for balance, accuracy, and coordination. One role of the cerebellum is coordination coherence in the sensorimotor system (McAfee *et al.* 2022). Cerebellum-based cueing utilizes this principle of coordinating coherence. Induce sensory stimulation to utilize sensorimotor control to drive the movement. Stimulating the sensorimotor system in a person living with PD assists in diverting the basal ganglion network. The dopamine depletion in the basal ganglion is responsible for impaired movement. By diverting the basal ganglion network, movement coordination, balance, and accuracy improve (Lanciego, Luquin, and Obeso 2012).

5. Back Rowing with thoracic rotation on Universal Reformer

Derivative of J. H. Pilates Rowing Back: Flat Back on Universal Reformer (NPCE Study Guide 2021, p. 53)

Intent
- Challenge pelvifemoral adaptation while challenging the shoulder girdle in a seated position

Gait reasoning
- Improves coordination throughout gait cycle
- Seated position to improve thoracic rotation

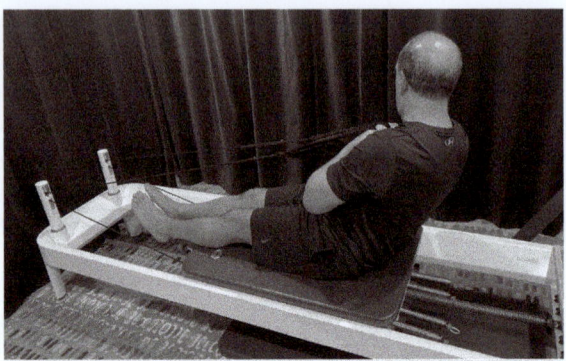

Figure 8.7

Set-up
- Footbar down
- Hand loops
- Medium spring

Starting position
- Seated with back toward footbar
- Legs extended resting on headrest
- Hold loops with fist grasp
- Elbows flexed with fists gently pressed together
- Torso organized to midline

Movement description
- Articulate flexion from pelvifemoral extension
- Posteriorly rotate pelvis
- Articulate to upright initiating from the atlanto-occipital joint
- Repeat 3 times
- Repeat roll-back
- Rotate thorax right to left in flexion
- Repeat 4 times each direction
- From atlanto-occipital joint initiate return to starting position
- Articulate flexion from pelvifemoral extension

- Posteriorly rotate pelvis
- Hold flexed position
- Extend elbows
- Extend shoulders
- Increase hip joint flexion leaning torso forward
- Maintain position
- Flex and extend elbows 5–8 times
- On last repetition extend elbows
- Abduct and externally rotate the humerus
- Hands reach for feet
- Articulate to upright initiating from pelvis
- Return to starting position
- Repeat 3 times

CUES

- Maintain the congruency of humeral head, thorax, and shoulder girdle
- Articulate the pelvifemoral motion during flexion
- Maintain femoral joint centration
- Inhale while articulating flexion to facilitate diaphragmatic expansion to allow ease of pelvifemoral glide

Author note

This exercise was a challenge for the client. The ability to co-ordinate the complex sequence increased his confidence. He reported he was not coordinated, so experiencing coordination in complex movements surprised him.

6. Swan on Wunda Chair with vestibulo-ocular reflex (VOR)

Derivative of J. H. Pilates Swan Front/Chest Press on Wunda Chair (NPCE Study Guide 2021, p. 73)
(See Editor note on VOR in exercise 4 above)

Editor note

The example in Figure 8.8 shows a different exercise—Mermaid on Universal Reformer (derivative of J. H. Pilates Seated Mermaid/Side Arm Sit on Wunda Chair, NPCE Study Guide 2021, p. 73)—rather than Swan on Wunda Chair to illustrate the VOR.

Intent
- Improve hip joint glide
- Activate non-moving LE

Gait reasoning
- Increase ability for pelvifemoral motion during extension for push-off
- Improve extension to facilitate eyes focusing on horizon rather than ground
- Maintain head balance and cervical extension and ability to move eyes
- Closed kinematic chain with feet against wall

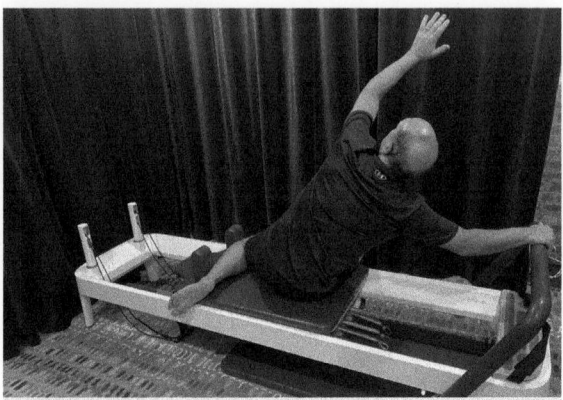

Figure 8.8

Set-up
- Heavy spring

Starting position
- Prone
- Hands on foot pedal
- Shoulder flexion, elbow extension
- Feet up against wall
- Set scapulae to optimal position on thorax

Movement description
- Find a visual point to focus on
- Flex the head and neck while maintaining focus on the point
- 3 repetitions
- Track eyes up
- Extend torso
- Keep eyes fixed on a point at the top
- Press pedal down while maintaining up eye position
- Return to the first point when eye tracking the up position is no longer possible
- Repeat 5 times

CUES
- ◆ Maintain scapulae contact with thorax during extension
- ◆ During VOR cue to nod yes while maintaining a point in visual field
- ◆ VOR to begin movement with the head nod down
- ◆ Reflexively move eyes into extension as preparation for the movement
- ◆ Be sure the client can track eyes up before performing the movement
- ◆ Demonstrate the VOR prior to starting position to minimize frustration and over-concentration that may increase any tremors in client's arms

7. Side lying lateral flexion on Wunda Chair

Derivative of J. H. Pilates Side Body Twist on Wunda Chair (NPCE Study Guide 2021, p. 77) and Star on Universal Reformer (NPCE Study Guide 2021, p. 61)

Intent
- ● Challenge lateral flexors
- ● Improve proprioception of hand-shoulder, girdle-thorax

Gait reasoning
- ● Activate laterality for weight transfer
- ● Encourage torso-pelvifemoral laterality for smoothing gait rhythm

Editor note
The term *laterality* refers to the preference for one side of their body over the other. Examples include left- or right-handed-ness and left- or right-footedness. It is task specific. It may also refer to the primary use of the left or right hemisphere in the brain.

Set-up
- ● Heavy spring

Starting position
- ● Lying with right side of pelvis on top of chair
- ● Place right hand on pedal
- ● Place left hand on top of chair or on handle
- ● Level the shoulder girdle

Movement description	• Head initiates lateral flexion as pedal moves up
	• Abduct left hip joint
	• Lower pedal by gently initiating from pelvifemoral
	• Adduct left hip joint
	• Hold torso mid-range
	• Flex and extend elbows, pumping arms
	• Count out loud 5 arm pumps maintaining mid-range position
	• Move to a different torso range
	• 5 arm pumps while counting backwards
	• Repeat on other side

CUES

- Use left hand under contralateral clavicle and gently lift the connective tissue
- Maintain shoulder girdle position on thorax during lateral motion
- While performing arm pumps use the top arm on the chair for balance so that the arm pumps are initiated from the hand

Author note

The client placed his arm slightly forward due to deformity at the elbow. Forcing an arm position would increase tremors. The hand on the contralateral clavicle gently drags the connective tissue toward the clavicle and medially toward the sternum. The client expected tremors; however, focusing on flowing through the movement made it fun for him, and the tremors were decreased.

8. Mermaid on Wunda Chair

Derivative of J. H. Pilates Seated Mermaid/Side Arm Sit on Wunda Chair (NPCE Study Guide 2021, p. 73)

Editor note

See Figure 8.8 which shows a different exercise—Mermaid on the Universal Reformer (derivative of J. H. Pilates Seated Mermaid Side Arm Sit on Wunda Chair, NPCE Study Guide 2021, p.73)—rather than Wunda Chair. The laterality is similar in both movements.

Intent	• Lateral torso flexion around shoulder girdle and hip joint
	• Improve pelvifemoral laterality

Gait reasoning	• Improve thoracic translation for one-leg stance balance
	• Enhance femoral glide through lateral and transverse pelvic motion
Set-up	• Heavy spring
Starting position	• Side seated on chair with right side toward pedal end
	• Right hip and knee joint flexion on chair side
	• Left hip and knee joint extension and abduction with foot flat on floor
	• Orientate the eyes and torso forward
	• Bilateral humeral abduction, elbows extended
Movement description	• Begin by adducting and abducting right UE
	• Repeat 3 times
	• On 3rd repetition place hand on pedal
	• Laterally flex torso to push pedal down 3–5 times
	• On the final repetition hold pedal in down position
	• Rotate torso to right
	• Left UE abducts and flexes reaching hand toward pedal
	• Rotate left to facing forward
	• Repeat 3 times
	• Return to starting position
	• Repeat on other side

CUES

- Hands-on cue for humeral head congruency is very helpful
- Place one hand on the scapula and the other on the superior aspect of humeral head maintaining congruency. This allows the torso lateral flexion to drive the pedal up and down
- If you are not able to be hands on, cue to lift the anterior axilla while laterally flexing

Author note

This exercise focuses on shoulder girdle congruency to increase the ROM of lateral flexion. The hands-on placement of the humeral head for congruency decreased the tremors, enabling the client to safely touch the pedal. To successfully meet the client's end range of lateral flexion, the pelvis had to rotate around the femur. Anchoring the extended femur into the floor enables the pelvis to rotate on the femur. To return to starting position, initiate by cueing angling the pubic bone toward the floor to provide articulation of the hip joints.

9. Standing Roll-Down on Wunda Chair with alternating single ankle plantar flexion

Derivative of J. H. Pilates Washer Woman/Hamstring 1 on Wunda Chair (NPCE Study Guide 2021, p. 73)

Editor note

This exercise requires the client to organize the torso at the midline while articulating alternating ankle plantar flexion and dorsiflexion. This may improve plantar flexion to mitigate the shuffle gait strategy.

Intent	● Challenge standing balance
	● Improve plantar flexion

Gait reasoning	● Coordinate standing balance with oppositional LE movements

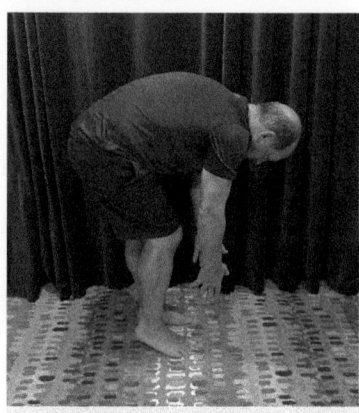

Figure 8.9

Editor note

This photo shows a non-equipment version of the Standing Roll-Down on Wunda Chair with alternating single ankle plantar flexion. The difference with the Wunda Chair is that the load force from the spring resistance of the foot pedal increases the challenge of balance.

Set-up	● Heavy spring

Starting position	● Standing 1 ft (30 cm) away from chair facing foot pedal
	● Right hip and knee joint flexion, ankle plantar flexion
	● Left hip and knee joint extension
	● Bilateral shoulder abduction for balance

Movement description
- Maintain push-off stance position
- Head initiates torso flexion
- Hands touch pedal pressing it down
- Reverse torso articulation initiating from pelvifemoral extension and pelvic posterior rotation
- 3 repetitions
- Repeat the movement while extending right knee during downward flexion
- Flex the knee to push-off position to return to starting position
- 3 repetitions
- Repeat series on other side

CUES
- Maintain thorax-shoulder-humeral head congruency throughout the exercise to decrease tremors
- If tremors occur, stand and march in place for 20 seconds
- Maintain pressure between bilateral feet
- Press tongue gently into the bottom of the mouth on the flexion down
- Embrace balance checks—they are integral to brain retraining

Author note
It was important to allow the client to hold the push-off position and let his body respond. His effort to control the wobbles increased his arm tremors. Understanding that training balance is to allow the body to wobble to find the righting reflex for improved balance decreased his tremors. During this exercise, breaks and marching in place were utilized to change the input. While the client was holding the push-off position, asking random questions helped to change the focus.

Author note
The tongue position creates a neurological complexity during movement due to the neuromyofascial continuity affecting the organization of the jaw and cervical region. Find a tongue placement of ease to lessen a possible inefficiency of movement. This may improve motor control and help establish new movement patterns (Koppele 2018).

Editor note
The dynamics of the tongue-mandible-hyoid system are managed by a dense and complex neural network which is not often found in other body structures (Pilat 2022). The author incorporates tongue movements to enhance motor control. Tongue articulation can fulfill the demands of phonation, breathing, swallowing, and chewing.

The journey to Session 11

Session 4/12
Client self-report

- Right knee and groin pain
- Fatigue scale 2
- Pain scale 3

Key changes observed

- Improved proprioception of left femoral centration improving pelvic orientation
- Improving foot and ankle articulation
- Able to glide bilateral femoral joints to improve torso organization

Reasoning behind choice of movements

- Improve foot loading to promote better femoral glide
- Increase weight-bearing load on left side to re-orientate pelvis toward left hip joint
- Standing movements for integration
- Review resistance band placement and the purpose of exercises
- Adjusted hip joint ROM to diminish torso effort over femoral-pelvic effort

Session movement sequence
1. Trapeze Table

- Seated push-through bar plantar flexion and dorsiflexion
- Side lying leg with spring from above
- Swan
- Breathing with pelvic rotations
- Roll-Down

2. Additional movements

- Lateral stepping
- Standing Roll-Down with alternating single ankle plantar flexion
- Standing Saw
- Standing push-off in tandem stance

Session 5/12
Client self-report

- Reported intense inguinal pain from prostate issues
- Difficulty urinating at night
- Had unpleasant visit with urologist prior to session
- Trouble walking
- Pain scale 3
- Fatigue scale 3

Key changes observed

- Significant pelvic shift toward left pubic bone
- Restricted pelvifemoral movement
- Observed gait with no arm swing or thoracic rotation
- After session, decrease in groin pain with pelvic reorganization

Reasoning behind choice of movements

- Facilitate right reflexive stability to improve left side organization
- Enhance reciprocal thoracic and pelvic movements for smoother gait cycle
- Reviewed side lying exercise to minimize tendency to laterally flex torso rather than abducting hip joint
- Placed client's hand on his pubic bone for sensory feedback to focus on pelvifemoral movement during abduction and adduction

Session movement sequence
1. Trapeze Table
- Bridge with roll-down bar
- Roll-Down
- Unilateral LE extension, abduction, flexion, adduction, both directions
- Swan without push-through bar
- Prone hip joint extension with no spring assistance
- Prone hip joint extension, abduction, adduction, flexion with no spring assistance

2. Standing

- Standing heel raises
- Standing heel raises with alternating knee flexion
- Standing push-off in tandem stance

Session 6/12
Client self-report

- Reported feeling great after last session
- Able to complete home program with no issues
- Pain scale 1
- Fatigue scale 2

Key changes observed

- Moving with more ease, smoothness, and confidence
- No inguinal pain
- Minimal knee pain due to an extended bike ride the day before
- No mention of tremors for the first time

Reasoning behind choice of movements

- Improve sensory integration of upper and lower body
- More unilateral movements to challenge coordination

Session movement sequence
1. Universal Reformer

- Single Leg Footwork
- Bridge with tongue movement

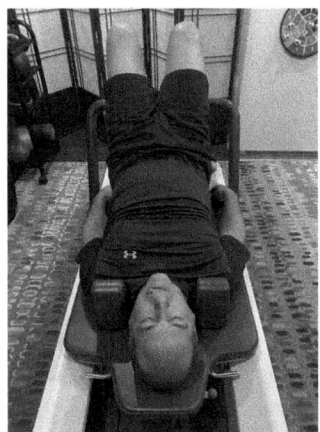

Figure 8.10

- Supine single arm with contralateral hip joint extension

2. Wunda Chair

- Swan
- Mermaid with rotation

3. Standing

- Standing heel raises
- Standing push-off in tandem stance with contralateral arm swing

Session 7/12
Client self-report

- Not feeling well after bad night's sleep and stress from work
- Pain scale 3
- Fatigue scale 4

Key changes observed

- Due to fatigue, simplified the routine by repeating previous session
- Increased cervical discomfort
- Increased number of breaks needed
- At the end of session, felt better and hoped for a better night's sleep

Reasoning behind choice of movements

- Eye and tongue warm-up exercises to help decrease limited cervical motion
- Added eye exercises to help ease cervical discomfort
- Pelvifemoral glide and articulation for improved motility of pelvic diaphragm and bladder
- Every exercise required to have ease of breath. If a slow deep breath was not possible, the movement was adjusted
- Challenge memory without increasing fatigue

Editor note

Neuromyofascial organization affects organ mobility. When the connective tissue is dehydrated, lacking the ability to glide between levels, the biotensegrity balance between tension and compression is restricted affecting organ function.

Organ motility is a normal intrinsic rhythm of an organ and movement that is inherent to the organ itself to allow for function. Motility can be reduced by an issue within the organ itself, such as inflammation or emotional concerns, or in relation to medication. Motility reduction may also be due to surrounding structures that have been binding an organ and impinging on its cellular motion (Barral Institute 2012).

Session movement sequence
1. Side Kick

- Explored Side Kick to find ease of breath

2. Universal Reformer

- Single Leg Footwork
- Bridge with tongue movement
- Supine single arm with contralateral hip joint extension

3. Wunda Chair

- Swan
- Mermaid with rotation

4. Standing

- Standing heel raises holding on to wall
- Standing push-off in tandem stance holding on to wall

5. Additional movements

- Began session with simple, smooth eye-tracking exercises
    - Eye tracking of a spoon, without head

motion, while spoon was moved in multiple directions

- Tongue exercise
  - Mouth closed, sliding tongue along all of the teeth
  - Repeated 3 times in each direction
- Tongue pressing into each cheek with gentle head turn in opposite direction of the tongue

Editor note

The dynamics of the tongue-mandible-hyoid system are managed by a dense and complex neural network which is not often found in other body structures (Pilat 2022). The author incorporates tongue movements to enhance motor control. Tongue articulation can fulfill the demands of phonation, breathing, swallowing, and chewing (see Figure 8.10).

Session 8/12
Client self-report

- Feeling better than at our previous session
- Ease with breathing
- Pain scale 1
- Fatigue scale 2

Key changes observed

- Improved breathing
- Discovered new multiple strategies during home program practice
- Change from stiff gait to ease and smoothness

Reasoning behind choice of movements

- Energy improved allowing to continue progressing sessions
- Improve coordination of reciprocal thoracic and pelvic movements

Session movement sequence
1. Universal Reformer

- Single Leg Footwork
- Single Leg Circles with contralateral arm circles in same direction
- Coordination
- Straps: feet in loops: extension and hip and knee joint flexion, knees extended, extension/abduction/flexion/adduction both directions
- Back and Front Rowing

2. Standing

- Standing heel raises

3. Additional movement

- Standing push-off in tandem stance with contralateral arm swing holding 3 lb (1.36 kg) hand weights

Session 9/12
Client self-report

- Fatigued but feels better after the sessions
- Pain scale 0
- Fatigue scale 3
- Recorded home program for economy of time and remembering cues

Key changes observed

- Observed client walk in from parking lot leading with head
- Increased confidence
- Walking without looking down
- Fatigue high, lessened intensity of session

Reasoning behind choice of movements

- Increase foot articulation

- Proprioception of feet throughout the day while walking
- Increase forward momentum from push-off

Session movement sequence
1. Universal Reformer

- Footwork: bilateral and unilateral with varied foot positions
- Supine arms with ankle circles
- Pulling Straps with added foot and ankle movement
- Seated Chest Expansion
- Seated rowing, bilateral and unilateral with thoracic rotation

2. Standing

- Standing calf raises
- Standing push-off in tandem stance with contralateral arm swing

3. Additional movements

- Standing Roll-Down with calf raises
- Included several questions during movements to test client's memory and ability to coordinate talking and moving

Session 10/12

- Client self-report
- Pain scale 0
- Fatigue scale 0

Key changes observed

- No longer identifies only as a Parkinson's patient
- More engaged and energetic
- Gait improved and less painful

Reasoning behind choice of movements
- Improve coordination of limbs
- Increase cadence of gait
- Introduce importance of grip strength

Session movement sequence
1. Added hanging from a pull-up bar with three different grips

- Bilateral supination
  - Right supination, left pronation
  - Left supination, right pronation

2. Universal Reformer

- Single Leg Footwork
- Arm straps
- Coordination
- Back Rowing and Front Rowing
- Pulling Straps
- Prone shoulder extension with elbow flexion holding risers

3. Standing

- Standing heel raises with alternative knee bends
- Standing push-off in tandem stance with contralateral arm swing

4. Additional movement

- Kneeling rotation in split stance

References

Barral Institute (2012) "Visceral motility testing." *Visceral Mobility and Motility Testing: Comprehensive Illustrated Collection of Visceral Motion.* [Standing Flip Chart]. Barral Productions, p. 1. barralinstitute.com.

Beh, S. C., Frohman, T. C., and Frohman, E. M. (2017) "Cerebellar control of eye movements." *Journal of Neuro-Ophthalmology, 37,* 1, 87–89.

Bexander, C. S., Mellor, R., and Hodges, P. W. (2005) "Effect of gaze direction on neck muscle activity during cervical rotation." *Experimental Brain Research, 167,* 3, 422–332.

Black, M. (2022) *Centered: Organizing the body through Kinesiology, Movement Theory and Pilates Techniques.* Edinburgh: Handspring Publishing, p. 209.

Breland, M. (2018) Understand Parkinson's: A guide for exercise professionals, patients, and caregivers. The Neuro Studio. [Video]. http://bit.ly/3ZCqOEF. [Accessed September 22, 2023].

Feng, Y. S., Yang, S. D., Tan, Z. X., Wang, M. M. *et al.* (2020) "The benefits and mechanisms of exercise training for Parkinson's disease." *Life Sciences, 245.* DOI: 10.1016/j.lfs.2020.117345.

Gilat, M., Bell, P. T., Ehgoetz Martens, K. A., Georgiades, M. J. *et al.* (2017) "Dopamine depletion impairs gait automaticity by altering cortico-striatal and cerebellar processing in Parkinson's disease." *Neuroimage, 152,* 207–220.

Goffart, L., Hafed, Z. M., and Krauzlis, R. J. (2012) "Visual fixation as equilibrium: Evidence from superior colliculus inactivation." *Journal of Neuroscience, 32,* 31, 10627–10636.

Hofheinz, M., Mibs, M., and Elsner, B. (2016) "Dual task training for improving balance and gait in people with stroke." *Cochrane Database of Systematic Reviews, 2016,* 10. DOI: 10.1002/14651858.CD012403.

Koppele Duffy, M. (2018) Understanding anatomy in action: Real life applications for muscular slings and 4-quadrant stability. The Neuro Studio. [Video]. http://bit.ly/3H86c4G. [Accessed September 22, 2023].

Koppele Duffy, M. (2022) Advanced Neuro Techniques Workshop. Workshop presented by The Neuro Studio, March 2022.

Kresge, C. and Elgelid, S. (2021) *The Feldenkrais Method.* Edinburgh: Handspring Publishing.

Lanciego, J. L., Luquin, N., and Obeso, J. A. (2012) Functional neuroanatomy of the basal ganglia. *Cold Spring Harbor, Perspectives in Medicine, 2,* 12. DOI: 10.1101/cshperspect.a009621.

McAfee, S. S., Liu, Y., Sillitoe, R. V., and Heck, D. H. (2022) "Cerebellar coordination of neuronal communication in cerebral cortex." *Frontiers in Systems Neuroscience, 15.* DOI: 10.3389/fnsys.2021.781527 ISSN=1662-5137.

Muthukrishnan, N., Abbas, J. J., Shill, H. A., and Krishnamurthi, N. (2019) "Cueing paradigms to improve gait and posture in Parkinson's disease: A narrative review." *Sensors (Basel), 19,* 24. DOI: 10.3390/s19245468.

NPCE Study Guide (National Pilates Certification Exam Study Guide) (2021) Miami, FL: National Pilates Certification Program, Inc.

Pilat, A. (2022) *Myofascial Induction: Volume 1—The Upper Body.* Edinburgh: Handspring Publishing, pp. 338–341.

Somisetty, S. M. and Das, J. (2022) Neuroanatomy, vestibulo-ocular reflex. [Updated 2022, July 25]. In: StatPearls [Internet]. Treasure Island (FL): StatPearls Publishing; 2022 Jan-. www.ncbi.nlm.nih.gov/books/NBK545297. [Accessed September 22, 2023].

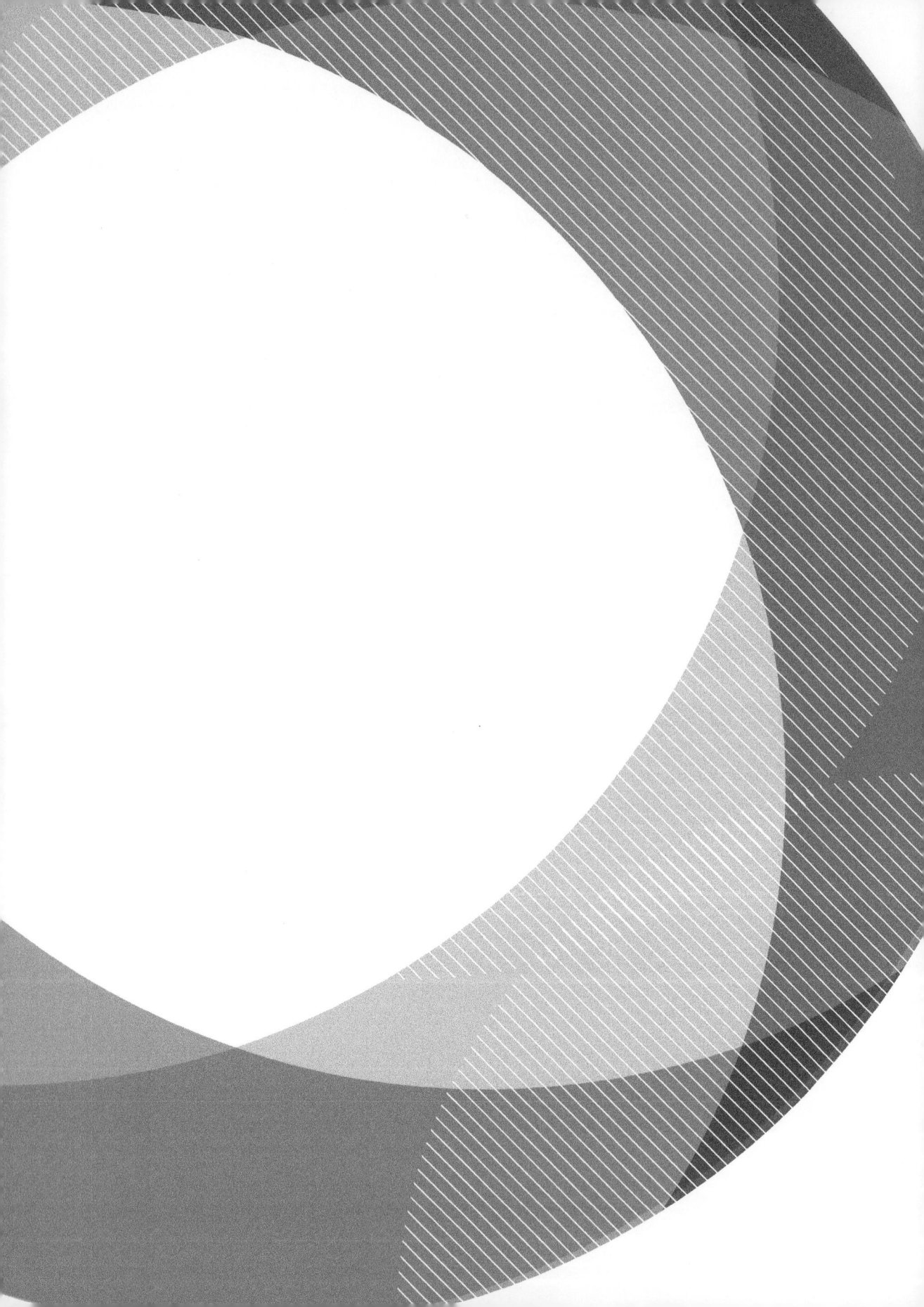

Pilates and Hypermobility and Ehlers–Danlos: Effect on Gait

Marylee Bussard

Hypermobile Ehlers–Danlos syndrome

Ehlers–Danlos syndrome refers to a group of connective tissue disorders that are classified into 13 subtypes. The most common of these is hypermobile Ehlers–Danlos syndrome (hEDS), the focus of this case report.

While joint hypermobility can be asymptomatic and even advantageous in some professions like ballet, it is not always the case that more flexibility is better. Those with hEDS are prone to a host of confounding and sometimes disabling symptoms, such as joint dislocations, pain and fatigue, compromised proprioception, and mast cell activation.

Prevalence

The prevalence of hypermobility spectrum disorders in general, and hEDS specifically, is unknown. Recent studies suggest that at least 1 in 5000 people have EDS and 80–90 percent of these individuals could have hEDS (Tinkle *et al.* 2017). Considering that up to 56 percent of patients with EDS are misdiagnosed, and many take years or even decades to receive a proper diagnosis, the true number is likely higher (Demmler *et al.* 2019).

Diagnosis

The classification for hEDS changed in 2017, making guidelines for diagnosis stricter, which helps avoid confusion with other EDS subtypes and different connective tissue disorders such as Marfan syndrome.

Unlike the other subtypes of EDS, hEDS has no known molecular or genetic basis.

Diagnosis is established using a set of criteria that—among other considerations such as symptomology, medical history, and family history—includes a Beighton scale score of ≥5 for adults, ≥6 for children and adolescents, and ≥4 for those over 50.

While generalized joint hypermobility is the common element among people with hEDS, a host of related symptoms—musculoskeletal, neurological, gastrointestinal, inflammatory—may be present. Often, the comorbidities in hEDS are more problematic than the joint issues. No two cases are alike (Jovin 2020).

Observable characteristics

The most common observable characteristics of hEDS include hyperextendable joints, such as elbows or knees, dropped foot arches, and somewhat softer, more fragile and stretchy skin than average (although not as pronounced as in other types of EDS).

Movement contraindications

A common risk for this group is the possibility of pain flare-ups, the cause of which can be complex and related to things other than exercise.

Use graded exposure when introducing new challenges and progress slowly.

The contraindications below are general guidelines for hEDS and not necessarily universal or permanent for every client. General contraindications and considerations include:

- End-range movements and stretches
- High-load, high-intensity activities can lead to flare-ups, hernias, or prolapses
- Open-chain exercises could result in nerve and joint discomfort
- Closed-chain movements are generally better tolerated by this population
- People with hEDS often struggle with stability and coordination

- Engender a sense of safety, which is holistic and trauma-informed
- Consider other common co-occurring conditions, such as:
  - Postural orthostatic tachycardia syndrome (POTS)—transitioning between body positions can cause light-headedness and fainting
  - Vascular EDS—heavy lifting and activities involving rapid acceleration and deceleration should be avoided due to weakened arteries
  - Digestive issues resulting in reflux, heartburn, abdominal pain, irritable bowel, and incontinence may impact the ability to sense and develop core control

Client description: 30-year-old biological female, identifies as female; successful attorney; mother of a small child

Dates of case report: Session 1: September 2, 2020; Session 12: October 27, 2020; in-person and virtual sessions due to pandemic interruption

Studio apparatus and props
Pilates equipment

- Universal Reformer
- Trapeze Table

Props used with equipment

- Dowel
- Mat

Home program props

- Soft 8 in. (20 cm) ball
- Medium resistance bands
- Dowel
- Mat

Methods and materials

Session 1/12
1. Health history interview

- Joint subluxations (hips, shoulders, elbows, lumbar region, etc.) identifiable since infancy
- Diagnosed with Ehlers–Danlos syndrome, hypermobility type, in 2020. (Had been diagnosed with classical EDS in 2008, before the guidelines changed in 2017)
- Left hip dysplasia
- Began doing Pilates at 13 years old to help with joint stability
- Near-fatal episode of appendicitis at 13 years old led to permanent scarring of her abdominal walls
- History of gastrointestinal, endocrine, autonomic,

and blood-related challenges secondary to EDS diagnosis. Is under the care of a range of physicians and has been proactive with exercise and rehabilitation

- Cardiologist ruled out vascular EDS, a serious and potentially life-threatening condition
- History of regularly dislocating the sacroiliac joints, most recently in 2017
- Gave birth in 2018 by C-section
- Endocrine: post-pregnancy thyroiditis; currently on Tirosint for hypothyroidism
- Other medications:
  - For pain: Lyrica, cyclobenzaprine, occasional use of OTC acetaminophen/ibuprofen
  - Albuterol inhaler (for asthma)
  - EpiPen (wheat allergy)
  - Claritin (for mast cell activation symptoms)
  - Dietary supplements: Vitamin C, B12, D3, iron (for anemia), CoQ10, pre-natal multi-vitamin, fish oil, magnesium
- Attended an intensive 4-month core rehabilitation physical therapy program at a leading rehab hospital, Shirley Ryan AbilityLab in Chicago, in 2019
- Set to begin another intensive program at Shirley Ryan AbilityLab just as our 12 sessions together ended; this one focused on chronic pain
- At the time of this study, client was also in physical therapy for wrist pain

2. Symptoms

- Flare-ups common. May be exercise- or hormone-induced during luteal phase of her menstrual cycle

- Nerve pain (especially affects hands when writing)
- Difficulty standing for long periods without pain and fatigue, impacting daily activities such as commuting to work, cooking, and socializing
- Chronic pain and inflammation in the hip joints, sacroliac joint issues
- Proprioception and balance challenges
- Autonomic challenges (low blood pressure, malabsorption of nutrients, gluten sensitivity, irritable bowel syndrome, past issues with temperature regulation)

3. Movement aids

- Uses mobility aids (canes, arm crutches) when commuting or to support long periods of standing at work, but not specifically during this exercise program

---

Final result of case report

Client reports significant improvement in functional movement including gait, balance, and climbing up and down stairs. Immediately after completing this series, she participated in an intensive physical/occupational therapy program for chronic pain, and MRI revealed a herniated disc. Presently reports near-total abatement of symptoms and is expecting her second child.

Session 2/12: Initial assessment

1. General observations of gait

◆ Holds right arm rigid

◆ Minimal thoracic rotation

◆ Right innominate drop during left stance phase

◆ Pelvis rotates left during right stance phase

◆ Foot position and stride length normal

2. Standing tests

◆ Full torso rotation

● Observations of inefficient side: left
■ Initially tentative with limited pelvis on femur internal rotation bilaterally, more limited on left
■ Right foot overpronation accentuated during left rotation

◆ Hemipelvis inferior motion

● Observations of inefficient side: both
■ Right
○ Unable to lower right innominate
○ Client fearful of potential subluxation of her left hip joint if she executes the movement fully
○ No left lumbar lateral flexion, pelvis rotates anteriorly and left
■ Left
○ Accompanied by right pelvic rotation, and with slight left thoracic rotation

◆ Hemipelvis superior motion

Session 12/12: Post-assessment

1. General observations of gait

◆ Both arms move freely in movement

◆ Thoracic rotation improved

◆ Right innominate drop during left stance phase improved

◆ Pelvis left rotation during right stance phase unchanged

2. Standing tests

◆ Full torso rotation

● Observations of inefficient side: left
■ Less tentative overall
■ Limited pelvis on femur internal rotation, unchanged
■ Right foot pronation unchanged

◆ Hemipelvis inferior motion

● Observations of inefficient side: both
■ Right: client continues to anteriorly tilt pelvis to protect her left hip joint from possible subluxation
■ Left: no change

◆ Hemipelvis superior motion

● Observations of inefficient side: left
■ Client anteriorly tilts pelvis and rotates pelvis left during left hemipelvis superior motion to avoid adduction and internal rotation of left LE, although slightly less than before, and she appears more comfortable attempting the movement

- Observations of inefficient side: left
  - Client anteriorly tilts pelvis and rotates pelvis left during left hemipelvis superior motion to avoid adduction and internal rotation of left lower extremity (LE), creating left lumbar and lower thoracic rotation
  - Appropriate heel lift and plantar flexion bilaterally

- Lateral pelvic shift

- Observations of inefficient side: left
  - Client reports that the lumbar region feels tight during this motion
  - Appropriate pronation and supination of the foot and ankle in both directions

3. Seated tests

- Hip joint and knee flexion

- Observations of inefficient side: right
  - Thorax translates right, flexion and rotation left
  - Client consciously engages the core to stay stable during this exercise, which she learned to do in past physical therapy training

Author note
Included dorsiflexion and knee flexion test. Both were efficient bilaterally. Included hip abduction with external rotation. Both were efficient bilaterally.

4. Sit and stand

- Lateral view

- Pelvis tilts anteriorly

- Anterior view

- Lateral pelvic shift

- Observations of inefficient side: left
  - Client reports she no longer experiences tightness during this movement
  - Appropriate pronation and supination of foot and ankle in both directions

3. Seated tests

- Hip joint and knee flexion

- Observations of inefficient side: right
  - Reduced right thoracic translation with hip flexion

Author note
Included dorsiflexion and knee flexion test. Both were efficient bilaterally. Included hip abduction with external rotation. Both were efficient bilaterally.

4. Sit and stand

- Lateral view
  - Pelvis tilts anteriorly

- Anterior view

- Thorax translates right, pelvis shifts left
- Right knee valgus motion with pro-nounced pronation in right foot and ankle

5. Standing balance

◆ Two-leg stance, eyes open

- 60 seconds
- Client reports her body must make "tons of microadjustments"

◆ One-leg stance, eyes open

- Right leg: easier than left, 60 seconds
- Left leg: very difficult, 60 seconds
- Client feels she is mostly working below the knee, with her "foot working super hard the whole time"

- Client moves with less pelvic and thoracic translation
- Right knee valgus motion and ankle pronation less pronounced

5. Standing balance

◆ Two-leg stance, eyes open
  - Client reports this feels "a lot better" than before and micro-adjustments are "much less"
  - 60 seconds

◆ One-leg stance, eyes open
  - Client reports that the right leg is still easier to balance on but that both legs feel easier than before
  - Right leg: 60 seconds
  - Left leg: 60 seconds

Session 3/12: Home program

Fatigue scale low grade

Pain scale low grade

Client self-report
- Excited to begin program

Author note

This client lives with chronic pain and stated up front that she feels frustrated by pain scales, stating that they are not helpful in communicating her true experience and, if anything, they downplay the pain she experiences as a daily part of her life. After some discussion, we opted for a more narrative description of her experience of pain and fatigue ("good" meaning pain was less than usual, low-grade pain, moderate pain, medium pain, and so forth).

Key changes observed by author at end of Session 3/12
- Client has extensive physical therapy and movement training in the past, including Pilates. In this session, she demonstrated solid awareness of torso activation without compensatory patterns (something she says she has worked hard at), although motor control shows room for improvement
- Unable to hold her legs in 90 degrees hip and knee flexion position for very long without triggering pain and tightness in her posterior torso and hip flexors. Client was able to intentionally redistribute the effort throughout her torso balancing the tensional forces
- Client committed to practice this at home
- It was more difficult to control excessive movement of the pelvis during leg circles with left leg

Reason behind choice of sequencing
- Assess and establish torso coordination and control in different positions
- Identify and build awareness of habitual patterns of excessive or compensatory movement strategies
- Identify notable movement strategies and begin working toward improving those strategies
- Establish how client's joints and tissues uniquely tolerate various movement challenges across different planes and positions to provide a safe and productive home exercise program

Session movement sequence

1. Pelvic tilts, "ha," windshield wipers

Intent
- Self-regulation and focus
- Pelvic proprioception
- Gauge client comfort and support her sense of movement safety
- Identify necessary adaptations

Gait reasoning
- Improve torso dynamic control and reduce discomfort
- Awareness of breath with torso activation
- Observe assessed movement patterns in all planes

Starting position
- Supine with knees flexed, feet flat on mat hip-distance apart
- Hands placed flat on stomach, heels of hands on ASIS, fingertips on pubic bone
- Breathe noticing the rise and fall of anterior abdominal wall beneath hands

Author note

In later sessions, the visualizations of the bony landmarks of the pelvis and interoception of tensional changes in the body brought increased awareness to sensations of effort and resting qualities. The author invited experimentation with differing qualities and patterns of torso activation.

Movement description
- Posteriorly rotate pelvis softly pressing posterior torso toward mat
- Return to starting position
- Repeat, observing how pubic bone moves toward the ceiling and then the floor
- Find a position where hands are parallel to ceiling
- Make the sound "ha," and observe how anterior abdominal wall pulls away from hands
- Try to gently recreate that drawing in feeling of the anterior abdominal wall without squeezing or bracing in other areas of body
- Next, bring arms to the side and slowly drop knees to the right, and then the left
- Repeat several times, as tolerated

2. Supine marching Derivative of Eve Gentry's knee folds (see Chapter 5, Gentry)

Intent
- Improve torso-pelvic proprioception
- Improve dynamic control
- Reduce excessive activation of hip flexors and posterior torso

Gait reasoning
- Improve dynamic control
- Reduce discomfort
- Support proprioception and motor planning

Starting position
- Supine with knees flexed, feet flat on mat hip-distance apart
- Prior to movement, place attention to expanse and weight of pelvis into mat

Movement description
- Slowly flex right hip lifting the foot and then lower
- Repeat on left side

Author note

Ask the client what they notice and build on this awareness. For example, if the client notes tightness in the hip flexors, stop the exercise and invite experimentation. Next, direct the client's attention toward any sensations that the pelvis is shifting on the mat with the initiation of the movement. Invite them to find a way to lift and lower the leg with little to no movement of the pelvis.

3. Modified Single Leg Stretch Derivative of J. H. Pilates Single Leg Stretch (NPCE Study Guide 2021, p. 46)

Intent
- Improve torso to LE connection and proprioception
- Improve dynamic control
- Reduce excessive activation of hip flexors and posterior torso
- Teach client to self-monitor and make appropriate adaptations while exercising

Gait reasoning
- Improved dynamic torso control
- Support proprioception and motor planning
- Build movement confidence

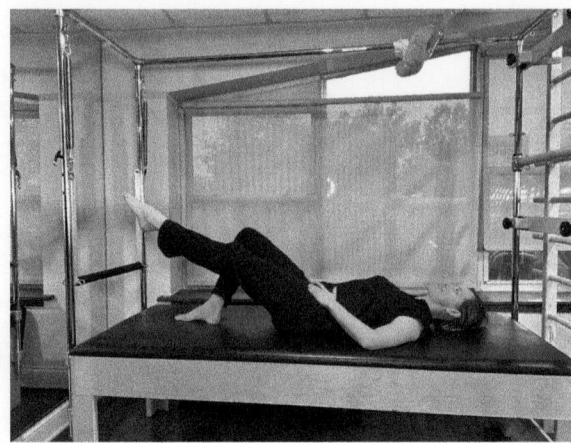

Figure 9.1

Starting position	● Supine on mat
	● Head down
	● Left knee bent with foot on mat
	● Right hip and knee flexed
Movement description	● Extend right LE very slowly to 45 degrees, return to starting position
	● Complete 5–6 repetitions on right side, taking about 6 seconds per repetition
	● Repeat on left side
	● Add repetitions over time, reaching 10–12 on each side

4. Modified Single Leg Circles Derivative of J. H. Pilates Single Leg Circles (NPCE Study Guide 2021, p. 46)

Intent	● Improve proprioception
	● Improve dynamic control
	● Reduce excessive activation of hip flexors and posterior torso
	● Teach client to self-monitor and make appropriate adaptations while exercising
	● Discover and address imbalances of strength and control
	● Reduce discomfort

Gait reasoning	• Improve dynamic control of hip joint for swing phase • Support proprioception and motor planning • Determine the comfort and availability of hip glide in all planes
Starting position	• Supine on mat • Left hip and knee flexed with foot on mat • Right LE extended above hip • Allow head of femur to sink into hip and sink into mat
Movement description	• Breathing normally • Right LE crosses midline, performing adduction/extension/abduction/flexion and returning to starting position • Count about 4 seconds per movement • Complete 5 repetitions before reversing • Right LE performs reverse abduction/extension/adduction/flexion and returns to starting position • Repeat with left LE • Add repetitions over time, completing 10 repetitions in each direction

5. Shoulder bridge with knees out 30 degrees

Intent	• Improve dynamic control • Improve articulation and reduce excessive bracing of torso • Activate hip extensors • Reduce excessive activation of hip flexors and posterior torso • Teach client to self-monitor and make appropriate adaptations while exercising • Reduce discomfort
Gait reasoning	• Improve dynamic control of hip extension with torso articulation • Support proprioception and motor planning • Assess hip extension, abduction, and flexion in supine position
Starting position	• Supine on mat, knees abducted 30 degrees • Feet lateral to ischial tuberosities • Take a moment to feel both feet fully in contact with mat

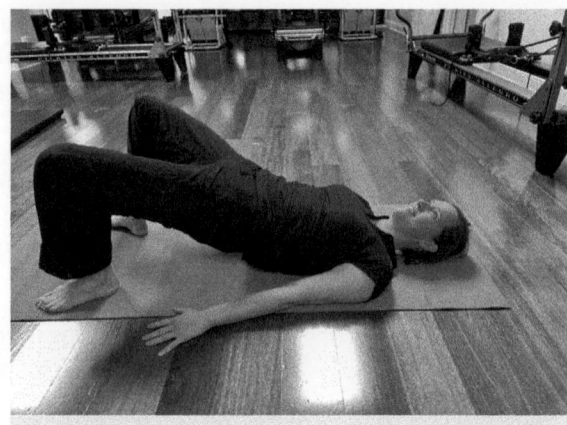

Figure 9.2

Movement description
- Inhale in position
- Exhale posteriorly, rotate pelvis, articulate torso from base to shoulders
- Do not lift so high as to excessively extend
- Hold, inhale
- Exhale, soften the sternum to initiate flexion articulation, rolling down to starting position
- Move slowly, taking 10–12 seconds per repetition
- Repeat 5 times
- Add repetitions over time, up to 18 repetitions
- Rest as needed

6. Ball squeeze

Intent
- Improve dynamic hip control
- Activate LE to torso with adduction and abduction movement
- Teach client to self-monitor and make appropriate adaptations while exercising
- Reduce discomfort

Gait reasoning
- Improved torso dynamic control in LE activation
- Support proprioception and motor planning
- Assess and activate hip joint medial and lateral glide

Starting position
- Supine on mat, hips and knees flexed with feet in line with ischial tuberosities
- Soft 8 in. (20 cm) ball placed between thighs

Movement description
- Gently squeeze ball for 5 seconds
- Release and repeat for a total of 15 times
- Add 1–2 repetitions every few days over time until you reach up to 30
- Rest as needed

7. Prone hip extension

Intent
- Activate hip extensors
- Improve torso dynamic control in hip extension
- Reduce excessive activation of hip flexors and posterior torso
- Teach client to self-monitor and make appropriate adaptations while exercising

Gait reasoning
- Support proprioception and motor planning in hip extension to reduce uncontrolled torso extension

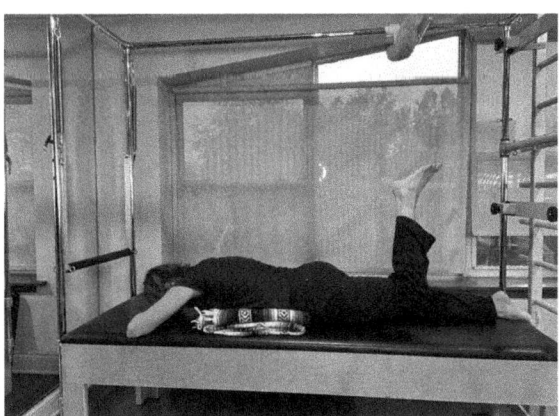

Figure 9.3

Starting position
- Lying prone on mat
- Hands under the forehead
- Press pubic bone into mat
- Draw anterior abdominals away from mat

Author note
Use a blanket under the abdominals and ASIS if excessive activation of the posterior torso is apparent.

Movement description
- Variation 1: straight leg
  - Lift right LE off mat
  - Pause, then lower
  - Only lift as high as you can without changing torso
  - Each repetition should take 3–4 seconds
  - Repeat 10 times
  - Change sides
  - Add 1–2 repetitions every few days over time until you reach 30 repetitions per side
  - Rest as needed
- Variation 2: knee flexion
  - Follow instructions as above with 100 degrees knee flexion, modifying for comfort

Author note

This movement was not possible for the client at the beginning, so she visualized the movement and isometrically contracted the LE until she could complete the movement.

8. 90/90 hip and knee flexion

Intent
- Improve dynamic torso control with LE in flexion
- Reduce excessive activation of hip flexors and posterior torso
- Build awareness of managing intra-abdominal pressure and avoiding hEDS risk factors such as hernias or organ prolapse during exercise and daily life (see Editor note on intra-abdominal pressure in Chapter 10)
- Teach client to self-monitor and make appropriate adaptations while exercising
- Reduce discomfort

Gait reasoning
- Improve torso dynamic in hip flexion
- Support proprioception and motor planning
- Increase movement confidence

Starting position
- Supine on mat
- 90/90 hip and knee flexion
- Feet in line with ischial tuberosities on mat

Movement description	● Flex right LE to 90 degrees with knee in 90 degrees flexion
	● Flex left LE 90 degrees with knee in 90 degrees flexion
	● Hold position for 30 seconds
	● Lower right LE to mat
	● Lower left LE to mat
	● Repeat as able, with the goal of being able to maintain the position without strain for up to 3 minutes

Author note

Because holding the LE in flexion was difficult for this client, I offered support: first, using my arms; second, using a support with a band; progressing to a third stage without support. By the end of the series, the endurance increased to 3 minutes without any aids. We progressed by incorporating Arm Springs using a resistance band wrapped around a doorknob.

9. Modified single leg lower lift with band

Intent	● Improve dynamic torso control with LE motion
	● Reduce excessive activation of hip flexors and posterior torso
	● Teach client to self-monitor and make appropriate adaptations while exercising
Gait reasoning	● Support proprioception and motor planning
Starting position	● Supine on mat
	● Left hip and knee flexion with foot on mat
	● Right LE hip flexion and knee extension
	● Use band

Author note

Because the client found it difficult to keep excessive activation of the hip flexors, we started with a resistance band and experimented with a heavier band to decrease hip flexor effort. We progressed to a lighter band requiring hip flexor activation, then performed the movement, unaided, with ease.

Movement description	• Inhale, extend right LE toward mat maintaining torso position
	• Exhale, flex right LE with knee extended
	• One repetition for 4–6 seconds
	• Repeat 6 times
	• Change to left side
	• Add 1–2 repetitions every few days as able, up to 30 per side
	• Rest as needed

10. Short Box Series variations in a chair (Flat Back, side bend, rotation, side to side)

Derivative of J. H. Pilates Reverse Swan/Torso Press Sit on Wunda Chair (NPCE Study Guide 2021, p. 73)

Editor note

In Short Box Series: Flat Back, the primary articulation occurs at the pelvifemoral joints. The spatial relationship of the thorax and pelvis is sustained throughout the pelvifemoral motion in the sagittal plane. Torso articulation is minimized.

Intent	• Improve articulation with control
	• Sense multi-directional structural strategies or palintonicity

Editor note

Palintonicity is derived from the Greek word *palintonos* meaning unity in opposition. The term is used in Rolfing to describe ideal posture as the balance of opposing forces and spatial relationships in movement, such as front/back, side to side, top to bottom, inside and outside (Martine 2018). Here, the author's intent is to bring a balance to opposing tensions within the whole body in all planes for dynamic stabilized functional movement and resiliency.

Gait reasoning	• Facilitate torso three-dimensional movement
	• Improve proprioception of torso motion
Starting position	• Sitting on the front edge of a chair or stool, feet on floor, hands resting on thighs
	• Parts of the series can be performed while standing

Movement description
- Repeat each of the following exercises slowly 3–4 times
- Flat Back
  - Inhale, rock back on the sitz bones maintaining torso organization
  - Exhale, return to starting position
- Side bend
  - Inhale, laterally flex to the right
  - Exhale, return to starting position
  - Repeat on left
- Side to side
  - Inhale, whole torso organization tilts to right, allowing opposite sitz bone to lift off box
  - Exhale, return to starting position
  - Repeat on left
- Rotation
  - Inhale, rotate to right
  - Exhale, return to starting position
  - Repeat on left
- Row the boat
  - Holding a dowel, inhale, reach arms to ceiling
  - Exhale, articulate flexion from top of head reaching toward toes
  - Inhale, trace dowel up the legs
  - Exhale, articulate in extension to midline orientation

11. Standing single leg balance and slow marching

Intent
- Increase strength and stamina during standing reducing dependency on aids

Gait reasoning
- Increase stamina during standing
- Build proprioception of foot continuity to torso
- Activation of standing on one leg for stance phase

Starting position
- Standing on both feet

Author note
Before progressing to the single leg balance, take a moment to feel the connection of the feet to the floor, visualizing roots from the bottom of the feet deep into the ground. Imagine a resistance band lifting from the arch of the feet creating a buoyancy continuity of the pelvic diaphragm, respiratory diaphragm, and through the roof of the mouth. Try to maintain this sense of buoyant lift throughout the balancing exercise.

Movement description	● Shift weight to one side and lift opposite foot, maintaining sense of buoyancy
	● Hold, observing the effort of the foot while keeping toes long, encouraging arch to lift
	● Slowly lower leg and change sides without over-shifting the weight, especially on right
	● Repeat several times on each side
	● Rest as needed

12. Self-observation during daily movements (e.g., walking, getting up from a chair)

Intent	● Provide education relevant to movement challenges setting in motion an iterative process of movement experimentation
	● Greater confidence, comfort, and ease in movement during daily life
	● Improved awareness and motor planning
Gait reasoning	● Awareness of whole-body motion during gait

Author note

During Session 5, a home-based Zoom session, we discussed movement patterns I had observed during her initial assessment. I shared visual educational materials explaining the role anatomy and structure plays in supporting posture and gait. We discussed which of these reflected her tendencies (both as she experienced them and as I observed them) and how these tendencies could relate to the fatigue and discomfort she was experiencing in daily life. We then took time for her to observe herself while walking, getting up from a chair, and standing on one leg and test out this newfound understanding in her body. She reported that connecting the dots in this way was one of the most impactful parts of the series.

Session 11/12: Studio Session

Fatigue scale	medium
Pain scale	medium

Client self-report
- Higher level than usual of bilateral hip and low back pain, which she described as her typical pattern of autoimmune over-reactivity. Made appointment with her rheumatologist
- Almost fainted getting out of a hot bath the previous day

Key changes observed by author at end of Session 11/12
- Client had been making consistent and steady progress until a medium-grade pain flare-up occurred between Sessions 10 and 11. While it is hard to pinpoint one specific factor, her perceived exertion in Session 10, specifically on new hip abduction exercises, was greater than in other sessions and may have played a role. Risk of flare-ups is inherent in serving clients with chronic pain, and not always within our control
- In Session 11, adjusted the effort, taking time to focus on self-regulation through breathing and relaxation. Reduced spring resistance
- Halfway through the session, client requested challenging movements attempted previously. After some discussion, I accommodated her request, trusting that she had the tools to know what was best for her body
- By Session 12, her level of pain was reduced to moderate

Reason behind choice of sequencing
- Self-regulation of nervous system
- Sense of movement optimism
- Sense of integration and achievement

Session movement sequence

1. Footwork on Universal Reformer   Derivative of J. H. Pilates Footwork on Universal Reformer (NPCE Study Guide 2021, p. 52) and J. H. Pilates Running (NPCE Study Guide 2021, p. 60)

Intent
- Gently move the body
- Improve proprioception
- Improve dynamic torso adaptability

Gait reasoning
- Support proprioception and motor planning
- Improve LE adaptation to ground forces

Set-up	● Springs: 2 heavy and 1 light ● Weight based on client feedback
Starting position	● Supine on carriage ● Feet on footbar
Movement description	● Feet positioned on footbar ● Pilates V 45 degrees external rotation ● Parallel arches ● Parallel heels ● Abducted, externally rotated heels ● Press feet on footbar and move carriage out and slowly return ● 8–10 repetitions ● Running ● 8–10 repetitions

CUES

- Due to the client experiencing a medium pain flare-up prior to beginning the exercise, I invited her into full-bodied, present-moment awareness with cues and inquiries
- Take several deep breaths. Observe the rise and fall of your stomach with each inhale and exhale
- Feel the back of your body supported by the carriage
- Try to relax any tension in your shoulders, jaw, etc.
- Allow your knees to slowly and gently drop to one side... and then the other. Stay here as long as you like
- How does this feel?
- Begin whenever you feel ready

Author note

Proprioception can be compromised with hEDS. These clients may find it challenging both to sense how their body is positioned and to gauge the appropriate amount of effort required for movement. Footwork on the Universal Reformer is invaluable for developing this awareness as it provides the opportunity to direct attention toward positioning and how the body adapts, and effort levels can be adjusted to meet the feedback provided by the springs.

2. Arm Springs: Circles Supine on Trapeze Table and Universal Reformer

Derivative of J.H. Pilates Mermaid on Universal Reformer (NPCE Study Guide 2021, p. 58) and derivative of J. H. Pilates Coordination on Universal Reformer (NPCE Study Guide 2021, p. 58)

Intent
- Integrate awareness of dynamic torso, three-dimensional breathing, and humeral head positioning in motion

Gait reasoning
- Improve torso adaptability to upper extremity (UE) movement for arm swing
- Support proprioception and motor planning

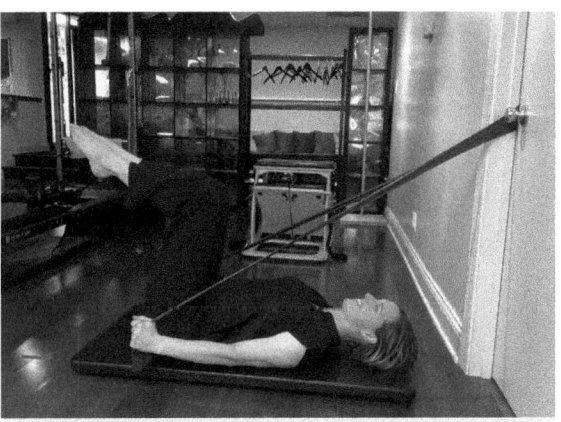

Figure 9.4

Editor note

Practitioner measured the needs of the client each session. Arm Springs were performed lying on the Trapeze Table using the springs in one session. Then practitioner varied the environment by using the Universal Reformer. The photo in Figure 9.4 shows a home version of this exercise.

Set-up
- Trapeze Table: light springs
- Universal Reformer: heavy spring

Starting position
- Trapeze Table and Universal Reformer
- Supine, 90 degrees hip and knee flexion

Movement description
- UE with elbows extended pull the straps
- Flexion and extension 3–6 times
- Abduction/adduction/flexion 3–6 times
- Extension/abduction/horizontal adduction 3–6 times
- Elbow flexion and extension with upper arm 3–6 times

CUES

- Exhale gently, allow abdominals to draw in
- How does it feel? If back or hip flexors feel tense, lower feet
- Exhale and soften the sternum. Try to maintain this feeling
- Direct breath toward low floating ribs in the back and side. Try to maintain that sense of fullness throughout breath cycle
- Collarbones wide
- Scapulae gliding down
- Press from the back and below the armpits, not from the chest
- Stay with the spring tension on the return

Author note

The Arm Springs exercise offers a challenging opportunity to introduce, and eventually integrate, multiple levels of proprioceptive awareness and control, contributing to a sense of strength and mastery.

3. Mermaid on Universal Reformer

Derivative of J.H. Pilates Mermaid on Universal Reformer (NPCE Study Guide 2021, p. 58)

Intent
- Torso lateral articulation
- Orientation around the midline
- Breath awareness
- Nervous system self-regulation

Gait reasoning
- Increase range of motion (ROM) in right UE
- Promote torso lateral flexion

Set-up
- Medium spring
- Footbar in top position

Starting position
- Seated sideways on Universal Reformer, right shin against shoulder stops, sole of left foot against right opposite thigh
- Left hand on footbar, thumb with fingers
- Right arm abducts/flexes toward ceiling

Movement description
- Inhale and laterally flex toward footbar
- Exhale, control carriage returning to starting position
- Repeat
- Variation: twist
  - Hands frame ends of footbar
  - Inhale, extend torso
  - Exhale, press carriage away from footbar lowering torso toward springs
  - Repeat

- Variation
  - Move right hand toward left hand on footbar
  - Press carriage out and breathe into this position
  - Walk the hand back to corner and return carriage to bumper
  - Repeat on other side

CUES

- During lateral flexion, draw the ribs away from footbar
- Breathe into any tightness sensed in reaching arm

Author note

Client had developed an unconscious habit of holding her right arm and shoulder rigid (presumably to provide added support to the weaker right side of the torso). These Mermaid variations helped bring awareness to this tension pattern.

4. Modified Knee Stretches and Knees Off on Universal Reformer	Derivative of J. H. Pilates Knee Stretch Series on Universal Reformer (NPCE Study Guide 2021, p. 60)
Intent	● Improve hip flexion and extension ● Improve proprioception and motor control, limiting uncontrolled torso movements during hip flexion and extension
Gait reasoning	● Promote balanced movement in hip joints ● Integration of torso control during hip joint movement ● Flexed position to challenge torso's strategy of hyperextension

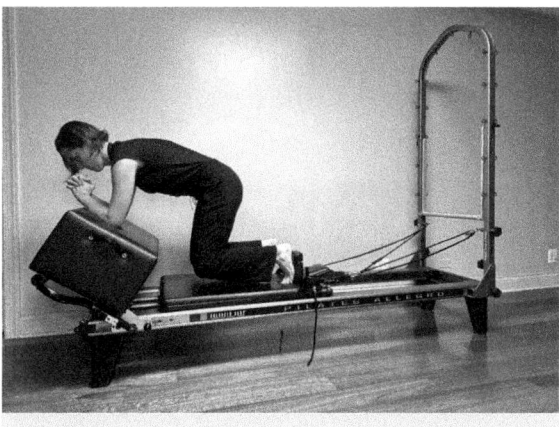

Figure 9.5

Set-up
- Springs: 1 heavy and 1 medium
- Footbar low
- Short box balanced on edge of footbar perpendicular to carriage

Starting position
- Kneeling on carriage
- Soles of feet against shoulder stops, metatarsals extended resting on carriage
- Forearms on box
- Torso in flexion for first set
- Torso in extension for second set

Movement description
- Press carriage out
- Control carriage on the way in, staying with the spring tension
- Repeat 5–6 times each variation
- Variation: Knees Off
  - Keep the carriage at home position
  - Hover the knees 2 in. (5 cm) above carriage while maintaining the flexed position

CUE
- Maintain balanced tensions within the torso to facilitate torso activation as the LE move into flexion and extension

Author note
Wrist pain is common for clients with hEDS. Using the box for a forearm variation allows them to experience the benefits of Knee Stretches without the pain.

5. Short Box Series on Universal Reformer: Flat Back, side bend, side to side, rotation, row the boat

Derivative of J. H. Pilates Short Box Series on Universal Reformer: Round Back, Flat Back, Twist (NPCE Study Guide 2021, p. 59)

Intent
- Facilitate torso three-dimensional movement
- Enhance proprioception of torso motion
- Improve palintonicity (see Editor note in Session 3/12, exercise 10)
- Control of upright torso for improved rotational pattern in gait
- Improve proprioception for sense of body moving through space during gait

Set-up
- 2 heavy springs to stabilize carriage
- Short box placed perpendicularly on carriage
- Client seated on box, feet under safety strap
- Dowel stored under legs in front of box

Starting position
- Flex torso
- Place hands on abdominal area

Author note

Taking a moment to orient the client to the feeling of the anterior abdominal wall pressing out into the hands on the inhale and drawing away from the hands on the exhale brings awareness of breath into the movement.

Movement description

Repeat each of the following exercises slowly 3–5 times
- Flat Back
    - Inhale, rock back on the sitz bones maintaining torso organization
    - Exhale, return to starting position
- Side bend
    - Inhale, laterally flex to right
    - Exhale, return to starting position
    - Repeat on left
- Side to side
    - Inhale, whole torso organization tilts to right, allowing opposite sitz bone to lift off box
    - Exhale, return to starting position
    - Repeat on left
- Rotation
    - Inhale, rotate to right
    - Exhale, return to starting position
    - Repeat on left
- Row the boat
    - Holding a dowel, inhale, reach arms to ceiling
    - Exhale, articulate flexion from top of head reaching toward toes
    - Inhale, trace dowel up legs
    - Exhale, articulate in extension to midline orientation

CUES
- Balance the tensions of the space between the crest of your pelvis and lower ribs
- Encourage awareness using touch cues at specific points of the torso where a translation off midline is apparent

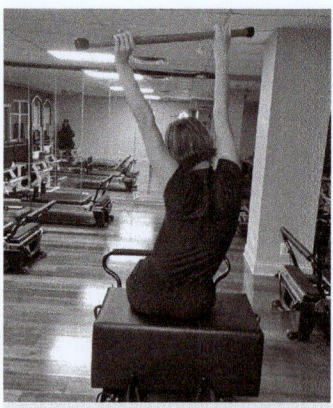

Figure 9.6

Author note

This is one of the most beneficial exercises in the Pilates series for building and refining proprioception of the torso as it can expose specific areas of challenge. In this client's case, a right arm restriction (also observed during gait) seemed to contribute to compensatory left rotation and right translation at the thoracolumbar junction. This exercise created opportunity to build awareness of this pattern.

6. Unilateral Leg Springs on Trapeze Table

Derivative of J. H. Pilates Leg Springs, Supine on Trapeze Table: Bicycle, Walking, Scissors, Circles (NPCE Study Guide 2021, pp. 67–68)
(See Chapter 5, Trier)

Intent
- Activate hip extensors
- Enhance dynamic torso control while extending hip
- Improve femoral joint glide
- Promote proprioception of LE especially the knee during light resistance

Gait reasoning
- Improve hip extension force from foot in push-off
- Improve control of rotation during hip extension
- Teach client to self-monitor and make appropriate adaptations while exercising

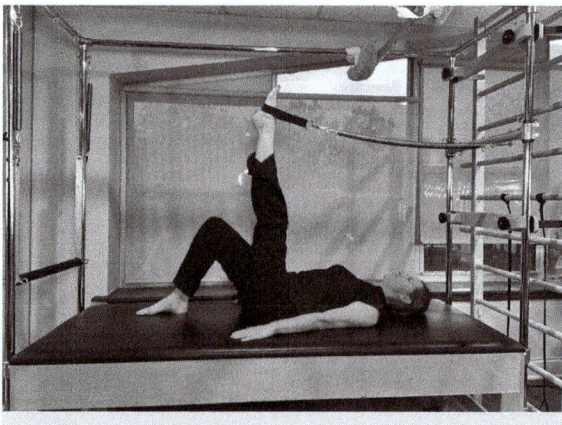

Figure 9.7

Set-up
- Light leg spring attached to the slider eye bolt on Trapeze Table

Editor note
The variety of Trapeze Tables have multiple eye bolts on the slider bar. The choice of placement of the leg spring will determine the angle of the variable resistance. The angle affects the dynamic pelvifemoral relationship. The training effect will vary according to the angle of the spring chosen.

Starting position
- Supine
- Right foot on table, hip and knee flexion
- Left foot in leg spring loop, flex hip and extend knee, foot toward ceiling
- Repeat on other side

Movement description
- Extend and flex hip
- 6 repetitions
- Hip joint rotation: continuous arcing motion of flexion to abduction, pulling down toward table, adduction to midline/flexion
- Repeat 4 times in each direction
- Hip abduction/external rotation with feet together
- 8 repetitions
- Press the LE into extension and flexion following the vector of the spring tension and slowly return

CUE
- Move slowly, maintaining congruency in the knee

Author note
Single leg spring exercises proved to be an appropriate and fruitful challenge for this client. I wanted to challenge her tendencies toward knee joint hyperextension, an issue she began therapy for as a teenager and which she had proactively managed during Footwork.

7. Side lying abduction, flexion, extension, and circumduction of the hip on a mat

Intent
- Improve proprioception and control of a range of gravity-resisted movements involving hip abduction
- Emphasize sensory awareness through exploratory movement

Gait reasoning
- Activate hip abductors to support right knee
- Improve dynamic torso control
- Foster greater ease and comfort during all movements
- Improve stamina in standing and single-leg balance
- Teach the client to self-monitor and make appropriate adaptations while exercising

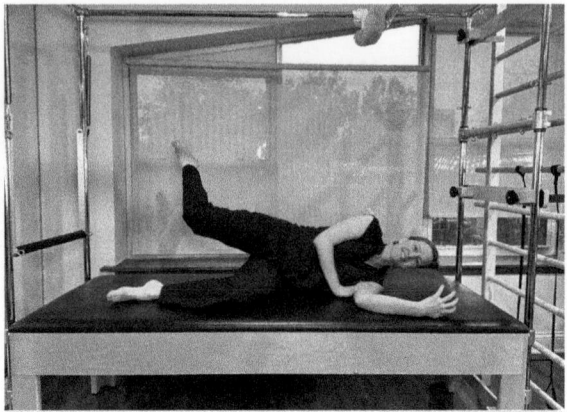

Figure 9.8

Editor note

The variety of Trapeze Tables have multiple eye bolts on the slider bar. The choice of placement of the leg spring will determine the angle of the variable resistance. The angle affects the dynamic pelvifemoral relationship. The training effect will vary according to the angle of the spring chosen.

Starting position
- Side lying on mat
- Head on a pillow
- Top hand on mat in front for added stability
- Knees flexed

Movement description
- Slowly raise top LE, exploring the space up and down, front and back, and in all directions
- Continue for 20–30 seconds, or as able
- Maintain the torso in side lying position with minimal anterior-posterior motion

CUES
- ◆ Imagine that your leg is an octopus tentacle
- ◆ Make your movements as slow and smooth as possible
- ◆ Explore as many kinds of movement with your leg as you can but try staying within a limited ROM
- ◆ Notice how this feels

8. Chest Expansion on Trapeze Table Derivative of J. H. Pilates Reverse Chest Expansion on Trapeze Table (NPCE Study Guide 2021, p. 67)

Intent
- ● Organization and integration of all previous learnings into gravity incorporating support of LE and feet
- ● Sense of meaningful progress and accomplishment

Gait reasoning
- ● Supporting proprioception and motor planning with multiple demands in gravity

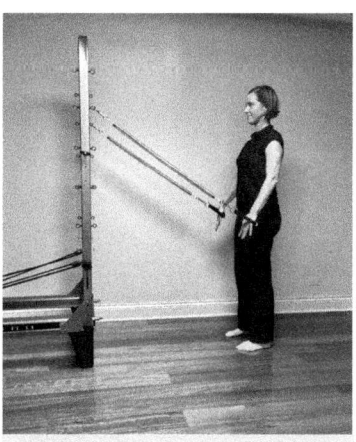

Figure 9.9

Set-up
- ● 2 light arm springs attached to outside of tower of Trapeze Table at roughly shoulder height

Author note
Fostering awareness of stance starting at the arches of the feet through the head gives a sense of being suspended. Awareness of expanding the breath into the side and back of the thorax and maintaining this expanse throughout the movement aims to promote proprioception and buoyant quality of movement.

Starting position	• Standing on floor an appropriate distance (for desired spring resistance) from tower end
	▪ Chest Expansion: facing Trapeze Table, elbows extended, LE by sides, palms in handles facing back
	▪ Reverse Chest Expansion: facing away from Trapeze Table, elbows extended, UE by sides, palms in handles facing front
	• Feet parallel or slightly turned out
Movement description	• Chest Expansion
	▪ Inhale, extend UE
	▪ Exhale, control UE in flexion
	▪ Repeat 5–6 times
	• Reverse Chest Expansion
	▪ Inhale, reach the palms up and forward to chest height
	▪ Exhale, slowly return arms down to sides
	▪ Repeat 5–6 times
	▪ Variation: lift heels on inhale, lower on exhale, as able

Author note

This exercise was introduced in the final session to integrate newfound awareness and reinforce multiple learnings in a standing position.

9. Washer Woman Over the Chair/ Hamstring 2 on Wunda Chair	J.H. Pilates Washer Woman Over the Chair/Hamstring 2 on Wunda Chair (NPCE Study Guide 2021, p. 77)
Intent	• Facilitate a feeling of ease and safety in lower back, where client was feeling some discomfort on this day
	• Reinforce torso control
Gait reasoning	• Closed kinematic chain activation from feet to head
	• Loading torso with the force of Wunda Chair into torso through UE
Set-up	• Medium spring
	• Build awareness of the feet supported by the ground and the torso articulating under load
Starting position	• Standing facing the pedal

Movement description
- From top down, flex occipitoatlantal joint, chin toward chest, articulate flexion through torso until heels of hands find pedal
- Press pedal down halfway
- Slowly control pedal up back to starting position
- Repeat 3 or 4 times
- Slowly roll up to extend the torso to standing

CUES
- Maintain a rounded torso and hinge from the hip joints only
- Notice how the legs and the torso work together to control the movement of the pedal

The journey to Session 11

Session 4/12
Client self-report

- Feeling better than last week
- Joints feeling more stable
- Pain: low grade
- Fatigue: no fatigue

Key changes observed

- Improved torso control during exercises
- Incorporating a feeling of buoyancy when walking
- Ability to organize without discomfort during Single Leg Springs

Reasoning behind choice of movements

- Building upon previous focus on dynamic torso control
- Introducing the feeling of activation in torso, palintonicity

Session movement sequence
1. Universal Reformer

- Footwork
- Shoulder Bridge
- Knee Stretches and Knees Off (on forearms using box)
- Short Box Series (Round Back, Flat Back, Twist, side bend, side to side)

2. Trapeze Table
- Single Leg Springs

- Arm Springs (feet on table/hip and knee to 90 degrees flexion)
- Chest Expansion
- Reverse Chest Expansion

Session 5/12
Client self-report

- Fairly sore from doing yard work
- Stamina is increasing in walking and standing
- Didn't have a "fatigue collapse" or use a mobility aid at work
- Pain: moderate
- Fatigue: moderate

Key changes observed

- Increased awareness of tension-holding and uncontrolled movement during exercise

● Ability to move torso with improved organization for gait patterning

Reasoning behind choice of movements

● Integrate and build upon previous gains in torso dynamic control
● Increase awareness of uncontrolled movement during walking
● Continue to increase stamina in standing and walking

Session movement sequence

1. Zoom session

● Marching
● Leg Circles
● Shoulder Bridge
● Prone hip extension
● Seated Short Box Series
● Standing marching

2. Self-observation during walking

Session 6/12
Client self-report

● Reported hips have been inflamed and tight for over 8 weeks, and it's more noticeable today
● Knees are red and warm, but she was able to walk to and from work without mobility aid
● "Other than gaining in strength and control, I think the biggest benefit I am getting so far is a much greater sense of movement awareness and improved motor planning. I think that more than anything will help me with daily life tasks and achieving the goals we discussed at the beginning of the program (standing longer, etc.)"
● Pain: moderate
● Fatigue: low grade

Key changes observed

● Increased ability to control hypermobility segments at thoracolumbar junction (T12–L1)

Reasoning behind choice of movements

● Integrate and build upon previous gains in dynamic torso stability
● Increase awareness of excessive tension and uncontrolled movement patterns during walking
● Build stamina in standing and walking

Session movement sequence

1. Universal Reformer

● Footwork (springs: 2 heavy, 1 medium)
● Arm Springs
  ■ 1 heavy spring
  ■ Legs in tabletop with rests in between sets
  ■ 7 presses, 5 circles in each direction, 10 triceps
● Shoulder Bridges (all springs)
● Knee Stretches and Knees Off on forearms using box (springs: 1 heavy, 1 medium)
● Short Box Series (Round Back, Flat Back, Twist, side bend, side to side)

2. Trapeze Table

● Chest Expansion
● Reverse Chest Expansion

3. Wunda Chair

● Washer Woman (1 medium spring)

Session 7/12
Client self-report

- Some hip and low back pain but "not too bad"
- Paying attention when walking and noticing areas of tension
- Alignment awareness is helping in day-to-day life, shoulders more relaxed
- Pain: low grade
- Fatigue: good

Key changes observed

- Improved strength and ROM in prone hip extension, especially on the limited (right) side

Reasoning behind choice of movements

- Incorporating three-dimensional breathing awareness with focus on both autonomic regulation and movement control
- Improve strength and mobility in hip flexion and extension

Session movement sequence
1. Zoom session

- Breathing awareness
  - Tabletop legs (with feet on wall)
  - Arm reaches maintaining neutral ribs
  - Shoulder Bridge with feet elevated—three-dimensional breathing
- Leg Circles: 5 each direction
- Marching review
- Prone hip extension
  - Variation 1: 10 each side
  - Variation 2: 10 each side plus extra set on the right side

2. Child's Pose breathing into the back

Session 8/12
Client self-report

- Has three doctor's appointments coming up to investigate hip inflammation, rule out possibility of ankylosing spondylitis, and regarding an intake into an intensive chronic pain program she will begin in a few weeks
- Pain: low grade
- Fatigue: good

Key changes observed

- Excellent concentration, slow deliberate movement, and awareness of placement of breath
- Ability to hold legs in tabletop without strain and incorporate arm springs for the first time
- Working to address the relative weakness in right leg and work around joint capsule instability in left hip
- Awareness of how right shoulder restriction leads to compensatory adjustments in torso during Short Box Series. Learning to make the torso "the anchor" that can serve to help stretch out the arm rather than the other way around

Reasoning behind choice of movements

- Continue to build torso control, axial elongation, and control in hip flexion and extension and breathing; integration of all of these
- Support ability to self-monitor and make appropriate adaptations during exercise

Session movement sequence
1. Trapeze Table

- Tabletop legs with push-through bar

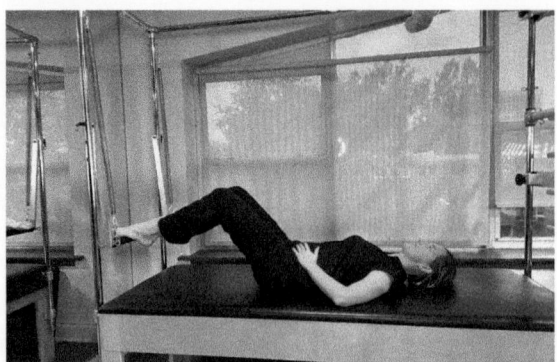

Figure 9.10

- Single Leg Springs
- Tabletop legs with Arm Springs

2. Wunda Chair

- Seated Footwork (2 medium springs)

3. Universal Reformer

- Shoulder Bridge with awareness of low back rib fullness (all springs)
- Knee Stretches, rounded torso: 6 slow repetitions (1 heavy, 1 medium spring)
- Knees Off: 3 sets 5 seconds each (1 heavy, 1 medium spring)
- Jackrabbit: 10 repetitions (1 heavy, 1 medium spring)
- Short Box Series (short box and dowel)

Session 9/12
Client self-report

- Had a cold and didn't exercise for a couple of weeks. Slept a lot
- Feeling stiff, but not in pain. Increase in pain medication has led to more strength
- Stamina in standing and motion in gait feel easier. Hip flexors less tight

- Pain: good
- Fatigue: good

Key changes observed

- Prone hip extension is becoming easier and gaining in ROM
- General strength and control has improved. She partly attributes this to the "virtuous cycle" of increased pain medication

Reasoning behind choice of movements

- Continue to build torso control, axial elongation, and control in hip flexion and extension, breathing, and integration of all of these
- Support ability to self-monitor and make appropriate adaptations during exercise

Session movement sequence
1. Zoom session

- Leg Circles, 10 each way
- Modified Single Leg Stretch, 10 each
- Tabletop legs—able to hold for 3 minutes while doing resistance band Arm Springs
- Roll-Back with resistance band
- Tabletop marching from above
- Inner thigh squeezes: 30 repetitions
- Shoulder Bridge knees out: 18 repetitions
- Prone hip extension
    - Variation 1: 30 each (increased ROM on right)
    - Variation 2: 20 each (ROM improved)

2. Standing Short Box: side bend, side to side, rotation

Session 10/12
Client self-report

- Feeling improved control in movements
- Pain: good

- Fatigue: good

Key changes observed

- Continued progress in general strength and control
- Weakness in modified right side plank (with knee down)

Reasoning behind choice of movements

- Continue to build torso control, axial elongation, and control in hip flexion and extension, breathing, and integration of all of these
- Support ability to self-monitor and make appropriate adaptations during exercise
- Introduction of hip abduction exercises

Session movement sequence
Zoom session

- Roll-Back with resistance band: 5 slow repetitions
  - Add 4 twists
- Leg Circles: 10 in each direction
- Tabletop legs with resistance band Arm Springs: 5 repetitions
- Shoulder Bridge: 18 repetitions
- Short Box Series: 3–4 repetitions each
- Mermaid: 3–4 repetitions
- Modified side plank on knee: 10 second hold on left side, unable to hold at all on right side
- Clams: 6 each side
- "Octopus tentacle": 15–20 seconds

References

Demmler, J., Atkinson, M., Reinhold, E., Choy, E., Lyons, R. A., and Brophy, S. T. (2019) "Diagnosed prevalence of Ehlers-Danlos syndrome and hypermobility spectrum disorder in Wales, UK: A national electronic cohort study and case-control comparison." *BMJ Open, 9.* DOI:10.1136/bmjopen-2019-031365.

Jovin, D. (Ed.) (2020) *Disjointed: Navigating the Diagnosis and Management of Hypermobile Ehlers-Danlos Syndrome and Hypermobility Spectrum Disorders.* San Francisco: Hidden Stripes Publications.

Martine, J. (2018) "Rolfing® structural integration." In: L. Chaitow (Ed.) *Fascial Dysfunction.* 2nd Ed. Edinburgh: Handspring Publishing, pp. 291–301.

NPCE Study Guide (National Pilates Certification Exam Study Guide) (2021) Miami, FL: National Pilates Certification Program, Inc.

Tinkle, B., Castori, M., Berglund, B., Cohen, H. *et al.* (2017) "Hypermobile Ehlers–Danlos syndrome (a.k.a. Ehlers–Danlos syndrome type III and Ehlers–Danlos syndrome hypermobility type): Clinical description and natural history." *American Journal of Medical Genetics Part C (Seminars in Medical Genetics), 175C,* 48–69. www.ehlers-danlos.com/pdf/2017-FINAL-AJMG-PDFs/Tinkle_et_al-2017-American_Journal_of_Medical_Genetics_Part_C-_Seminars_in_Medical_Genetics.pdf. [Accessed September 24, 2023].

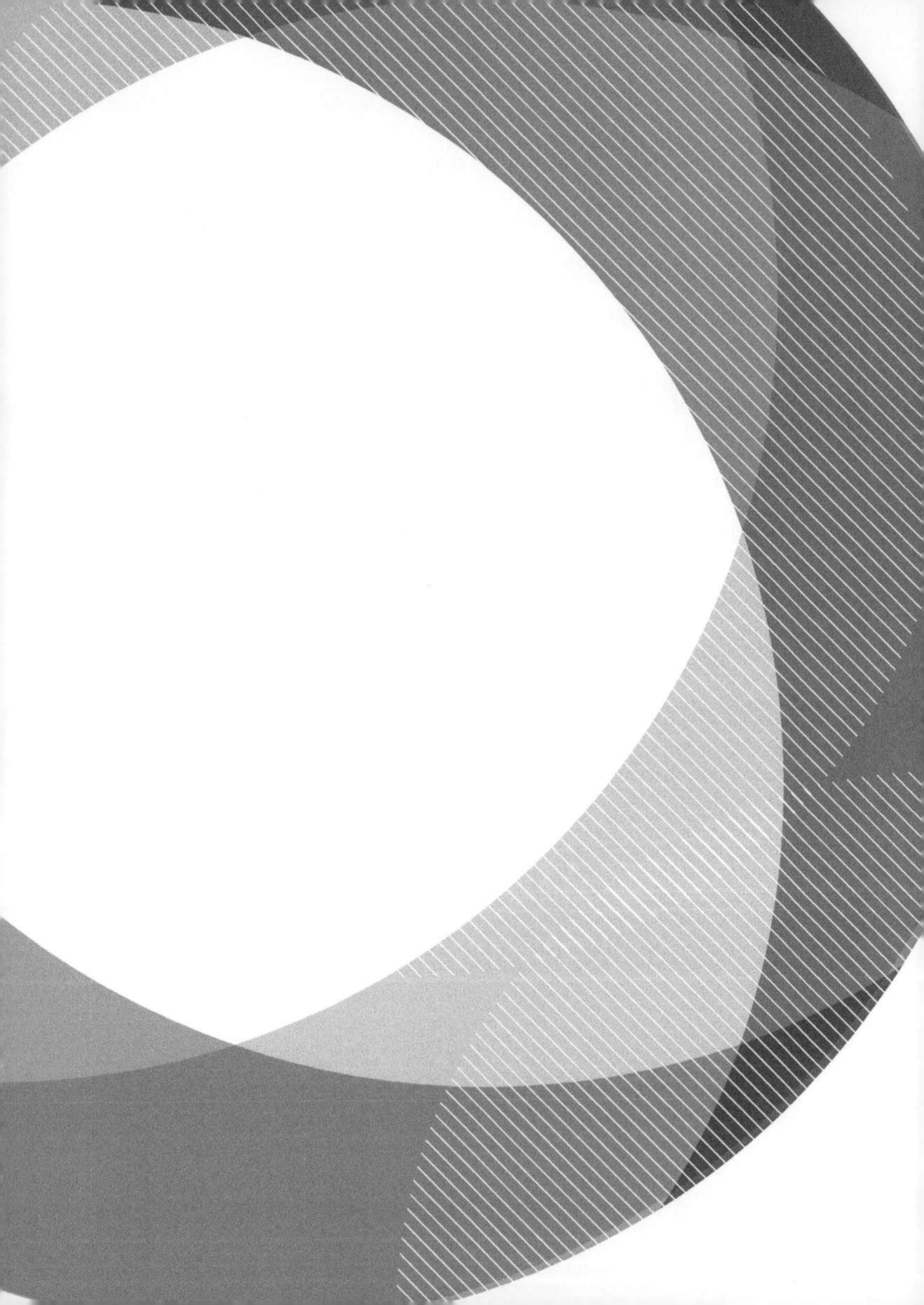

Pilates and Lyme Disease: Effect on Gait

Amy Hershey

Lyme disease is a bacterial infection that is transmitted to humans through the bite of an infected tick. The spiral-shaped bacteria, known as a spirochete, has many different strains with the most common being Borrelia burgdorferi. Although likely around for centuries, it was formally identified during the 1970s after an unexplainable outbreak of juvenile arthritis in Lyme, Connecticut. Today, cases of Lyme disease have been confirmed in all 50 US states and in over 80 countries worldwide. According to the CDC, there are 300,000 reported new cases of Lyme disease annually in the US; however, due to its difficulty being recognized and diagnosed, some estimates have that number as closer to 3 million new cases annually (CDC 2024). Approximately 60 percent of early acute infections are missed and 75 percent of individuals do not recall seeing the tick that bit them. When early and acute infections are missed, Lyme disease will disseminate throughout the body and can present with over three dozen different potential symptoms, some of which are neurological. Neurological Lyme disease, neuroborreliosis, is not a different type of Lyme disease but merely a classification of symptoms that are neurologically based (Ross Russell *et al.* 2018). Collectively, different symptoms of Lyme disease also account for over 300 other illnesses, which is why it is often referred to as "the great imitator." Most commonly, Lyme disease is misdiagnosed as rheumatoid arthritis, lupus, fibromyalgia, or chronic fatigue syndrome and/or multiple sclerosis.

When the Borrelia spirochete enters the body, it possesses the unique ability to change its shape and appearance in order to penetrate different cells within the body (Chaconas, Castellanos, and Verhey 2020). One common location where the spirochete tends to congregate is in collagen-based structures, especially because collagen is avascular and thus the spirochete can evade the body's natural immune response. For example, tendons and the interior portion of the menisci are avascular and frequent areas of pain. Lyme disease very commonly manifests as arthritis (Stanek and Strle 2018). There is limited research regarding Lyme disease and fascia; however, we can deduce that if collagen is a common site of congregation for the Borrelia spirochete, then fascia is almost certainly affected. Furthermore, Lyme disease can induce an inappropriate immune response by activating the release of cytokines, which are proteins involved in regulating the immune system (Buhner 2015). Triggering over-production of cytokines leads to an over-stimulated immune system and, consequently, Lyme disease has elements of an autoimmune disease.

Lyme disease has dozens of potential symptoms; therefore, it is imperative for a Pilates instructor to conduct a thorough health history prior to commencing a program. Common symptoms include: neck pain, joint pain, muscle weakness, migraines, vertigo, confusion (also known as "brain fog"), and balance challenges (Mead 2015). Instructors should be aware that POTS is a potential symptom and, if present, should avoid any exercises that move from a supine to seated position. Treatment for Lyme disease involves heavy rounds of antibiotics that can cause increased exhaustion and nausea. Not all Lyme cases will display the same symptoms, and symptoms can shift daily; therefore, programs should be adjusted appropriately to address (or avoid) current issues. Spring tension and positional considerations should be monitored closely to avoid over-exertion. It may be easy to attribute any presenting pain or discomfort to Lyme disease; however, it is important to remember that not all sources of pain are related to the disease and any new symptom should always be cleared by a physician.

Client description: 26-year-old biological female, identifies as female; research technician

Dates of case report: Session 1: July 12, 2020; Session 12: August 20, 2020

Studio apparatus and props
Pilates equipment

- Trapeze Table
- Wunda Chair
- Universal Reformer

Props used with equipment

- 22 in. (55 cm) ball
- 10 in. (25 cm) resistance band, medium to heavy
- Non-skid rubberized mat
- Mat

Home program props

- 10 in. (25 cm) stretch band loop, heavy resistance
- Yoga block
- 10 in. (25 cm) Overball, inflated
- Rotational disc
- 2 small face towels
- Larger hand towel
- Long box
- Couch or wall
- Floor-length mirror
- Mat

Methods and materials

Session 1/12
1. Health history interview

- Symptoms began in 2015, initially with fatigue and joint pain
- By 2016 had 25 headaches per month, excruciating joint and neck pain, dizziness, brain fog, extreme exhaustion (would not get out of bed some days)
- Saw various specialists and tried different meds, which often times exacerbated symptoms
- Diagnosed with Lyme disease in 2019
- Currently undergoing treatment which involves going off and on antibiotics supplemented with different herbal remedies and supplements
- Symptoms flare up with stress, environmental changes, and poor diet
- Client is naturally hypermobile

2. Symptoms

- Joint pain (most commonly in the knees)
- Neck pain
- Migraines
- Fatigue
- Vertigo

3. Movement aids

- None

> **Final result of case report**
> The client displayed significantly more control of her body with less movement compensations noted in post-assessment. She reported a noticeable decrease in knee discomfort. Although there are still gait abnormalities present, there is more vertical lift, which would imply improved push-off and reduced movement. Improvements in arm swing suggest greater ability of rotation of the thorax. Fatigue levels are slightly improved on good days; however, fatigue is still present and unpredictable, which is a hallmark of Lyme disease.

Session 2/12: Initial assessment

1. General observations of gait

◆ Minimal arm swing; slightly more arm swing on right

◆ Right hemipelvis superior motion coupled with left translation of ribcage

◆ Right leg circumduction present

◆ Lateral shifting of pelvis

◆ No thoracic rotation as evident by the lack of arm swing

◆ Excessive pronation in stance phase on both feet

◆ Low force production ability in push-off

2. Standing tests

◆ Full torso rotation

● Observations of inefficient side: left
  ■ Compensatory excessive scapula motions
  ■ Minimal internal rotation of hip joint on both sides
  ■ Compensatory contralateral hemi-pelvis inferior motion observed when rotating left
  ■ Limited left supination and right pronation

◆ Hemipelvis inferior motion

● Observations of inefficient side: left
  ■ Left innominate anteriorly rotates
  ■ Thorax rotates right
  ■ Displays more "range" on left side but with significantly more movement compensations

◆ Hemipelvis superior motion

Session 12/12: Post-assessment

1. General observations of gait

◆ Gait is more natural and freer

◆ Increased arm swing and subsequent thoracic rotation

◆ Right leg circumduction is still present

◆ Still pronates on right foot, less visible on left

◆ Less lateral pelvic shift

◆ More force production in push-off phase evident by faster pace

2. Standing tests

◆ Full torso rotation

● Observations of inefficient side: left
  ■ Less compensatory movement in scapula and thorax attributed to improved body awareness and control
  ■ Increased internal rotation of right femur when rotating right
  ■ Minimal internal rotation of left femur when rotating left
  ■ No compensatory hemipelvis inferior motion observed
  ■ More pronation on right foot

◆ Hemipelvis inferior motion

● Observations of inefficient side: left
  ■ No significant anterior pelvic rotation on left
  ■ Reduced right thoracic rotation

◆ Hemipelvis superior motion

● Observations of inefficient side: left

- Observations of inefficient side: left
  - Thorax translates right
  - Left innominate anteriorly rotates
  - Less left plantar flexion

◆ Lateral pelvic shift

- Observations of inefficient side: left
  - Limited left lateral shift
  - Left femoral joint lacks abduction
  - Right femoral joint lacks adduction
  - Thorax translates right
  - Minimal functional movement of feet, lacks left supination and right already in pronation

3. Seated tests

◆ Thoracic rotation

Author note

The subject was not diagnosed with Ehlers–Danlos syndrome but does score a 9 on the Beighton score. She presents with hyperextended knees and elbows as well. Her hypermobility presents some unique movement compensatory patterns and strategies that may not exist for other people. Essentially, her joints allow for movement beyond a range that she can support and therefore her flexibility does not translate to having good mobility.

Editor note

The Beighton scoring system measures joint hypermobility on a 9-point scale. The range of movement is measured using a goniometer, an instrument that measures the joint angle. If one does not have a goniometer, using observation will be sufficient to determine the possibility of a positive finding. The joints tested are: metacarpal joint of both 5th phalanges beyond 90 degrees; base of both thumbs touching the forearm; elbows and knees extended an extra 10 degrees; and the torso being able to touch

- Thorax translates right
- Pelvis laterally shifts to right instead of anteriorly rotating
- Limited left plantar flexion

◆ Lateral pelvic shift

- Observations of inefficient side: left
  - Both sides appear equal
  - Improved femoral joint abduction and adduction
  - Client reports mild discomfort on right femoral joint during left sway
  - No noticeable thoracic translation

3. Seated tests

◆ Thoracic rotation

- Observations of inefficient side: both
  - Ribs translated slightly to the right from initial assessment toward center
  - Sitz bones weighted equally

◆ Hip joint and knee flexion

- Observations of inefficient side: left
  - Thorax translates to the right
  - Left ischial tuberosity increases weight distribution when attempting to lift left

the floor without flexing the knees (The Ehlers–Danlos Society 2023).

- Observations of inefficient side: both
  - Before initiating movement, ribs are already translated slightly left
  - Sitting more heavily on left sitz bone
  - Rotating left, ribs translate to right righting the thorax toward center
  - Rotating left, pelvis shifts to become more balanced on sitz bones equally
  - Neither of these self-correcting shifts occur when rotating right and pattern exaggerates

◆ Hip joint and knee flexion

- Observations of inefficient side: both
  - Right: thorax translates slightly to left
  - Left: weight shifts heavily onto left ischial tuberosity and thorax translates to right

4. Sit and stand

◆ Lateral view

- No movement compensations noted

◆ Anterior view

- Asymmetrical weight shift to right
- Knee valgus observed on both sides, more on right

5. Standing balance

◆ Two-leg stance, eyes open

- Successful: 60 seconds

◆ One-leg stance, eyes open

- Right leg: 24 seconds
- Left leg: 40 seconds
- In left leg stance right hemipelvis inferior motion and pelvis rotates forward

4. Sit and stand

◆ Lateral view

- No compensations noted

◆ Anterior view

- No asymmetrical shift noted
- Knee valgus right side only

5. Standing balance

◆ Two-leg stance, eyes open

- 60 seconds

◆ One-leg stance

- Right leg: 39 seconds
- Left leg: 53 seconds
- On left side, right hemipelvis inferior motion

Session 3/12: Home program

Fatigue scale	2
Pain scale	6
Client self-report	• Excited to begin • High energy
Key changes observed by author at end of Session 3/12	• Good body awareness when body is contacting surfaces • Difficulty with proprioception when no external feedback surface is provided
Reason behind choice of sequencing	• Starting with feet and working up the closed kinematic chain • Progress from simple to more complex and integrated movements • Integrating movement in all planes • Exercises in different orientations to gravity for challenge of proprioception (prone, supine, side lying, seated, and standing)

Session movement sequence

1. Breathing

Intent	• Increase capacity of expansion and rib mobility • Improve thoracic mobility in all planes
Gait reasoning	• Rib articulation to allow rotation during gait • Bring awareness of inefficient side
Starting position	• Seated on mat or on a chair with torso upright • Legs can be in any comfortable position • Place each hand on lower lateral ribcage

Movement description	• Inhale to the fullest capacity
	• Exhale completely
	• Use hands to feel ribcage motions
	  ■ Expansion on inhale, notice if one side expands more
	  ■ On exhale, sense how ribs return to starting position
	• Repeat at least 10 times
	• Practice sending the breath into one side of the ribs (see Chapter 5, Gentry: bellows breathing)

2. Doming the foot with towel

Intent	• Improve doming action of the foot
	• Reduce over-pronation of both feet
Gait reasoning	• Address over-pronation observed during gait
	• Force production of the push-off phase can be reduced by over-pronation
Starting position	• Seated upright on chair with hips and knees at 90 degrees
	• Spread towel on floor
	• Place one foot flat on towel
Movement description	• Dorsiflex the foot with calcaneus on floor lifting forefoot off the towel
	• Articulate from rear foot to mid-foot to forefoot placing whole foot on towel
	• Initiate from medial aspect of foot and drag towel inward toward heel increasing plantar arch. All metatarsals remain in contact with floor
	• Repeat 5 times
	• Initiate from 1st metatarsophalangeal joint and drag towel toward medial heel
	• Focus on lifting medial arch as towel is pulled
	• Once foot is no longer able to drag towel further, dorsiflex and lift mid-foot and forefoot off towel extending the phalanges
	• Articulate through the foot flexing phalanges through mid-foot and place plantar surface of foot on towel
	• 8 repetitions

Author note

If the doming is hindered from a position of dorsiflexion, extend the knee slightly and move the foot forward. Starting in a plantar flexed position places the arch in supination and allows for more lift of the arch.

3. Banded knee openers and knee folds

Derivative of Eve Gentry knee folds (see Chapter 5)

Intent	• Activation of hip in sagittal and coronal planes
	• Balance hip flexors and extensors with lateral and medial hip activation

Gait reasoning
- Reduce excessive lateral pelvic movements during gait
- Improve torso and hip joint control to allow for more fluid motion during gait

Starting position
- Supine on mat with both knees flexed and feet flat on floor
- Heels in line with ischial tuberosities
- Position the stretch band loop around both femurs at approximately mid-point
- Abduct slightly to tauten band
- Place hands on the anterior superior iliac spine (ASIS) to feel for unwanted pelvic movements

Movement description
- Right lower extremity (LE) abducts
- Ipsilateral foot will roll to the lateral edge to follow motion of right LE
- Move right LE to a range where there is no additional torso movement
- Slowly return the right LE to starting position
- Maintain tension on loop throughout movement
- Repeat on left LE
- 8 repetitions on each side
- Return to starting position
- Flex right hip with knee in line with center of ipsilateral hip joint
- Slowly lower to starting position while maintaining tension in strap
- 8 repetitions each side

4. Supine flexor activation

Intent
- Coactivation of torso and LE flexors
- Coordinated movement of upper extremity (UE) and contralateral LE

Gait reasoning
- Activate flexors of torso and LE to improve proprioception of LE to torso continuity
- Maintain torso control through dynamic leg movements

Starting position
- Supine in 90 degrees hip and knee flexion, feet off mat
- Ankles dorsiflexed
- Place hands flat on distal, anterior surface of thigh
- Press legs away slightly so elbows extend

Movement description	• From starting position, actively press hands and thighs against each other with maximal effort
	• Do not allow the shape of the starting position to change
	• Hold the maximal-effort isometric contraction for 10 seconds, then release contraction while maintaining the position for 10 seconds.
	• Repeat 5 times
	• Rest
	• Assume starting position
	• Actively press right hand into right LE as the left LE lowers to floor, taps floor, and returns to starting position
	• Repeat, actively pressing left hand into left LE as right LE lowers to floor, taps floor, and returns to starting position

5. Shoulder bridges

Intent	• Synergistic activation of extensors and flexors
Gait reasoning	• Develop torso adaptability
	• Potentiation of posterior hip for force production in push-off phase
	• Increase range of motion of thorax and shoulder girdle for better arm swing
Starting position	• Supine with feet flat on mat and knees flexed
	• Heels in line with ischial tuberosities
	• Place arms by sides, palms down
Movement description	• Beginning with ischial tuberosities, posteriorly rotate pelvis
	• Sequentially articulate torso off mat
	• Move from flexion through extension to reach top of bridge
	• Press arms down into mat and keep head and neck alignment
	• Feel activation from arms into shoulder girdle and extensors
	• Slowly roll back down sequencing from superior to inferior, articulating the torso
	• Return to starting position
	• 8 repetitions

6. Swan preparation with rotation (Black 2022)

Intent
- Synergistic activation of extensors and flexors
- Integrate upper and lower body movements

Gait reasoning
- Bilateral activation of extensors for midline orientation
- Contralateral patterning

Starting position
- Prone on mat
- Elbows flexed with right hand stacked on top of left hand
- Place forehead on top of hands
- Roll 2 small hand towels and place under anterior surface of each femur
- Gently press into each towel to maintain hip extension throughout movements

Movement description
- Head and both UE lift off mat while keeping forehead on top hand
- Pause at top range and hold for 3 seconds before slowly lowering back to starting position
- Repeat 5 times
- With right hand still on top, rotate head to right with left zygomatic arch on dorsal side of right hand
- Keeping left UE and hand on mat, lift right UE and head moving into thoracic right rotation and extension
- Repeat 5 times
- After 5 repetitions, add straight lift of contralateral leg
- Repeat 5 times

7. Wall quadruped leg with arm lifts

Intent
- Loading UE
- Increase shoulder activation
- Sensing UE and LE continuity with torso
- Integration of torso activation from distal support of hands and knees

Gait reasoning
- Oblique continuations of UE to opposite LE, both anteriorly and posteriorly
- Contralateral movement coordination
- Torso control during dynamic limb movements

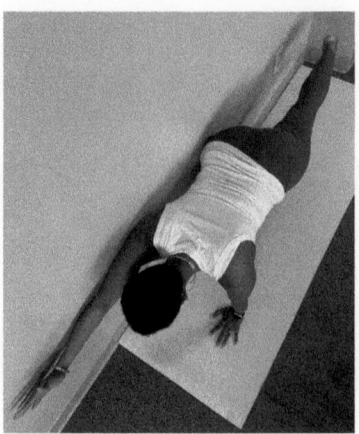

Figure 10.1

Starting position
- Quadruped position on mat
- Maintain mid-range torso position, neither flexed nor hyperextended
- Position lateral hip and leg against the side of a wall (or couch)

Author note
Do not lean against the wall—it is a guide to help facilitate motor learning and control.

Movement description
- Slide contralateral foot to the leg positioned against wall along the mat into hip and knee extension, foot remains on the floor
- Simultaneously, slide wall-side arm forward, elbow extended, fingers on floor
- While maintaining starting position of torso, extend LE and flex UE
- Hip and LE against wall maintain position against wall, avoiding any lateral weight shift
- Repeat leg and arm lift 10 times
- Return to starting position to switch sides

8. Quadruped rotation with ball

Intent ● Increase thoracic articulation and rotation

Gait reasoning ● Facilitate thoracic articulation and rotation from midline while minimizing rib translation
● Improve arm swing and torso amplitude in gait

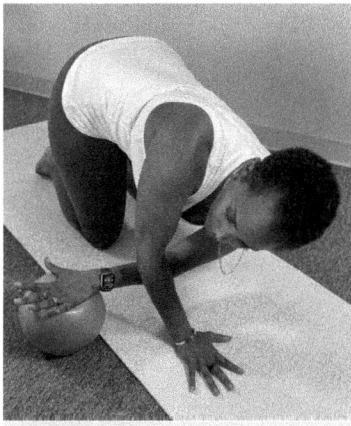

Figure 10.2

Starting position ● Quadruped position on mat with hands placed slightly in front of shoulders
● Place right wrist on Overball

Movement description ● Roll ball to left while allowing left elbow to flex
● Torso will follow into left rotation
● Repeat 5 times and then switch sides

9. Seated rotational disc

Intent ● Oppositional control of torso and head in transverse plane

Gait reasoning ● Coordinate oppositional rotation allowing for better transfer of weight from foot to foot
● Bring awareness of inefficient side
● Facilitate alignment of thoracolumbar junction with S2 while rotating

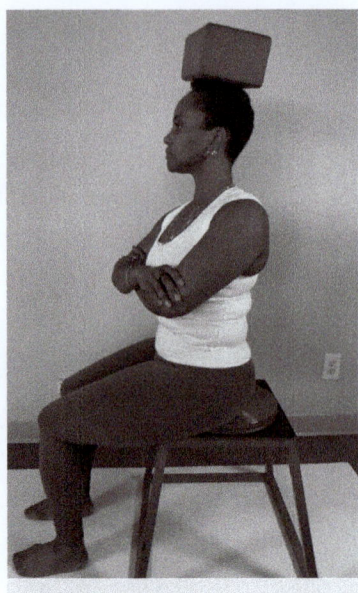

Figure 10.3

Starting position
- Place rotational disc on flat, hard surface of chair or bench
- Sit on disc with both feet on floor
- Knees and hips at 90 degrees
- Overball placed between thighs
- Yoga block balanced on head
- Arms crossed and placed on chest with hands directly inferior to the coracoid process

Author note
Overball is used for proprioceptive feedback and directional assistance, not squeezing.

Movement description
- Slide right knee forward allowing pelvis and disc to rotate left
- Maintain position of thorax and head forward
- Alternate sides for 5 repetitions
- Rotate from top down maintaining position of disc and head forward
- Focus eyes forward maintaining gaze to front
- Repeat, alternating sides 5 times
- Maintain position of torso and disc
- Rotate head alternating sides while keeping yoga block balanced on head
- Final movement pattern is to maintain head position, rotating upper torso region to lower torso
- Repeat coordinated movement 5 times on each side

Author note

For each segment, match the ranges on each side. Do not go to maximum range if ranges differ on right and left.

10. Heel lifts and lowers

Intent
- Articulate feet in plantar flexion and dorsiflexion
- Organize torso during movement from feet

Gait reasoning
- Increase force production during push-off phase of gait
- Balance of standing leg for mid-stance phase of gait
- Weight transfer from the ground

Starting position
- Stand in parallel stance position in front of a mirror

Movement description
- Lift both heels maintaining pressure on medial ball of foot
- Use mirror to ensure foot does not move into supination and inversion
- Heel should stay behind leg and not become visible in mirror
- Slowly lower the heels on a 3 count back to floor
- Repeat 5 times
- Transition to single-leg variation

Author note

The client is hypermobile so therefore over-moves in her mid-foot and externally rotates the tibia to achieve heel lift. Not allowing the heel to become visible trains the proper range for optimal foot to torso coordinated effort.

11. Standing single-leg swings

Intent
- Use gravity and momentum to promote free motion of leg swing

Gait reasoning
- Develop motor control for swing phase
- Arm swing potential
- Stance leg support

Starting position
- Place stance foot on first step of stairs or on a box
- Facing side of staircase, allow contralateral lower limb to hang freely
- Hands placed on top of pelvis to help find level starting position

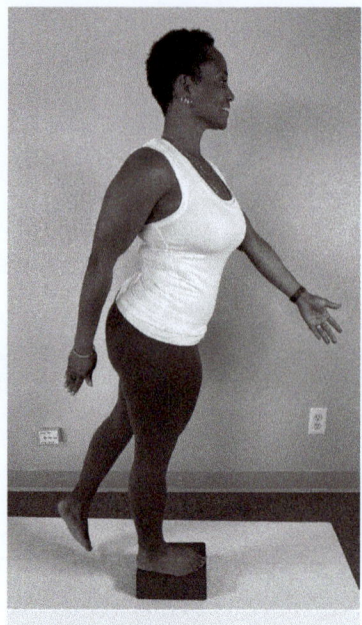

Figure 10.4

Movement description
- Begin by allowing leg to swing forward and back
- Release hands and swing arms freely to replicate gait motion
- 10 leg swings of each leg

12. Step-ups

Intent
- Organize the body in standing upright position
- Awareness and control torso through dynamic leg movements
- Coordination of multiple movements

Gait reasoning
- Stance leg support
- Develop controlled flexion and extension of the hip, knee, and ankle joints

Starting position
- Place right foot on box with hip and knee flexed, ankle dorsiflexed
- Place left foot on floor behind box, hip and knee extended, ankle dorsiflexed
- Hands on hips

Movement description
- With left hip and knee extended, elevate left calcaneus into plantar flexion with metatarsals on mat
- Lift calcaneus into plantar flexion, metatarsals on mat
- Transfer weight over right foot to extend right hip and knee as the left LE leaves the floor
- Stand on right LE leg and balance for 2 seconds
- Slowly flex right knee and hip and lower left LE, placing metatarsal arch on floor, foot in plantar flexion
- Slowly move into dorsiflexion
- Repeat 5 times for each leg

Session 11/12: Studio session

Fatigue scale 5

Pain scale 3

Client self-report
- Feeling sad that case study is concluding
- Energy is low

Key changes observed by author at end of Session 11/12
- Client displayed significantly improved proprioceptive awareness of her body in space
- Energy level was higher
- Improved mood

Reason behind choice of sequencing
- Move in different body positions with different relationships to gravity
- Complete all the exercises that were progressively added throughout the program

Session movement sequence

1. Footwork with push-through bar on Universal Reformer Derivative of J. H. Pilates Parakeet on Universal Reformer (NPCE Study Guide 2021, p. 64)

Intent
- Articulate ankle, knee, and hip joints in a coordinated and dynamic movement pattern
- Perform Footwork for client whose vestibular function is disturbed by Universal Reformer carriage movement
- Work bilaterally and unilaterally

Gait reasoning
- Coordination of flexion and extension of knee, hip, and ankle joints
- Unilateral challenges for adaption of torso with leg movements
- Increase articulation from foot to torso

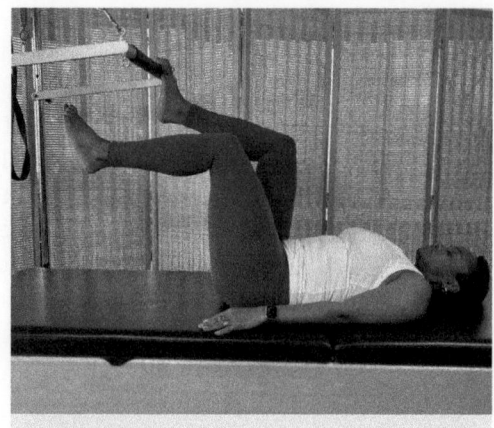

Figure 10.5

Set-up
- 2 medium springs from above (for bilateral)
- Medium spring from above (for unilateral)
- Use non-slip wrap on bar

Starting position
- Supine with feet toward push-through bar, feet apart, metatarsal heads on the push-through bar
- LE parallel, hips and knees extended

Movement description
- Ankles move through plantar flexion and dorsiflexion slowly with extended hips and knees
- 10 repetitions
- Plantar flex feet
- Dorsiflex with knee and hip flexion to approximately 90 degrees
- Slowly extend the hips and knees
- 10 repetitions
- Single-leg variation (remove 1 spring)
- Parallel LE, one foot with mid-foot on bar
- Knee and hip flexion to range attained in bilateral movement
- 5 repetitions with contralateral leg straight on carriage
- 5 repetitions with contralateral leg held in tabletop position

CUES
- Observe coordinated movement of foot to torso and any changes of torso position
- S2 posterior thorax and occiput remain in contact with carriage throughout the movement

Author note

This client is hypermobile and lacks the proprioceptive aware-ness of when her knees hyperextend. To bring awareness, place a resistance band on the posterior aspect of the knees and hold. As the legs extend, apply gentle pressure with the band to keep the knees from hyperextending while activating the posterior hip. This technique may be used on the Universal Reformer with Footwork.

2. Shoulder bridge with push-through bar on Universal Reformer

Derivative of J. H. Pilates Parakeet on Universal Reformer (NPCE Study Guide 2021, p. 64)

Intent
- Torso articulation with hip flexion and extension coordination
- Control of hip flexion and extension
- Activation of torso and hip extensors and flexors
- Generate movement from feet

Gait reasoning
- Activate extensors of torso and LE for propulsion phase
- Sagittal plane articulation assists in reorganizing torso allowing for ability to adapt without excessive translatory movement

Set-up
- Medium spring from above on the push-through bar

Starting position
- Supine on carriage with feet toward push-through bar, feet apart, metatarsal heads on push-through bar
- LE parallel, knees and hips extended
- Bar low but not past vertical frame poles
- Place Overball between knees for positional assistance, not to squeeze

Movement description
- Flex knees and hips to move bar inward and upward
- Once bar begins to move upward, allow knees to extend slightly
- Do not allow knees to extend fully
- Maintaining position of bar, begin to lift pelvis and articulate torso off mat
- Slowly articulate down, returning torso to mat and bar to starting position
- Repeat 5 times

CUES

+ To initiate the lift-off, visualize lifting the ischial tuberosities up toward the ceiling facilitating movement of hip extension
+ Press UE firmly down on the mat at the top range allowing the thorax to extend
+ Inhale fully at the top range, exhale slowly to articulate down to starting position

Author note

This exercise is traditionally done with a straight leg pressing the bar up for the lift-off. Due to the tendency for this client to hyperextend, this was modified to keep the knees slightly flexed and to hold the bar relatively still during lift-off. Maintaining a flexed knee position increases the tension generated from the feet.

3. Mermaid on Trapeze Table

Derivative of J.H. Pilates Mermaid on Universal Reformer (NPCE Study Guide 2021, p. 64)

Intent
- Movement in frontal plane
- Intentional rib translation from organized center line
- Selective control of shoulder girdle on thorax

Gait reasoning
- Orientate torso to midline
- Focus on thoracic translation to inefficient side
- Lateral flexion necessary for swing-through phase

Set-up
- Medium spring from above on the push-through bar
- Long box

Starting position
- Sit with right side toward push-through bar with feet on long box
- Right hand on push-through bar with elbow extended, UE at approximately 60 degrees abduction
- Left hand behind occiput with elbow flexed
- A single non-skid rubberized mat is placed under left ischial tuberosity (see Author note)

Movement description
- Laterally flex torso toward push-through bar allowing bar to move passively
- Maintain equal weight on sitz bones
- Contralateral elbow reaches up to ceiling to facilitate length tension from pelvis to head
- Gently press head into hand to maintain proper head alignment
- Return to starting position

CUES

- ◆ Cue rib translation on inefficient side
- ◆ When laterally flexing to the right, verbally cue to gently press the ribs and waistline to the left. This reflects how the client was presenting at the onset of the exercise and indicates the client presented with more weight distributed on her right ischial tuberosity with a slight right translation of the thorax
- ◆ The single non-skid rubberized mat under the left ischial tuberosity gives proprioceptive feedback to shift the weight to the left ischial tuberosity, allowing more ability to translate the thorax to the left and improving right lateral flexion

Author note

The hypermobile client has many different strategies to correct a misalignment, which often lead to more misalignments. Since this client lacks good proprioception, the props help to facilitate the feedback necessary for developing proprioception.

4. Foot-ankle on Wunda Chair

Derivative of J. H. Pilates Achilles Stretch on Wunda Chair (NPCE Study Guide 2021, p. 79)

Intent
- ● Improve ankle plantar flexion and dorsiflexion
- ● Organization of vertical torso in relation to gravity while articulating ankle
- ● Balance standing on one leg

Gait reasoning
- ● Heel strike for force absorption
- ● Plantar flexion for force production and propulsion forward
- ● Talocrural joint in sagittal plane, improving talar glide
- ● Stance phase balance

Set-up
- ● Wunda Chair with 2 springs on medium setting

Starting position
- ● Stand facing chair with one foot placed on foot pedal
- ● Metatarsal arch is on foot pedal
- ● Knee flexed leaning against edge of chair directly inferior to patella
- ● Hands on either side of chair
- ● Torso extended

Movement description	<ul><li>Press through forefoot to press foot pedal down slightly moving into plantar flexion</li><li>Maintain equal pressure through entire metatarsal arch</li><li>Slowly allow foot pedal to lift back up moving ankle into dorsiflexion</li><li>Once movement is established, move hands to hips and stand upright relative to standing leg</li></ul>

Author note

The spring tension is heavy. Increased recruitment occurs with increased load, so finding the right balance is instrumental to develop adaptations. This client experiences Lyme symptoms in her knees and can present with hesitation in her movement when the load is heavy. However, with the knee in a fixed position this exercise provides a good opportunity to increase the load and target the LE.

5. Standing Leg Pump on Wunda Chair

Derivative of J. H. Pilates Standing Leg Pump: Front on Wunda Chair (NPCE Study Guide 2021, p. 79)

Intent
- Coordinated timing of hip, knee, and ankle flexion and extension
- Balance development of standing leg
- Awareness of torso adaptability with dynamic leg movements

Gait reasoning
- Timing sequential movement of hip, knee, and ankle joints
- Correlation of single-leg balance with dynamic movement of contralateral leg

Set-up
- 2 springs on medium setting

Starting position
- Stand facing Wunda Chair in parallel stance with right foot metatarsals on foot pedal and left foot on small box on floor
- Foot pedal is all the way down, extending both hips and knees
- Hands are on hips or holding on to handles if needed for balance

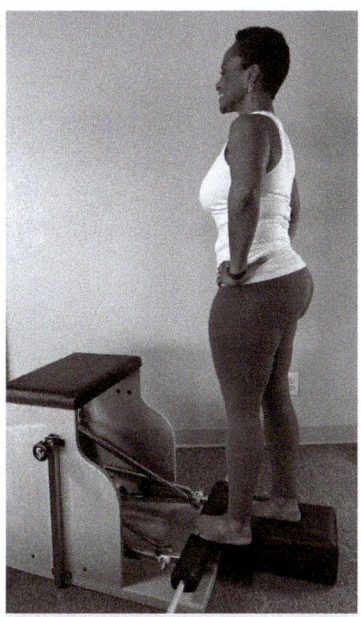

Figure 10.6

Movement description
- Lift right heel so ankle moves into plantar flexion with slight flexion of knee and hip
- While maintaining upright torso, flex hip and knee of right foot slowly allowing foot pedal to lift while keeping ankle in plantar flexion
- Press down through metatarsals of foot
- Return foot pedal to starting position
- Repeat 8 times
- Next, lower heel so ankle is in dorsiflexion
- Repeat the pumping motion while maintaining dorsiflexion

CUE
- Maintain consistent contact of the foot on the foot pedal throughout the movement

Author note
Standing on a small box allows for the foot pedal leg to press into full knee and hip extension.

6. Standing Leg Pump: Crossover on Wunda Chair — Derivative of J. H. Pilates Standing Leg Pump (NPCE Study Guide 2021, p. 79)

Intent
- Maintain torso organization through multi-planar movements

Gait reasoning
- Activation of posterior-lateral hip for stance leg
- Balance challenge against force vectors from Wunda Chair

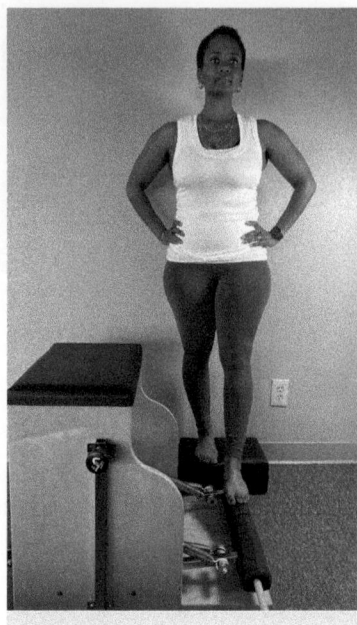

Figure 10.7

Set-up
- Wunda Chair with 2 medium springs

Starting position
- Stand on side of chair in parallel position
- Inside standing leg positioned at corner of foot pedal
- Outside leg will cross over and press foot pedal all the way down

Movement description
- Slowly allow foot pedal to lift, flexing hip and knee while LE adducts
- Maintain upright torso placement throughout lift phase
- Return foot pedal to starting position
- Leg will abduct while hip and knee extend
- Repeat 8 times on each leg

Author note
Similar to Standing Leg Pump, an addition is to stand the client on a small box so the foot pedal leg has the ability to be completely extended through the hip and knee while maintaining a level pelvis.

7. Prone arm press on Wunda Chair with extension added

Derivative of J. H. Pilates Swan Front/Chest Press on Wunda Chair (NPCE Study Guide 2021, p. 73)

Intent
- Proprioception of UE and LE to torso continuity
- Activate extensors in a different position relative to gravity

Gait reasoning
- Develop coordination of torso in sagittal plane with UE movement
- Facilitate a supported upright stance
- Challenging movement in a different orientation relative to gravity

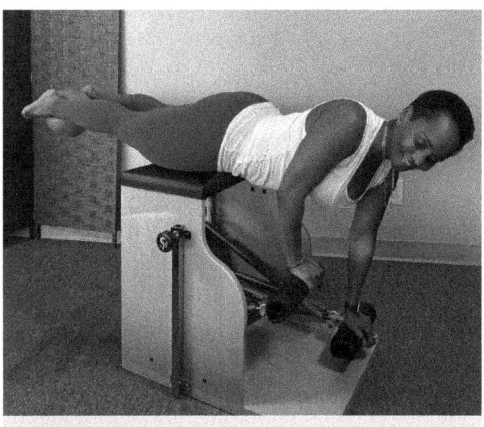

Figure 10.8

Set-up
- Spring on high setting

Starting position
- Lying on top of chair in prone position with pelvis positioned on chair
- Hands on foot pedal with arms extended straight
- Legs fully extended with Overball between ankles

Movement description
- Maintaining prone position, lift foot pedal approximately 1 in. (2.5 cm) from ground
- Flex elbows allowing foot pedal to lift while maintaining torso position
- Extend elbows to push foot pedal back to starting position
- Repeat 5 times
- Move into extension by lifting the gaze, allowing the torso to sequentially extend
- Move to a range where legs maintain leg position
- Do not allow Overball to lower during extension
- Return to starting position
- Repeat 5 times

Author note

Similar to Standing Leg Pump, an addition is to stand the client on a small box so the foot pedal leg has the ability to be completely extended through the hip and knee while maintaining a level pelvis.

8. Side Arm Twist on Wunda Chair

Derivative of J. H. Pilates Side Arm Twist (NPCE Study Guide 2021, p. 75)

Intent
- Improve torso rotation bilaterally
- Challenge multi-planar movement of torso against gravity
- Closed kinematic chain of hand to torso

Gait reasoning
- Continue focus of improving torso rotation
- Dynamic movement of torso against resistance

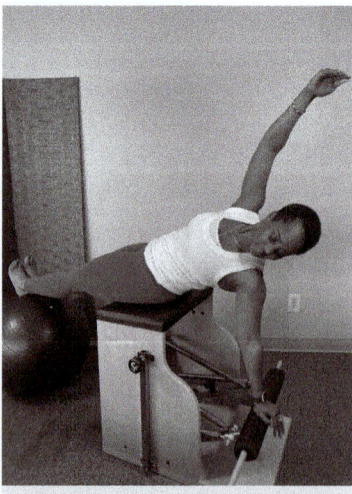

Figure 10.9

Set-up	• Spring on medium setting
Starting position	• Sit on chair facing backward with feet placed on 22 in. (55 cm) ball for stability • Knees extended • Feet plantar flexed • Both hands placed behind head, elbows flexed
Movement description	• Right torso rotation while maintaining equal pressure on ischial tuberosities • Keep ball still • Release right arm and place hand on foot pedal • Press foot pedal down while sequentially moving into slight flexion • Repeat, moving foot pedal up and down 5 times • Return to starting position • Repeat on other side

9. Knee Stretch on Universal Reformer	J. H. Pilates Knee Stretch (NPCE Study Guide 2021, p. 60)
Intent	• Integrated movement incorporating loading UE, LE, and torso with coordinated movement • Developing proprioception of LE to torso connections • Promotes quality hip joint actions
Gait reasoning	• Sagittal plane movement patterning • Selective control of torso with dynamic leg movement
Set-up	• 2 medium springs • Footbar in high position
Starting position	• Kneel on the carriage in quadruped position • Arms straight and hands placed on footbar • Ankle in dorsiflexion with feet pressing against the shoulder stops • Torso in mid-range of optimal position
Movement description	• Press legs back to open carriage moving hip and knee into extension • Control carriage back to starting position as hip and knee move back into flexion • 8 repetitions

CUE

◆ Maintain the position of the torso and arms throughout the leg movements

Author note

The Universal Reformer was avoided predominately due to the vertigo and migraine symptoms. However, in Knee Stretch, the head is not on the moving carriage and remains stable throughout the duration of the exercise. The client was able to tolerate the Universal Reformer with Knee Stretch without episodes of vertigo.

The journey to Session 11

Session 4/12
Client self-report

● Mild soreness in right knee
● Fatigue scale 5
● Pain scale 4
● Reported wrist pain in quadruped leg lift

Key changes observed

● Better awareness of body movements

Reasoning behind choice of movements

● Beginning with introduction of simple movements of LE
● Explore these movements in various planes and directions
● Work on how the torso relates to these different variations
● Adjust exercise to hold initial set-up in quadruped to adapt to wrist, then drop to forearms for leg lift component
● Add opposite leg-arm movement to supine flexor activation

Session movement sequence
1. Trapeze Table

● Footwork

2. Wunda Chair

● Foot-ankle (hands on chair)
● Standing Leg Pump Front (hands on handles)

3. Universal Reformer

● Knee Stretch

Session 5/12
Client self-report

● Reports elevated anxiety
● Pain scale 5
● Fatigue scale 3
● Reduced to no wrist pain in quadruped position
  ■ Resumed hand position for leg lift component
● Add knee extension movement to banded knee folds
● Client reports losing yoga block in rotational series
  ■ Review entire series in-studio

Key changes observed

- Breathing more controlled and slower as session progressed
- More ability to find midline before initiating movements

Reasoning behind choice of movements

- Exercises selected that provide support and direct feedback to the torso

Session movement sequence
1. Trapeze Table

- Footwork
- Seated Mermaid

2. Wunda Chair

- Standing Leg Pump
- Standing Leg Pump Crossover

3. Additional movement

- Washer Woman Over the Chair/Hamstring 2 (NPCE Study Guide 2021, p. 77)

Session 6/12
Client self-report

- Fatigued and experiencing mild headache
- Extra-fatigued due to high humidity levels
- Fatigue scale 7
- Pain scale 2

Key changes observed

- Although movements were slow, organization of motor skills improving

Reasoning behind choice of movements

- Minimize positional changes due to headache
- Minimize unwanted head motion

Session movement sequence
1. Side lying hip abduction with knee flexion added to home program, including on Trapeze Table

2. Trapeze Table

- Footwork
- Parakeet
- Side lying top-loaded push-through bar

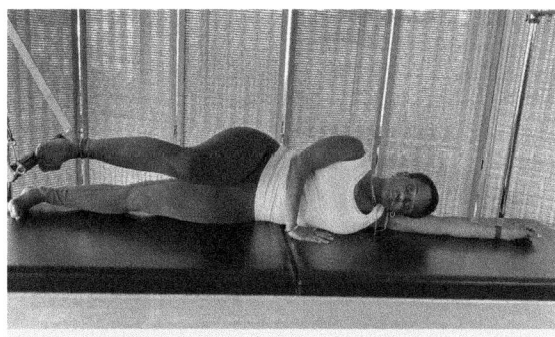

Figure 10.10

3. Wunda Chair

- Standing Leg Pump
- Standing Leg Pump Crossover

Session 7/12
Client self-report

- Recovered from migraine episode, good energy
- Bilateral soreness in lateral hip
- Fatigue scale 3
- Pain scale 3

Key changes observed

- Improved torso organization
- Increased proprioception in balance work
- Client self-adjusts positively without direction

Reasoning behind choice of movements

- Introduce more complex movements
- Work in different body positions in relation to gravity

Session movement sequence

1. Full step-up added

- Alternate legs for each repetition

2. Wunda Chair

- Foot-ankle
- Standing Leg Pump
- Standing Leg Pump Crossover
- Swan Front
- Side Arm Twist

Session 8/12
Client self-report

- Increased work demands
- Fatigue scale 5
- Pain scale 2

Key changes observed

- Gait pace increased and with more intention
- Less visible pelvic lateral shift
- Improved arm swing

Reasoning behind choice of movements

- Continue to work on progressions

- Review new exercises introduced in previous session

Session movement sequence
1. Trapeze Table

- Footwork
- Parakeet
- Seated Mermaid

2. Wunda Chair

- Swan Front
- Side Arm Twist

Session 9/12
Client self-report

- Reports noticeably decreased body aches
- Fatigue scale 3
- Pain scale 0

Key changes observed

- Client moves more confidently, references midline
- Demonstrates a command of the choreography
- Anticipates her own movement compensation tendencies and adjusts

Reasoning behind choice of movements

- Progress exercises to increase balance challenges

Session movement sequence
1. Wunda Chair

- Foot-ankle, arms reach overhead
- Standing Leg Pump, hands behind head
- Standing Leg Pump Crossover, hands on hips

2. Universal Reformer

- Knee Stretch
- Single Leg Knee Stretch
- Standing lunge position, one foot on shoulder stop, hands on footbar, torso natural curvature, pressing carriage back into hip extension

> **Editor note**
> The Single Leg Knee Stretch is also known as Scooter or Eve's Lunge. In this case, the author focused on the torso relationship to LE movement in the sagittal plane—a derivative of Eve's Lunge (see Chapter 5, Gentry).

Session 10/12
Client self-report

- Neck pain reported
- Elevated overall tension
- Fatigue scale 3
- Pain scale 5

Key changes observed

- Significantly less compensatory movements throughout torso
- Sitz bones weighted equally when seated

Reasoning behind choice of movements

- Work on entire movement progression

Session movement sequence
1. Home program review

- Presented some additional variations to incorporate into home program

- Client plans to continue home sessions after completion of program
- Added plank variations and side kick variations

2. Wunda Chair

- Foot-ankle
- Standing Leg Pump
- Standing Leg Pump Crossover
- Swan Front
- Side Arm Twist

References

Black, M. (2022) *Centered: Organizing the Body through Kinesiology, Movement Theory and Pilates Techniques.* Edinburgh: Handspring Publishing, pp. 129–130.

Buhner, S. (2015) *Healing Lyme.* 2nd Ed. Silver City, NM: Raven Press.

CDC (Centers for Disease Control and Prevention) (2024) Lyme Disease Surveillance and Data. www.cdc.gov/lyme/data-research/facts-stats/index.html. [Accessed June 27, 2024].

Chaconas, G., Castellanos, M., and Verhey, T. B. (2020) "Changing of the guard: How the Lyme disease spirochete subverts the host immune response." *The Journal of Biological Chemistry, 295,* 2, 301–313.

Mead, P. S. (2015) "Epidemiology of Lyme disease." *Infectious Disease Clinics of North America, 29,* 2, 187–210.

NPCE Study Guide (National Pilates Certification Exam Study Guide) (2021) Miami, FL: National Pilates Certification Program, Inc.

Ross Russell, A. L., Dryden, M. S., Pinto, A. A., and Lovett, J. K. (2018) "Lyme disease: Diagnosis and management." *Practical Neurology, 18,* 6, 455–464.

Stanek, G. and Strle, F. (2018) "Lyme borreliosis—from tick bite to diagnosis and treatment." *FEMS Microbiology Reviews, 42,* 3, 233–258.

The Ehlers–Danlos Society (2023) Assessing Joint Hypermobility. The Beighton Scoring System. www.ehlers-danlos.com/assessing-joint-hypermobility. [Accessed June 27, 2024].

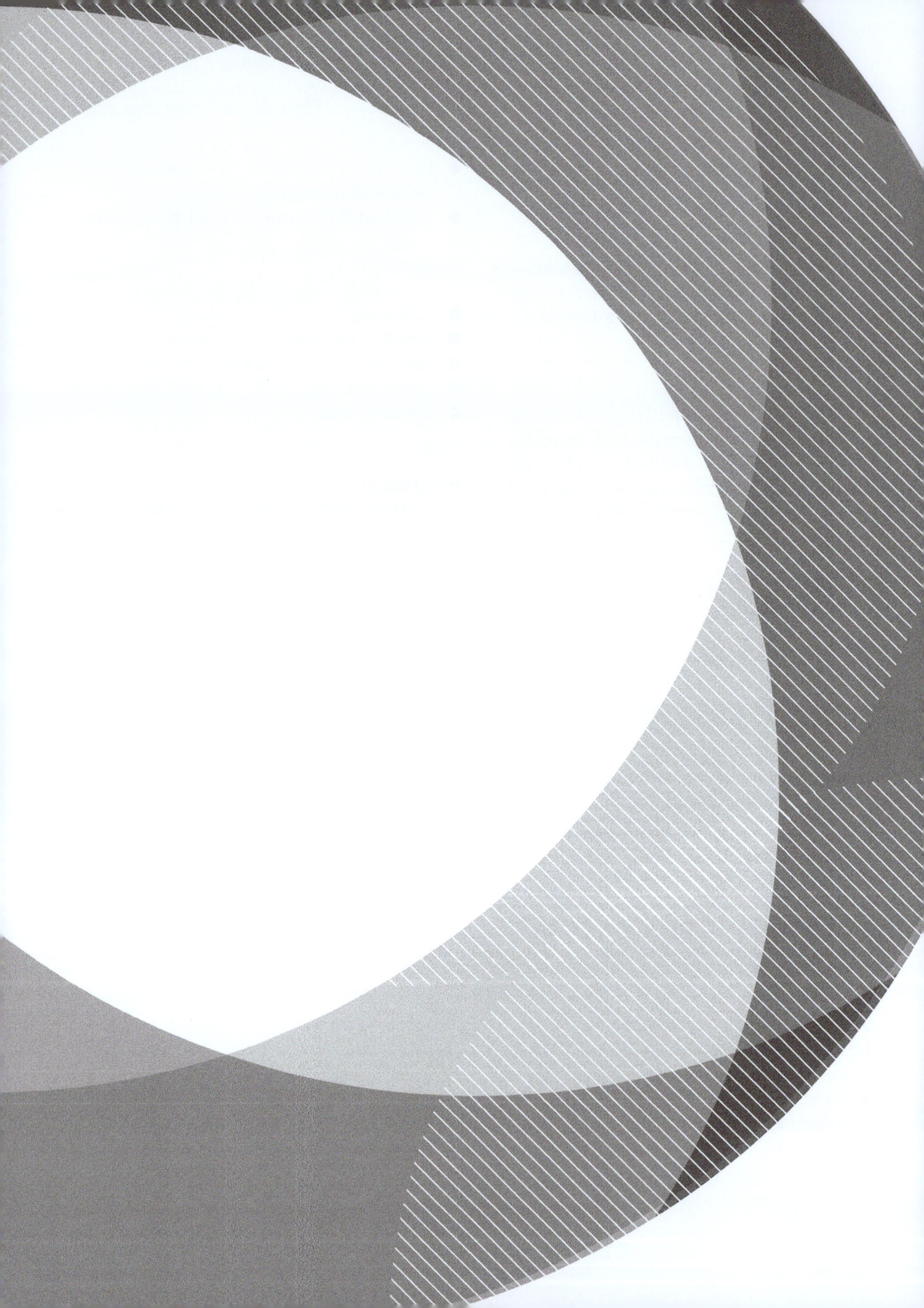

Pilates for Trauma Related Stress and Anxiety: Effect on Gait

Jojo Bowman and Jessie Lee

Most people will at some point in their lives experience some form of trauma. This can be in the aftermath of an accident, injury, illness, or overwhelming events such as personal loss, divorce, or hardship (Benjet *et al.* 2016). Life is no longer predictable or controllable and some may experience feelings of helplessness and fear.

According to the polyvagal theory, the body and mind engage in three fundamental physiological states in a threatening event (Porges 2021). The social engagement system will look for safety first and, if this is not met, then mobilization with fight or flight, and finally immobilization and dissociation (van der Kolk 2014). In most circumstances the nervous system will return to homeostasis once the danger has passed (Payne, Levine, and Crane-Godreau 2015). An event becomes traumatic (Porges 2017) when the entire organism becomes overwhelmed and fails to reset, leaving the body, mind, and spirit stuck and continuing to behave as if there is danger in the present moment, even though the event has passed (Heines 2016). Left unresolved, it can lead to an acute or chronic stress response, eventually resulting in post-traumatic stress with symptoms such as dissociation, neuromuscular tension, shivering, shallow breathing, depression, and anxiety (Substance Abuse and Mental Health Services Administration 2014).

While psychological and narrative therapies can be extremely beneficial, a somatic approach, with guided attention to proprioceptive, interoceptive, and kinesthetic experiences, also plays an important role in recovery (van der Kolk 2014). The vagus nerve with its many branches bridges the gap between mind and body. The ventral vagal pathways send signals to the heart and lungs to help slow down heart rate and breath, restoring a sense of calm (Porges 2021). Paying attention to breath (Chaitow 2014), safely, and tactile sensory feedback with the use of external stimulus such as heat, different textured surfaces, and appropriate touch (Schleip and Stecco 2021) are all part of a support process toward regulation of the nervous system.

Sensory imprints of trauma generate a full spectrum of body sensations from uncomfortable to painful (Payne *et al.* 2015). Significant alterations of interoceptive processing have been linked to anxiety and depression (Schleip and Stecco 2021). Awareness of interoceptive and proprioceptive sensations help improve body perceptions (Payne *et al.* 2015). Educating the client to notice a sudden muscular tensioning, or how a breath is held, helps them to see the sensations for what they are: patterned reflexes in response to feeling unsafe or afraid in anticipation of pain (van der Kolk 2014). Graded exposure to new movements as well as repeating and returning to key exercises that promote positive bodily sensations of comfort and ease help to create a safe base to move forward from (Heines 2016).

Establishing an environment where it is safe to move (Porges 2017) and investigating new ways of breathing and moving will slowly allow the nervous system to reorganize itself into new patterns, thereby restoring ownership of physical reactions and gaining a sense of mastery over self (Levine 2008).

Considerations:

- Contact clinical practitioner regarding client medicine intake. Some psycho-pharmaceuticals cause excessive fatigue

and affect body sensations and mental alertness

- Observe emotional states. If the client exhibits signs of self-harm or suicidal thoughts, always refer the client to a higher level of care (Substance Abuse and Mental Health Services Administration 2014)

Client description: 53-year-old biological female, identifies as female; CEO and mother of two children

Dates of case report: Session 1: February 17, 2020; Session 12: June 24, 2020. All sessions in-person, with 13-week pandemic interruption between Sessions 5 and 6

Studio apparatus and props
Pilates equipment

- Trapeze Table
- Wunda Chair with split pedal

Props used with equipment

- Large wedge or flat pillow
- Roller or rolled blanket
- 2 SmartSpine™ triangles
- SmartSpine™ globe

Home program props

- Firm, spikey ball, 4 in. (10 cm)
- 2 soft, air-filled balls, 4 in. (10 cm)
- Partially deflated ball, 8.5 in. (22 cm)
- Half roller
- Weighted eye mask (optional)

Author note

Heat in the therapeutic range, with temperatures up to 40 degrees C, contributes to relaxation of fascial stiffness in relation to myofascial dysfunction (Chaitow *et al.* 2018). The SmartSpine system uses the fascial properties of thermoreception, interoception, and proprioception as an effective delivery system to increase movement potential as well as movement ease, improving the fascial hydrodynamic ability (Schleip and Stecco 2021).

Methods and materials

Session 1/12
1. Health history interview

- Living in long-term stressful life conditions
- Early 2017: car accident, causing whiplash syndrome and concussion

- Late 2017: increased pain and reduced range of motion (ROM) in both shoulders—treated with two cortisone injections
- Left eye had a vitreous collapse causing blurry vision
- A full medical check prior to beginning case study, to receive medical permission to participate in gait-focused Pilates training
- Since 2017: experiences fatigue and reoccurring shivering with cold or feverish symptoms in relation to exercise and periods of stress
- All client medical test results were clear and normal

2. Symptoms

- Easily fatigued, frequent headaches, dizziness, nausea, and connective tissue pain
- Cognitive issues, pain in neck, shoulders, and lumbar region
- Influenza, cold, or feverish symptoms (no measurable fever), and connective tissue pain when exercising or with physical exertion. Alleviated by several hot showers daily

- Stress and reoccurring anxiety
- Feels disconnected from her body
- Reduced neck movement
- Limited torso flexion with increased tonicity and stiffness

3. Movement aids

- None

Final result of case report

The client was able to walk with fluidity, midline orientation, and ease. Hard heel strike was reduced. Pain in the lumbar and cervical regions was diminished. She no longer experienced influenza symptoms post-sessions. She reported feeling an increased connectivity and awareness of body with improved coping strategies to handle stress and anxiety.

Session 2/12: Initial assessment

1. General observations of gait

◆ Excessive lumbar lordosis

◆ Hard heel strike

◆ Propulsion phase: plantar flexion minimal on both sides

◆ No apparent thoracic rotation

◆ Pendulum arm swing with elbow flexion, right arm less active than left

◆ Limited pelvic motion

◆ Limited foot loading through forefoot

◆ Gait asynchronous

2. Standing tests

◆ Full torso rotation

● Observations of inefficient side: left
  ■ Unable to sequentially articulate from thorax to pelvis
  ■ Minimal pelvifemoral motion
  ■ Right foot small degree of pronation, left foot no supination

◆ Hemipelvis inferior motion

● Observations of inefficient side: both
  ■ Lowering of hemipelvis and associated lumbar lateral flexion restricted bilaterally
  ■ Rotation of thoracolumbar junction (TLJ) to right

Session 12/12: Post-assessment

1. General observations of gait

◆ Improved lumbar curve in sagittal plane

◆ Softer heel strike

◆ Propulsion phase: plantar flexion accessible

◆ Improved thoracic rotation

◆ Balanced arm swing with decreased elbow flexion

◆ Visible counter-rotation of pelvis and thorax

◆ Foot loads from heel through forefoot

◆ Able to walk with fluidity, midline orientation, and ease

2. Standing tests

◆ Full torso rotation

● Observations of inefficient side: left
  ■ Visible sequential articulation from thorax to pelvis
  ■ Improved pelvifemoral motion
  ■ Right foot increased pronation, improved left foot supination

◆ Hemipelvis inferior motion

● Observations of inefficient side: left
  ■ Improved lowering of right hemipelvis with associated lumbar lateral flexion
  ■ Limited lowering of left hemipelvis with associated lumbar lateral flexion
  ■ Decreased rotation of TLJ to right

Editor note

Restriction in one plane may result in movement compensation in another plane. A restriction of lumbar lateral flexion in the coronal plane tends to create a rotation in the transverse plane.

◆ Hemipelvis superior motion

● Observations of inefficient side: both
  ■ Right
    O Right rotation of TLJ
    O Left lateral thoracic translation
    O Left scapula protraction and internal rotation of left humeral head
  ■ Left
    O Limited
    O Inability to transfer pelvis over right foot

◆ Lateral pelvic shift

● Observations of inefficient side: both
  ■ Right
    O Left thoracic lateral flexion
    O Right rotation of TLJ region
    O Limited medial and lateral hip glide

Editor note

The combined motions of thoracic translation toward the weighted right leg and the lowering left innominate with left lumbar translation is an efficient gait pattern. In this test, right lateral pelvic shift, the thorax would translate right. The finding of left lateral thoracic translation is not preferred. Lateral flexion is a paired motion with an oppositional translation and rotation.

  ■ Left
    O Right thoracic lateral translation
    O Limited medial and lateral hip glide

◆ Hemipelvis superior motion

● Observations of inefficient side: left
  ■ Right
    O TLJ midline with respect to sacrum
    O Decreased left lateral thoracic translation
    O Improved shoulder girdle and left scapula adaptation relative to thorax, left humeral head congruent
  ■ Left
    O Less limited with improvement of ability to transfer pelvis over right foot

◆ Lateral pelvic shift

● Observations of inefficient side: left
  ■ Right
    O Decreased left thoracic lateral flexion
    O TLJ and S2 organized to midline
    O Improved medial and lateral hip glide
  ■ Left
    O Less right thoracic translation
    O Less limited ability to laterally shift pelvis
    O Improved bilateral hip glide, on left more than right

3. Seated tests

◆ Hip joint and knee flexion

● Observations of inefficient side: right
  ■ Left thoracic lateral translation
  ■ Right rotation of TLJ
  ■ Right pelvic rotation

Author note

Included dorsiflexion and knee flexion test. Left was inefficient. Limited left knee flexion and dorsiflexion, left femur adducts. Included hip abduction with external rotation. Right was inefficient. Left thoracic lateral translation with right rotation of TLJ region.

4. Sit and stand

◆ Lateral view

● Increased lordosis in cervical and lumbar regions

◆ Anterior view

● In sit to stand right femur adducts
● In stand to sit right foot pronates

5. Standing balance

◆ Two-leg stance, eyes open

● 60 seconds

◆ One-leg stance, eyes open

● Slow, continuous cervical rotations throughout, aiming for 30 seconds
  ■ Left leg: 26 seconds
  ■ Right leg: 24 seconds

3. Seated tests

◆ Hip joint and knee flexion

● Observations of inefficient side: right
  ■ Decreased left thoracic lateral translation
  ■ Right rotation of TLJ
  ■ Reduced right pelvic rotation

Author note

Included dorsiflexion and knee flexion test. Left was inefficient. Left femur in optimal position for the task. Increased dorsiflexion. Included hip abduction with external rotation. Right was inefficient. TLJ and S2 orientated to midline, no apparent translation.

4. Sit and stand

◆ Lateral view

● Ability to modulate torso organization for improved lordosis

◆ Anterior view

● In sit to stand right femur in optimal position for the task
● In stand to sit decreased right foot pronation

5. Standing balance

◆ Two-leg stance, eyes open

● 60 seconds

◆ One-leg stance, eyes open

● Slow, continuous cervical rotations throughout, aiming for 30 seconds
  ■ Left leg: 27 seconds
  ■ Right leg: 30 seconds

Session 3/12: Home program

Fatigue scale	6
Pain scale	7
Client self-report	● Pain from mid-back to head ● Sore swollen eyes
Key changes observed by author at end of Session 3/12	● Fewer exercises than planned ● Focus on body sensations provokes nausea, dizziness, and feelings of overwhelm and sadness ● Perceives a state of danger when physically moving and responds with a freeze response and increased stress ● Shivering and cold with influenza symptoms at end of session
Reason behind choice of sequencing	● Verticality organizing to midline ● Lumbopelvic femoral articulation ● Challenge adaptability in standing, supine, and quadruped positions ● Prone and side lying omitted as they cause neck discomfort, pressure on shoulder impingement, and dizziness

Session movement sequence

1. Standing tactile foot rolling

Intent	● Tactile stimulation to shift attention from mind to body ● Sensory input into feet
Gait reasoning	● Stimulate sole of foot to improve proprioception of foot loading ● Increase ankle articulation
Starting position	● Parallel stance with one foot placed on 4 in. (10 cm) diameter spikey ball with knee flexed ● Hold a bar for balance
Movement description	● Roll ball on plantar side of one foot ● Plantar flex rolling ball forward and dorsiflex rolling back to starting position ● Standing firmly on supporting foot ● 10 repetitions with each foot ● Focus on rhythm and gentle nasal breathing

Author note

As the client experiences new movements through painful areas, that have been exposed to trauma, feelings of discomfort, nausea, or overwhelm can occur. Help them to reorientate and self-regulate by bringing their attention and awareness back to the present. Ask them to sit or stand and walk around the room focusing on the surroundings (Payne *et al.* 2015). Create a personal grounding strategy that provides a feeling of safety, such as noticing the support of the ground or tactile feedback from a spikey ball on the soles of the feet or surfaces of the hands (Linden 2016).

2. Seated foot articulations

Intent	• Sensory input into feet
	• Foot articulation in all three planes
	• Improve proprioception
	• Flexion and extension of knee and ankle
Gait reasoning	• Dorsiflexion and plantar flexion for heel strike and forward propulsion
	• Foot adaptability for ground surfaces
Starting position	• Sitting on edge of Trapeze Table or a stable chair, pelvis slightly higher than knees
	• Both feet on floor in parallel hip-distance apart
	• Right foot dorsiflexed with heel on floor with a soft, air-filled ball, 4 in. (10 cm) in diameter, under metatarsal arch
Movement description	• Dorsiflex and plantar flex
	• Pressing gently into ball, roll ball forward extending knee
	• Plantar flex right foot flexing phalanges to floor
	• Dorsiflex right foot flexing knee
	• Return heel to floor
	• Return to starting position
	• 8 repetitions
	• Repeat with left foot
	• Eversion/inversion
	• Maintain heel on floor, roll ball laterally initiated by 1st phalange everting the calcaneus
	• Maintain heel on floor, roll ball medially initiated by 5th phalange inverting the calcaneus
	• Knee will move slightly with the movement
	• 8 repetitions
	• Repeat with left foot

3. Supine anterior-posterior pelvic rotations

Intent
- Introducing gentle nasal breathing to help self-regulate
- Coordinate breathing with a rhythmic movement
- Introducing pelvifemoral rhythm

Gait reasoning
- Facilitating reorganization of torso
- Stimulating lumbopelvic-femoral articulation

Starting position
- Supine with knees in flexion, feet in line with ischial tuberosities
- Place 2 soft, air-filled balls, 4 in. (10 cm) in diameter, on lateral sides of the sacrum
- Upper extremities (UE) along sides resting on mat

Editor note

The placement of the two balls, one on each side of the sacrum laterally, will be approximately at S2. Fine-tune the placement allowing for ease in both anterior and posterior rotations.

Movement description
- Exhale, rocking the pelvis into posterior rotation
- Inhale, rocking the pelvis into slight anterior rotation
- Create a gentle and rhythmic movement
- 10–15 repetitions

Author note

The fight-flight-freeze response seen in trauma-related stress and anxiety can affect movement and breathing patterns (Gilbert 2014). [NEW] [Is this chapter reference 2014a or 2014b? See EQ document, page 1 query.] This client exhibited shallow breathing and a rigid quality of movement. The organization from the neuromyofascial response presented as mid- to lower thorax posterior rotation, increasing the anterior costal angle and placing the thorax anterior to the pelvis. To help regulate the intra-abdominal pressure for improved breathing, emphasize organizing the dome of the diaphragm relative to the pelvis (Milanesi and Caregnato 2016) (see Author note on intra-abdominal pressure in Chapter 10).

Soft cranial-sacral rocking motions (Meert 2012) increase the fascial glide of the dura mater and nerve pathways (Upledger and VredeVoogd 2019), releasing the fascial restrictions of the TLJ and improving the three-dimensional aspects of the thorax, restoring optimal breathing patterns (Kolar *et al.* 2014).

4. Sagittal lumbopelvic femoral series

Intent
- Facilitating proprioception of hip joints in flexion and extension
- Posterior pelvic rotation to counter anterior pelvic rotation strategy
- Lower extremity (LE) motor control in the sagittal plane

Gait reasoning
- Torso organization with LE flexion and extension
- Increase ROM of hip joint flexion and extension

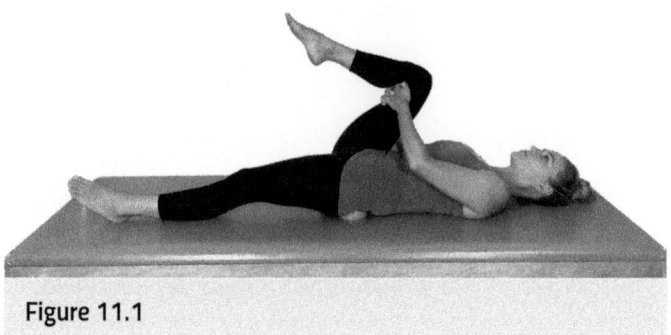

Figure 11.1

Starting position
- Supine with 2 soft, air-filled balls, 4 in. (10 cm) in diameter, placed on lateral sides of sacrum
- Right LE softly flexed toward chest with both hands supporting under the knee
- Left LE extended in parallel, heel on mat

Movement description
- Hold starting position
- Exhale, to rock pelvis into posterior rotation
- Inhale, to rock pelvis into slight anterior rotation
- Initiate rocking motion from pelvis
- Allow flexed right LE to follow the movement
- Keep extended left LE parallel and heel anchored into mat
- 5 repetitions
- Repeat on other side
- LE flexion and extension
- Flex the left extended knee and draw the foot in toward ischial tuberosity
- In a continuous motion, left knee extends increasing hip joint flexion with plantar flexion

- Extend left hip joint with dorsiflexion
- Lower to the starting position
- Complete 1 full cycle
- 5 repetitions
- Repeat on other side

5. Small pelvic bridge

Intent
- Adduction of LE for midline orientation
- Increasing lumbopelvic-femoral articulations in posterior pelvic rotation

Gait reasoning
- Improve extension and forward propulsion
- Facilitating verticality

Starting position
- Supine with knees in flexion, feet on mat in line with ischial tuberosities
- Soft, half-inflated, 8.5 in. (22 cm) diameter ball placed between superior aspect of femurs
- UE along sides resting on mat

Movement description
- Exhale, rotate pelvis posteriorly, activating lightly around ball
- Sequentially articulate from the coccyx into bridge position
- Reach knees over toes for ankle dorsiflexion
- Inhale at the top
- Exhale, articulate from thorax to pelvis returning to starting position
- 10 repetitions

6. Supine cervical flexion, extension, and rotation on half roller

Intent
- Breathing to a rhythmic movement
- Proprioceptive awareness of head and cervical region, while safely visiting an area of trauma (whiplash)
- Stimulating cervical flexion, extension, and rotational motions
- Addressing neuromyofascial continuity from occiput to sacrum
- Vestibular stimuli

Gait reasoning
- Improve transference of ground forces to soften heel strike to head
- Facilitating verticality

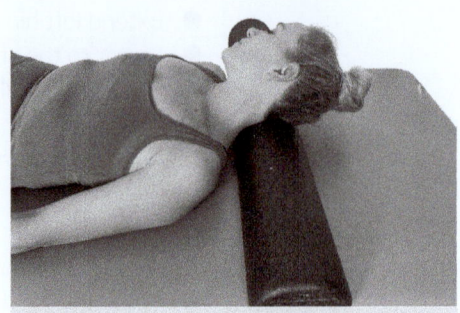

Figure 11.2

Starting position

- Supine with knees in flexion, feet on mat in line with ischial tuberosities
- UE along sides resting on mat
- Head placed on half deflated, soft ball, 8.5 in. (22 cm) in diameter, cradling the parietal region
- Eyes can be open with a soft gaze or closed according to client's preference

Movement description

- Flexion and extension
  - Exhale, roll the ball superiorly nodding chin down toward sternum
  - Inhale, roll ball inferiorly nodding chin away from sternum
  - Repeat as client prefers
- Cervical rotation
  - Roll head slowly laterally right and left
  - Eyes can be open or closed
  - Repeat as client prefers

Author note

If discomfort is experienced with dizziness or nausea, the movements can be done without the soft ball in the beginning, to accustom the vestibular system to the movement. A firm surface can increase stimuli facilitating a different proprioceptive experience. A half roller was used as an alternative to the ball or mat for the head rotation, with the head placed on the apex of the roller.

7. Quadruped breathing

Intent	● Activation of abdominal region against gravity while maintaining midline orientation
	● Shoulder girdle organization relative to torso and cervical-head region
Gait reasoning	● Organizing pelvis and thorax with breathing
	● Activation of flexors and extensors
Starting position	● Quadruped position
Movement description	● Prepare with inhale and exhale while maintaining quadruped position
	● Inhale, expand the posterior thorax allowing the abdominals to move while maintaining quadruped position
	● Exhale, gently feel abdominal wall move posteriorly, maintaining quadruped position
	● Continue for 5 breathing cycles
	● Keep breathing patterns soft

8. Torso flexion and Child's Pose

Intent	● Reorganize unconscious holding of torso
	● Facilitate flexion and lumbopelvic femoral articulations
	● Learn pelvifemoral rhythm and coordination
Gait reasoning	● To improve upright orientation for improved thorax and pelvic rotation
Starting position	● Kneel in quadruped position
Movement description	● Exhale to initiate sequential flexion from coccyx to head
	● Inhale into posterior thorax as coccyx moves toward sternum
	● Exhale, return to starting position
	● 5 repetitions
	● Finish in yoga pose Balasana, known as Child's Pose

9. Supine rotations

Derivative of J. H. Pilates Mat Spine Twist and Corkscrew (NPCE Study Guide 2021, pp. 48–49)

Intent	● Facilitate sensory awareness of torso through feet
	● Activating transverse plane torso motion
Gait reasoning	● Improve thoracic rotation and counter-rotation of pelvis
	● Adduction of the LE improving load transfer

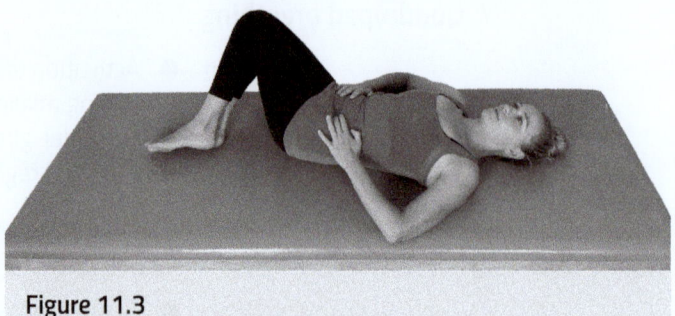

Figure 11.3

Starting position	• Supine with knees in flexion, feet on mat
	• Knees and feet together at midline
	• Hands on inferior abdominal region
	• Elbows resting on the mat

Starting position
- Supine with knees in flexion, feet on mat
- Knees and feet together at midline
- Hands on inferior abdominal region
- Elbows resting on the mat

Movement description
- Rotate pelvis aiming knees to left
- Maintain bilateral scapulae on mat
- Knees and feet stay together
- Initiate the return from right thorax rotation articulating through pelvis
- Knees and feet return last to starting position
- 5 repetitions
- Change to right rotation

Session 11/12: Studio session

Fatigue scale   2

Pain scale   4

Client self-report
- Positive report after Session 10. No shivering cold or influenza symptoms or need for usual hot showers post-session

Key changes observed by author at end of Session 11/12
- Improved movement efficiency with no discomfort during session
- Improved organization from sitting to standing
- Midline organization in all three planes resulting in improved verticality
- Increased stride length

Reason behind choice of sequencing
- Completing a session without onset of physical symptoms such as shivering, nausea, and dizziness
- Breathing with ease during movement
- Increasing interoceptive awareness
- Home program sequence consistent with small adjustments to gently challenge but not overload
- Support self-regulation

Session movement sequence

1. Constructive rest with heat

Editor note

Constructive rest position (CRP) is a position described by Dr. Lulu Sweigaard in her 1974 publication *Human Movement Potential* as a position to allow the neuromyofascial system to integrate toward rest. CRP promotes slower breathing and has a calming effect (Black 2022).

Intent
- Enhance awareness prior to moving or at end of session
- Weighted eye mask is optional and optimal at end of session to lessen over-stimulation through the eyes
- Heat to facilitate parasympathetic state before or after the session to minimize freeze response

Gait reasoning
- Facilitate a softer and mindful gait pattern through embodiment

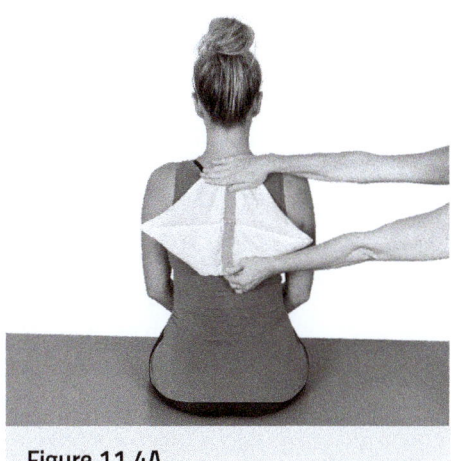

Figure 11.4A

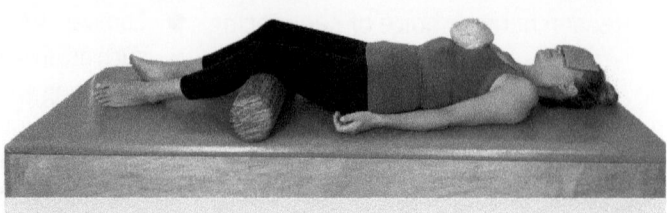

Figure 11.4B

Set-up	● 2 SmartSpine triangles and a SmartSpine globe
	● Rolled blanket or foam roller
	● Weighted eye mask

Starting position	● Supine
	● Hip and knee extension in a relaxed state with heels on mat
	● Place a rolled blanket or foam roller under knees
	● Lie on 2 heated SmartSpine triangles placed in a horizontal diamond shape under the region between the TLJ and cervicothoracic junction
	● Heated SmartSpine globe on sternum

Movement description	● Relaxation-guided body scan
	■ Sense the breath into heat of triangles and relax body
	■ Allow weight of heated globe to soften sternum toward sacrum
	■ Focus on gentle nasal breathing, letting the breath flow in and out
	■ Suggested time 5–10 minutes

Author note

The client has difficulty with regulation of body temperatures (homeostasis) (Schleip and Stecco 2021) and feels cold and shivery during and after exercising. The heated SmartSpine helps minimize the onset of these symptoms, refine interoceptive awareness, and has a calming effect on the nervous system. Warmth is a component of interoception. Interoception is processed in the limbic area of the brain, which is in communication with and triggers the parasympathetic nervous system (Schleip and Stecco 2021).

Use heat with caution avoiding use on open wounds, acute inflammatory diseases, peripheral neuropathy/vascular disease, and skin sensation impairments (Klingler 2021).

CUES

- Suggestions for guided relaxation and body scan:
  - Let the breath flow naturally in and out
  - Let the eyes feel heavy in the eye sockets
  - Let the tongue and jaw relax
  - Pay attention to any areas of tension and allow the breath to enter
  - Allow any areas of holding to feel the heat
- Begin scan of body from feet and up:
  - Feel the heels in contact with the mat, the back of the LE, the soft tissues of the pelvis, and the sacrum
  - Notice which areas of the body are in contact with the mat
  - Allow the sternum to soften and slide toward the sacrum
  - Feel the scapulae sink into the mat and widening
  - Sense the weight of the head

2. Repeat of home program

Intent
- Continuous repetition of Home Program is essential to measure the physical reactions, prior to adding additional exercises

Gait reasoning
- Facilitating verticality and orientation to midline
- Improve the force transmission and vector from heel strike to head
- Improve dorsiflexion and plantar flexion
- Improve rotation and counter-rotation

Author note

- Breathing patterns are introduced gradually to allow the body to become accustomed. Deep breathing and over-cueing the breath may increase symptoms of nausea, dizziness, and hyperventilation. Gentle nasal breathing allows the client to naturally integrate the breath with the rhythm and movement of the exercises
- A breathing pattern focusing on inhale through the nose and exhale through the mouth is first introduced in quadruped and seated positions, where client feels most comfortable

3. Supine leg slides   Derivative of Eve Gentry leg slides (see Chapter 5, Gentry)

Intent
- Coordination of breathing and LE movements
- Pelvifemoral and knee to ankle flexion and extension
- Sensory awareness of abdominal region during breathing

Gait reasoning
- Torso adaptation with hip extension
- Motor control pelvifemoral and knee to ankle flexion and extension

Set-up
- 2 SmartSpine triangles and a SmartSpine globe

Starting position
- Supine with knees in flexion, feet on mat in line with ischial tuberosities
- Hands placed on inferior abdominal region with flexed elbows on the mat
- Lying on 2 heated SmartSpine triangles under the region between the TLJ and cervicothoracic junction
- Heated SmartSpine globe on sternum

Movement description
- Inhale posteriorly into heat of triangles, as abdominal region expands under fingertips
- Exhale slowly allowing the abdominal wall to move posteriorly
- The sternum softens towards the sacrum with the weight of the globe
- 5 repetitions
- Inhale posteriorly into heat of triangles
- Exhale, slide right LE along mat to extend right hip and knee joint
- Inhale, dorsiflex right ankle
- Exhale, slide right LE back to starting position
- 5 repetitions
- Change sides

CUE
- On the exhale, imagine the abdominal region as a woven net under the umbilicus

4. Supine torso rotation

Intent
- Improve rotation of thorax and pelvis
- Activate transverse plane torso movement
- Activate external rotation of glenohumeral joint
- Articulate costal sternal joints

Gait reasoning ● Counter-rotation of thorax and pelvis

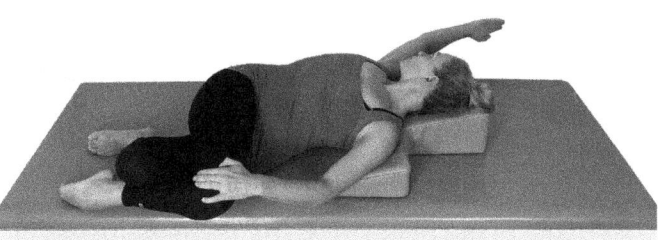

Figure 11.5

Set-up ● Mat
● Sloped wedge or flat pillow

Starting position ● Supine with knees in flexion, feet on mat, head resting on wedge or flat pillow
● UE resting on mat at 45° angle palms down

Movement description ● Cross right LE over left LE with knee to knee
● Rotate knees, pelvis, and lumbar region left while head rotates to right
● Stay in position
● Place left hand on right knee
● Externally rotate and abduct right UE sliding along the mat to 135° abduction
● Stay in position for 1–3 breaths reaching out through right phalanges
● Return to starting position rotating right initiating and articulating from thorax, pelvis, and knees
● Slide right UE to starting position
● 2 repetitions on each side

CUES

◆ Allow the pelvis to rotate with the weight of the LE to the left, as the thorax rotates in opposition
◆ Breathe into left ribs to laterally translate to left as thorax rotates right
◆ Imagine a light shining from sternum up and to the right
◆ Gently anchor right scapula and find the rotation from thorax with a continuum into right arm

Editor note

Elevating the thorax with the sloped wedge helps bring the lumbar region posterior allowing the thorax to rotate anteriorly. This position allows for ease in movement of the diaphragm and lung mobility through changing the relationship of the thorax and pelvis. The diaphragm has complex fascial connections which link it to many other structures.This position supports synchronization of cardiac and respiratory rhythms(Pilat 2022).

5. Weight shifting seated and standing

Intent
- Proprioception and awareness of whole body in space
- Verticality for improved three dimensional motions
- Improving vestibular function with weight shift and awareness of center of mass

Gait reasoning
- Facilitate the feeling of uprightness
- Improve organization of TLJ with S2
- Improve vestibular function and ease of head and balance

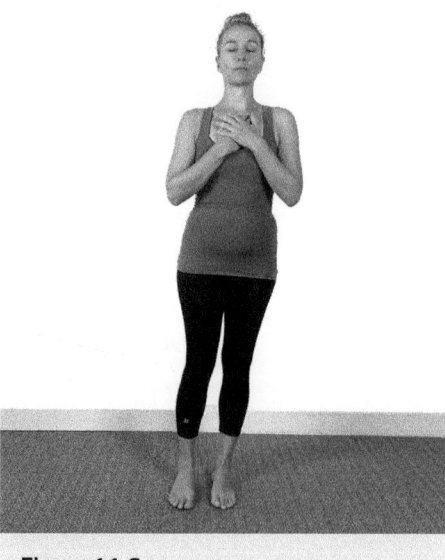

Figure 11.6

Set-up
- Chair or Trapeze Table

Starting position
- Seated version
  - Seated on edge of the Trapeze Table or a chair with both ischial tuberosities evenly loaded on the seat. Hips slightly higher than knees. Both feet planted on floor
  - Place one hand on top of the other on manubrium
- Standing version
  - Stand in parallel stance, placing an even weight distribution on the feet
  - Place one hand on top of the other on manubrium

Movement description
- Seated
  - Shift weight of the ischial tuberosities anteriorly
  - Return to starting position
  - Shift weight of the ischial tuberosities posteriorly
  - Return to starting position
  - Shift weight laterally to left ischial tuberosity
  - Return to starting position
  - Shift weight laterally to right ischial tuberosity
  - To return to center feeling the midline and verticality
  - Notice the TLJ in midline with S2
  - Notice an ease of breath
- Standing
  - Shift weight anteriorly to the metatarsal arches
  - Return to starting position
  - Shift weight posterior to posterior aspects of the calcaneus
  - Return to starting position
  - Laterally shift weight to left allowing feet to adapt
  - Return to starting position
  - Laterally shift weight to right allowing feet to adapt
  - To return to center, feel the alignment of the diaphragms stacked over one another

6. Wunda Chair Leg Pumps   Derivative of J. H. Pilates Wunda Chair Double Leg Pumps: Parallel, Heels (NPCE Study Guide 2021, p. 72)

Intent
- Articulation and activation of ankle, knee, and hip joints in seated position in sagittal plane
- Awareness and motor learning of LE movement patterning in flexion and extension
- Utilize the variable spring resistance of the Wunda Chair to assist a continuum of spring resistance for proprioceptive coordination (see Chapter 6)
- Gait reasoning
- Torso dynamic stability challenge during LE movement

Set-up
- 2 springs on third hook from top

Starting position
- Seated at front edge of seat
- Place the foot on the pedals where the cuboid meets the calcaneus in line with ischial tuberosities
- UE along sides

Movement description
- With dowel through foot pedal
- Press into heels lowering foot pedal
- Maintain ischial tuberosities central contact
- Return foot pedal resisting spring tension
- Repeat 5 times
- Remove dowel from foot pedal
- Place one foot on corresponding foot pedal
- Press evenly into heels lowering foot pedals of the chair, remain at the same level
- Maintain ischial tuberosities central contact
- Return foot pedal resisting spring tension
- Repeat 5 times
- Alternating LE flexion and extension
- Press into right foot at the cuboid calcaneal contact point lowering foot pedal
- As right foot rises increasing flexion, left foot at the cuboid calcaneal contact point lowers foot pedal
- Repeat 5 times

7. Sit to stand half squat

Intent
- Increasing load specifically targeting pelvifemoral, knee flexors, and extensors
- Improve LE coordination of flexion and extension
- Sagittal plane organization during sitting to standing

Gait reasoning ● Improve transfer of force and adaptability from feet through body

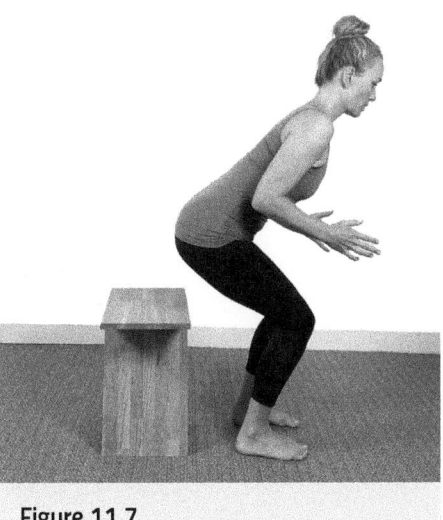

Figure 11.7

Set-up ● Chair or Trapeze Table

Starting position ● Sitting on edge of Trapeze Table or a stable chair, hip joints slightly higher than knees
● LE parallel stance
● UE alongside, elbows flexed at 90 degrees

Movement description ● Lean spine forward folding into hip flexion, keeping head in central axis
● Load the feet from the cuboid-calcaneal through mid-foot with forefoot contact
● Extend the LE to stand
● Initiate descent to sitting by ischial tuberosities moving posterior for hip flexion, gliding femoral head posterior and inferior
● Foot loads toward cuboid-calcaneal contact to sit
● 5 repetitions

8. Standing roll-down bar press down

Intent
- Stimulate torso midline orientation and proprioceptive coordination through variable spring resistance from the roll-down bar
- Whole-body integration in standing

Gait reasoning
- Adaptability with extensor activation for forward propulsion phase
- Integrate movement of the foot and lower limb with ground force reaction
- Improve push-off, swing, and stance

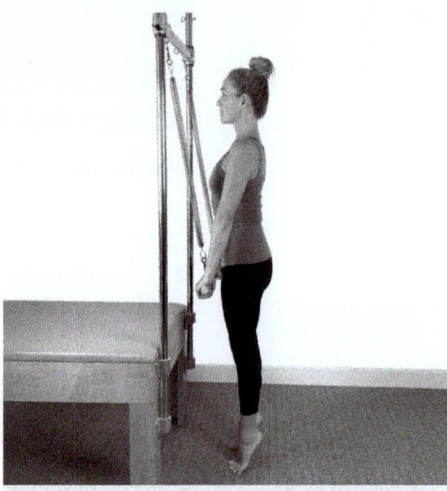

Figure 11.8

Set-up
- Trapeze Table with roll-down bar attached at horizontal sliding bar set 4" (10 cm) from top
- 2 very light short springs

Starting position
- Standing on the floor facing the roll-down bar in parallel stance, 1 ft (30.5 cm) away
- Hands hold outer edge of roll-down bar
- Elbows flexed and abducted
- No tension in the springs

Movement description
- Extend elbows pressing roll-down bar towards feet
- Maintain torso midline orientation as the elbows extend
- Flex elbows, return to starting position
- 5 repetitions
- Extend elbows, simultaneously plantar flex while pressing the roll-down bar towards feet
- Maintain torso midline orientation as the elbows extend
- Lower feet, dorsiflexion
- Flex elbows, return to starting position
- 5 repetitions

9. Seated UE abduction/ external rotation

Intent
- Articulation of glenohumeral joint, integrated coordinating with cervical, thoracic, scapulae, and clavicular movement
- Improve tissue glide of UE stimulating glide of thorax and cervical regions

Gait reasoning
- Organization of shoulder girdle for UE swing
- Improve proprioception of central axis through thoracic extension and rotation

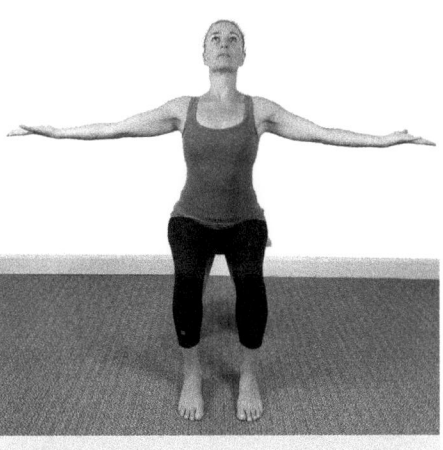

Figure 11.9

Set-up
- Chair or Trapeze Table

Starting position ● Seated on edge of Trapeze Table or chair
● Feet in contact with floor, slightly wider apart than hip joints
● UE 45 degrees abduction, palms down

Movement description ● Inhale to prepare
● Exhale leading with thumbs, externally rotate glenoid humeral joint to 90 degrees abduction
● As hands rise, gently extend upper thorax
● Inhale, continue to feel the manubrium moving, slight posterior rotation and external rotation of UE
● Exhale to return to starting position
● 2 repetitions

CUES

◆ During gentle upper thoracic extension and manubrium movement, maintain integrity of the lumbopelvic organization
◆ Cue the movement to be performed gently and slowly

The journey to Session 11

Session 4/12
Client self-report

● Strong influenza, shivering, and cold symptoms after Session 3, which offset a feeling of being overwhelmed and sad
● Fear of not being able to cope
● Fear of moving and doing the home program again
● Fatigue scale 5
● Pain scale 5

Key changes observed

● Strong reactions to moving with nausea and dizziness
● Shallow breathing

Reasoning behind choice of movements

● Began upright with feet for tactile and proprioceptive feelings to minimize the nausea and dizziness
● Applying heat SmartSpine to refine interoceptive skills, ease tension and the sensation of shivering and cold in the body
● Gentle torso movements of flexion, extension, and rotation close to the midline to stimulate neuromyofascial resiliency to ease discomfort
● Home program only to be executed once a week to decrease onset of cold and influenza symptoms; fewer repetitions of each exercise
● Removed cervical flexion and extension, added cervical rotation on soft partially inflated ball 8.5" diameter
● Removed small pelvic bridge

Session movement sequence
1. Repeat of home program

2. Mat sequences

- Supine leg slides
- Weight shifting seated and standing

3. Wunda Chair

- Leg Pumps

4. Mat

- Supine constructive rest with heat

Session 5/12
Client self-report

- Feeling exhausted and stressed due to personal circumstances
- Had a strong reaction after Session 4 of feeling sad and wanting to cry
- Feels more conscious about the relation between the body and mental states
- Fatigue scale 8
- Pain scale 5

Key changes observed

- Due to extreme tiredness session was shortened
- Applying heat has a relaxing effect and reduces the feeling of cold and influenza symptoms
- Has less nausea reactions and is more present

Reasoning behind choice of movements

- Reduced program allowing the body to feel safe and adapt to the movements

Session movement sequence
1. Repeat of home program

2. Mat sequences

- Supine leg slides
- Weight shifting seated and standing

3. Wunda Chair

- Leg Pumps

Session 6/12
Client self-report

- First session after COVID-19 lockdown
- Understands the impact a stressful lifestyle has on her body
- Refined awareness of internal listening skills and improved ability to not overload daily life
- Fatigued after being back at work after lockdown from increased stress, sadness, poor sleep patterns
- Fatigue scale 8
- Pain scale 8

Key changes observed

- Initially presented with dominant torso extensor tone, an anterior pelvic rotation, and excessive lumbar sagittal curvature
- As session progresses the excessive tone was less dominant
- Improved breathing pattern with thorax orientation relative to the pelvis
- Reasoning behind choice of movements
- Improve breathing and lessening of excessive anterior-posterior curvature for ease in gait
- Synchronizing torso rotation with alternating LE movement
- Felt sense of midline, evenly loaded ischial tuberosities in sitting for vestibular stimuli
- Felt sense right and left foot loading in standing for vestibular stimuli

Session movement sequence

1. Repeat of home program

2. Mat sequences

- Repeat of home program
- Constructive rest with heat
- Supine leg slides
- Supine rotations
- Weight shifting seated and standing

Session 7/12
Client self-report

- Very tired after the last session, achy sensations
- Feels positive about progression despite reactions
- Coping with the feeling of being overwhelmed
- Improved awareness of unconscious holding and ability to shift stiffness through the home program
- Fatigue scale 4
- Pain scale 3

Key changes observed

- Good integration of the pelvic series achieving more coordination and range of movement
- Sudden onset of nausea during the cervical rotation supine on half roller
- Session was shortened with less exercises than planned
- Reasoning behind choice of movements
- Repetition of a reduced program so as not to induce feelings of overwhelm
- Recognition of the same exercises to create a sense of safety

Session movement sequence

1. Repeat of home program

2. Mat sequences

- Constructive rest with heat
- Repeat of home program
- Supine leg slides
- Supine rotations
- Weight shifting seated and standing

Session 8/12
Client self-report

- Symptoms of shivering and cold after Session 7, but felt relaxed and had deep uninterrupted sleep
- An increased awareness of the stress affecting movement patterns
- Kinesiophobia head and neck
- Acceptance of the traumas that reside in the body and grateful to be guided to a better place
- Fatigue scale 4
- Pain scale 4

Key changes observed

- Improved organization when supine overall and during supine anterior-posterior pelvic rotations exercise
- Experience of micro neck movements facilitated an emotional reaction of crying with memories of the car accident
- Reasoning behind choice of movements
- Repetition of key exercises from Sessions 6 and 7 to progress at a slow pace, to test if repetition and recognition of the program will give less symptoms of shivering and cold

Session movement sequence

1. Repeat of home program

2. Mat sequences

- Constructive rest with heat

- Repeat of home program
- Supine leg slides
- Supine rotations
- Weight shifting seated and standing

Session 9/12
Client self-report

- Feels on the right track with a reduction of shivering and cold symptoms post-session
- Feels heavy in the body with sore eyes and fuzzy head
- The exercises are experienced deep in the body
- Fatigue scale 7
- Pain scale 6

Key changes observed

- Improved somatic understanding
- Able to move through the program with less overwhelm
- Increased ROM of the shoulder girdle without pain

Reasoning behind choice of movements

- Constructive rest at beginning and end of session to help self-regulation and reduce symptoms of cold and influenza
- Repetition of key exercises with increased focus on gentle breathing
- Continue to find ease movements with cervical flexion and extension; cervical rotation and weight shifting seated and standing
- Facilitate newfound ROM of the shoulder girdle into unconscious consciousness
- Observing the symptoms that arise, but not reacting to them

Session movement sequence
1. Repeat of home program

2. Mat sequences

- Supine constructive rest with heat
- Repeat of home program
- Supine rotations
- Seated arm and chest opening
- Weight shifting seated and standing
- Supine constructive rest with eye mask

Session 10/12
Client self-report

- Heaviness in the body with deep sleep after previous session with no symptoms of cold and influenza
- Feeling of progression and a better somatic understanding during exercises and in daily life
- Feels relieved and lighter
- Fatigue scale 2–3
- Pain scale 2–3

Key changes observed

- Improved organization of LE patterning during flexion and extension in Sit to stand half squat
- Fluid integration of key exercises
- Right hip flexor unable to sustain movement in sagittal lumbopelvic femoral series

Reasoning behind choice of movements

- Repetition of key exercises with the new additions to develop confidence
- Added squat series to improve endurance and organization during flexion and extension

Session movement sequence
1. Repeat of home program

2. Mat sequences

- Supine constructive rest with heat

- Repeat of home program
- Supine rotations
- Weight shifting seated and standing
- Sit to stand half squat
- Seated arm and chest opening

References

Benjet, C., Bromet, E., Karam, E. G., Kessler, R. C. *et al.* (2016) "The epidemiology of traumatic event exposure worldwide: Results from the World Mental Health Survey Consortium." *Psychological Medicine, 46,* 2, 327–343.

Black, M. (2022) *Centered: Organizing the Body through Kinesiology, Movement Theory and Pilates Techniques.* Edinburgh: Handspring Publishing, p. 184.

Chaitow, L. (2018) "Removing obstacles to recovery: Therapeutic methods, mechanisms and fascia." In: L. Chaitow (Ed.) *Fascial Dysfunction: Manual Therapy Approaches.* 2nd Ed. Edinburgh: Handspring Publishing, p. 127.

Gilbert, C. (2014a) "Interaction of psychological and emotional variables with breathing dysfunction." In: L. Chaitow, D. Bradley, and C. Gilbert (Eds.) *Recognizing and Treating Breathing Disorders: A Multidisciplinary Approach.* 2nd Ed. Edinburgh: Churchill Livingstone Elsevier, pp. 82–83.

Gilbert, C. (2014b) "Psychological assessment of breathing problems." In: L. Chaitow, D. Bradley, and C. Gilbert., (Eds.) *Recognizing and Treating Breathing Disorders: A Multidisciplinary Approach.* 2nd Ed. Edinburgh: Churchill Livingstone Elsevier, pp. 129–136.

Heines, S. (2016) *Trauma Is Really Strange.* London: Singing Dragon, pp. 3, 24–28.

Klingler, W. R. (2021) "Temperature effects on fascia." In: R. Schleip and J. Wilke (Eds.) *Fascia in Sport and Movement.* 2nd Ed. Edinburgh: Handspring Publishing, pp. 22–23.

Kolar, P., Kobesova, A., Valouchova, P., and Bitnar, P. (2014) "Dynamic neuromuscular stabilization: Developmental kinesiology: Breathing sterotypes and postural–locomotion function." In: L. Chaitow, D. Bradley, and C. Gilbert (Eds.) *Recognizing and Treating Breathing Disorders: A Multidisciplinary Approach.* 2nd Ed. Edinburgh: Churchill Livingstone Elsevier, p. 15.

Levine, P. (2008) *Healing Trauma.* Boulder, CO: Sounds True, p. 31.

Linden, D. J. (2016) *Touch: The Science of Hand, Heart, and Mind.* New York: Penguin Random House, p. 63.

Meert, G. F. (2012) "Fluid dynamics in fascial tissues." In: R. Schleip, T. W. Findley, L. Chaitow, and P. A. Huijing (Eds.) *Fascia: The Tensional Network of the Human Body.* Edinburgh: Churchill Livingstone Elsevier, p. 179.

Milanesi, R. and Caregnato, R. C. (2016) "Intra-abdominal pressure: An integrative review." *Einstein (Sao Paulo, Brazil), 14,* 3, 423–430.

NPCE Study Guide (National Pilates Certification Exam Study Guide) (2021) Miami, FL: National Pilates Certification Program, Inc.

Payne, P., Levine, P. A., and Crane-Godreau, M. A. (2015) "Somatic experiencing: Using interoception and proprioception as core elements of trauma therapy." *Frontiers in Psychology, 6,* 93. DOI: 10.3389/fpsyg.2015.00093.

Pilat, A. (2022) *Myofascial Induction: Volume 1—The Upper Body.* Edinburgh: Handspring Publishing, pp. 440–441.

Porges, S. W. (2017) *The Pocket Guide to the Polyvagal Theory.* New York: W. W. Norton & Company, pp. 112–114.

Porges, S. W. (2021) *Polyvagal Safety: Attachment, Communication, Self Regulation.* New York: W. W. Norton & Company, pp. 72–74, 173–176.

Schleip, R. and Stecco, C. (2021) "Fascia as sensory organ." In: R. Schleip and J. Wilke (Eds.) *Fascia in Sport and Movement.* 2nd Ed. Edinburgh: Handspring Publishing, pp. 176–177.

Substance Abuse and Mental Health Services Administration (2014) "Trauma-Informed Care in Behavioral Health Services." Treatment Improvement Protocol (TIP) Series 57. HHS Publication No. (SMA) 13-4801. Rockville, MD: Substance Abuse and Mental Health Services Administration, pp. 4–7, 128.

Upledger, J. E. and VredeVoogd, J. D. (2019) *Craniosacral Therapy.* 35th Ed. Seattle, WA: Eastland Press, pp. 133–136.

van der Kolk, B. (2014) *The Body Keeps the Score: Brain, Mind, and Body in the Healing of Trauma.* London: Allen Lane, pp. 80–83, 86, 100–101.

Pilates and Long COVID With Underlying Condition of Cushing's Disease: Effect on Gait

Rosa Marimba Gold-Watts

This client contracted SARS COVID-19, which subsequently became long-haul COVID-19. Long-haul COVID or post-COVID symptoms are a wide range of symptoms that present at least four weeks after having had the disease, and can appear with varying degrees of severity even when initial symptoms are mild (see box below). COVID-19 is associated with an increase of inflammation in the body, or mast cell activation (see box below), as well as joint and muscle pain. It was impossible in this case to identify whether increased joint and muscle pain was due to symptoms of COVID-19 or long-term complications of having Cushing's disease (a pre-existing condition), as there is extensive overlap in both symptoms and common presentation, as well as in the evolution of both diseases.

Symptoms reported by the client of long-haul COVID have included:

- Tachycardia
- Extensive numbness, cold, and tingling primarily in the right side of her body
- Increased systemic inflammation
- An increase in previous Cushing's symptoms, including thoracic pain and muscle spasms, inflammation, and mast cell activation

Long-haul COVID interacts with pre-existing conditions to amplify the symptoms. In this case, Cushing's disease preceded COVID-19. Cushing's disease is a rare disease most often characterized by an increased level of cortisol due to a pituitary adenoma. Increased cortisol may impact a number of areas of the body, with symptoms as wide-ranging as hip joint and shoulder weakness, chronic swelling, osteoporosis, fatigue, impaired immunological function, and poor concentration, as well as symptoms that are specific to each patient (Mayo Clinic Staff 2023a). The effects of Cushing's disease are extremely challenging to identify as they share many things in common with other health conditions. A definitive diagnosis was made only after a lengthy period of time, and unfortunately, due to the delay, the disease had progressed significantly. The client in this case report had a tumor removed from her pituitary gland three years prior to our sessions, and has been recovering from the long-term effects of excessive levels of cortisol. Diagnostic imaging usually shows a tumor in roughly half of the diagnosed patients, even when one has been confirmed through other methods such as surgery or bloodwork.

In addition to these issues, the client has a number of other chronic degenerative issues which make immune function and physical recovery challenging. All of the practitioners involved with this client's recovery have found it impossible to differentiate between issues caused by COVID and Cushing's disease and normal degenerative changes of the body, as both diseases seem to exacerbate all pre-existing conditions.

While working with the client, she was not always able to build on previous work due to the long COVID and Cushing's symptoms, so our progression was not linear. Additionally, when the client was having major symptoms of tachycardia, the movement program was significantly reduced with limited positional changes and transitions, and therefore some weeks contain considerably more exercises than others. Lastly, the client experienced a back injury unrelated to these sessions before Session 6, which caused some setbacks and resulted in some significant changes in our final assessment.

Movement contraindications and considerations for this client:

- Extreme flexion and extension
- Transitions between exercises and on or off equipment due to dizziness or tachycardia
- Back injury unrelated to our sessions sustained before Session 6

(See Editor note on long COVID at the beginning of Chapter 13.)

Client description: 57-year-old biological female, identifies as female; Pilates teacher

Dates of case report: Session 1 (February 10, 2021); Session 12 (May 27, 2021). All sessions were virtual over Zoom. They were not continuous because of client's heart symptoms and tachycardia due to long COVID-19

Tachycardia

Tachycardia is a rapid heart rate (over 100 beats per minute) that may or may not be irregular and is not in proportion with the level of exertion or activity being performed. Symptoms include chest palpitations and the sensation of a racing heart, dizziness, a rapid pulse, shortness of breath, and in some cases fainting (Mayo Clinic Staff 2023b).

Props such as the sling and deflated 9 in. (23 cm) ball were used to simulate proprioceptive feedback.

Postural orthostatic tachycardia syndrome (POTS)

Postural orthostatic tachycardia syndrome (POTS) is a type of tachycardia related to positional changes of the body, most commonly seated to standing or lying down to standing. This is particularly relevant in a Pilates setting where a client is being asked to change positions on equipment frequently. In this case, I tried to limit big transitions such as floor to standing, instead using progressions that could be performed slowly and with minimal change in level, for example seated to supine, supine or prone to side lying, etc.

Author note

Although not optimal, the sessions were virtual due to both geographical location and limitations to in-person sessions because of the pandemic. However, in-person sessions would have been preferable in this case, both for the challenges of transitions between equipment when the client was experiencing pain and tachycardia symptoms and for the option of using hands-on cueing to aid in proprioception.

Mast cell activation syndrome

Mast cell activation syndrome (MCAS) is an immunological condition in which mast cells become hyper-responsive and cause a wide range of chronic symptoms that are similar to an allergic response. It is considered a mast cell activation disorder and is associated with both COVID-19 and Cushing's syndrome. Symptoms can include tachycardia, flushing, hives, headaches, abdominal cramping and diarrhea, nausea, respiratory symptoms, and hypotension (Walker 2021).

Studio apparatus and props
Pilates equipment

- Trapeze Table
- Universal Reformer
- Wunda Chair
- Pilates Arc
- Magic Circle

Props used with equipment

- Sling
- 9 in. (23 cm) partially deflated ball
- 3 in. (8 cm) ball
- 4 in. (10 cm) yoga block
- Long box
- Mat

Home program props
Home program includes equipment because client teaches Pilates and has access to equipment

- Trapeze Table
- Stability sling
- 9 in. (23 cm) partially deflated ball
- Mat

Methods and materials

Session 1/12
1. Health history interview

- Long COVID-19
- Chronic right side numbness and tingling due to COVID-19
- Cushing's disease
- Degenerative disc disease (cervical and lumbar) associated with persistent back pain
- Spinal stenosis, cervical, L5/S1
- POTS
- Inguinal hernias on right and left; right is more severe
- 60 percent tear in right rotator cuff
- History of frozen shoulder
- Chronic right shoulder pain

2. Symptoms

- Shortness of breath
- Tachycardia/POTS
- Dizziness
- Excessive production of cortisol
- Persistent lumbar and pelvic pain

3. Movement aids

- None, except for occasional use of a sacroiliac joint (SIJ) belt introduced right before our last session

Final result of case report
Despite experiencing back pain in our last 6 sessions, due to an injury sustained outside of this case report, the client demonstrated notable improvement in the assessments of hemi-pelvis superior motion, hip translation, gait lower extremity (LE) swing mechanics, increased thoracic rotation, and breathing capacity. The client had fewer episodes of dizziness due to consistent breathing practice.

Session 2/12: Initial assessment

1. General observations of gait

◆ Short stride length with limited LE extension and no lateral pelvic shift

◆ Excessive movement of right innominate

◆ Limited movement of left innominate

◆ Left heel strike to stance phase: right innominate elevates and mid- to lower thorax side bends creating momentum to transfer weight onto right leg

◆ Abducts LE through frontal plane rather than moving through flexion/sagittal plane

◆ Limited arm swing, especially the right, due to an adaptation for rotator cuff injury

◆ Thoracic rotation limited to the thoracolumbar junction (TLJ)

2. Standing tests

◆ Full torso rotation

● Observations of inefficient side: left
  ■ Lacks ocular, cervical, and upper thoracic rotation
  ■ Left rotation: right scapula abducts, left scapula adducts
  ■ Rotation occurs at TLJ
  ■ Right hemipelvis superior motion on left pelvis rotation
  ■ Left foot lacks supination, right foot pronates

◆ Hemipelvis inferior motion

Session 12/12: Post-assessment

1. General observations of gait

◆ Longer stride length with improved LE extension and lateral pelvic shift on both sides equally

◆ Less movement of right innominate

◆ Improved movement of left innominate

◆ Left heel strike to stance phase: less right innominate elevation, less mid- to lower thorax side bending

◆ Improved LE motion from frontal plane to sagittal plane motion

◆ Improved arm swing on both sides

◆ Thoracic rotation similar to initial assessment

2. Standing tests

◆ Full torso rotation

● Observations of inefficient side: right
  ■ Greater ease of motion bilaterally despite inefficient side changing from left to right
  ■ Right rotation: right scapula adducts, left scapula abducts
  ■ Rotation occurs at TLJ
  ■ Right hemipelvis superior motion on right and left rotation
  ■ Right rotation foot pronation not as supple as original assessment

- Observations of inefficient side: left
  - Right lateral lumbar flexion limited
  - Left thoracic translation
  - Excessive extension at TLJ

◆ Hemipelvis superior motion

- Observations of inefficient side: left
  - Right thoracic translation excessive relative to hemipelvis superior motion
  - Right lumbar lateral flexion limited
  - Limited right hip adduction

◆ Lateral pelvic shift

- Observations of inefficient side: right
  - Consistent with both right hemipelvis superior motion and restricted thoracic range of motion (ROM)
  - Less control and loss of balance
  - TLJ shifts left
  - Upper thoracic right translation

3. Seated tests

◆ Thoracic rotation

- Observations of inefficient side: left

Author note

The right side became inefficient due to left SIJ and right upper thorax pain. The client experienced pain in the pelvis on the left side of the SIJ with right rotation.

◆ Hemipelvis inferior motion

- Observations of inefficient side: left
  - Right lateral lumbar flexion limited
  - Thorax still translates left
  - Less extension at TLJ
  - Increased thoracic left translation with lumbar right lateral flexion

Author note

This finding may have been influenced by pain of the left SIJ due to an injury sustained outside of our sessions before Session 6.

◆ Hemipelvis superior motion

- Observations of inefficient side: left
  - Right thoracic translation less excessive relative to hemipelvis superior motion
  - Right lumbar lateral flexion limited
  - Slight improvement in right hip adduction

◆ Lateral pelvic shift

- Observations of inefficient side: right
  - More ease on left
  - More control and better balance
  - TLJ remains stable
  - Less upper thoracic right translation

3. Seated tests

◆ Thoracic rotation

- Observations of inefficient side: right

- Lacks thoracic rotation
- Adducts left scapula to increase ROM
- Abducts right scapula to increase ROM

◆ Hip joint and knee flexion

● Observations of inefficient side: right
   - Generally good hip flexion bilaterally, right exhibited more effort
   - Shifted weight to left ischial tuberosity with lumbar lateral flexion

Author note

Included dorsiflexion and knee flexion test. Right was inefficient. Limited dorsiflexion and plantar flexion. Included hip abduction with external rotation. Right was inefficient. Limited hip abduction and external rotation.

4. Sit and stand

◆ Lateral view

● Efficient knee, hip joint flexion, and ankle dorsiflexion
● Thoracolumbar junction extension when moving from sit to stand

◆ Anterior view

● Rises evenly without any notable weight shift or lateral translation
● Efficient knee, hip joint flexion, and ankle dorsiflexion
● Maintains LE organization throughout

- Lacks thoracic rotation
- Adducts right scapula to increase ROM
- Abducts left scapula to increase ROM

Author note

This was a change from our initial assessment. The lack of tissue glide created a pinching sensation when rotating right. This was consistent with the post-assessment findings in standing rotation.

◆ Hip joint and knee flexion

● Observations of inefficient side: right
   - Improvement in right hip joint flexion
   - Weight on ischial tuberosities even with no lumbar lateral flexion

Author note

Included dorsiflexion and knee flexion test. Right ankle dorsiflexion improved despite right being more limited than left. Included hip abduction with external rotation. Improved right hip abduction and external rotation.

4. Sit and stand

◆ Lateral view

● Efficient knee, hip joint flexion, and ankle dorsiflexion
● Thoracolumbar junction extension when moving from sit to stand

◆ Anterior view

● Rises evenly without any notable weight shift or lateral translation
● Efficient knee, hip joint flexion, and ankle dorsiflexion
● Maintains LE organization throughout

5. Standing balance

◆ Two-leg stance, eyes open

● 60 seconds
● Relative ease standing with fatigue at the end of 60 seconds
● Feels mild posterior torso strain when standing

◆ One-leg stance, eyes open

● Right side is unstable
● Fatigued on right side

5. Standing balance

◆ Two-leg stance, eyes open

● 60 seconds
● More ease when standing
● Significant improvement in stamina
● Improved balance and midline orientation
● Feels less strain when standing, despite chronic pain in recent weeks

◆ One-leg stance, eyes open

● Significant improvement in right leg stance: less fatigue, improved balance

Session 3/12: Home program

Fatigue scale	4
Pain scale	5

Client self-report
- Significant brain fog and nerve sensitivity on right side, including down the right leg

Key changes observed by author at end of Session 3/12
- Standing more upright
- Calmer and more present
- Increased ROM of hip joints
- Improved torso articulation

Reason behind choice of sequencing
- Increase torso and hip joints articulation
- Coordination of pelvifemoral movement
- Improve torso activation through variety of load distribution
- Improve upper extremity (UE) ability to swing freely with thoracic rotation
- Improve push-off

Session movement sequence

1. Mermaid on Trapeze Table   J.H. Pilates Mermaid on Universal Reformer (NPCE Study Guide 2021, p. 64)

Intent
- Amplify coupled movement of translation and rotation
- Tissue glide restriction due to inflammation associated with both COVID and Cushing's disease
- Improve breathing with introducing elastic movement quality and glide of the structures and surrounding tissues in torso

Editor note
Tissue glide is restricted with an increased systemic inflammation due to the viral toxins and cytokine storm (Pilat 2022) associated with COVID. Cushing's disease is a state of chronic glucocorticoid excess that is associated with increased inflammation (Shah *et al.* 2017). In both diseases, improving gentle tissue glide helps the client move without excess resistance, increasing the ability to exercise.

Gait reasoning
- Improve torso's ability to laterally flex
- Increased counter-rotation of the thorax and pelvis
- Improve rib osteokinematics for respiration patterning to increase stamina (Lee 2018)

Set-up
- Bar top-loaded with 1 medium spring

Starting position	• Sitting sideways on the Trapeze Table near push-through bar
	• Feet supported on box
	• Holding bar with hand nearest to bar with resting spring
	• Other hand behind head
Movement description	• Pull bar down and extend elbow
	• Push bar away to laterally flex toward the bar
	• Opposite hemipelvis is weighted on table
	• Return to starting position through articulation from bottom to top

2. Unilateral Leg Springs on Trapeze Table	Derivative of J. H. Pilates Leg Springs: Bicycle, Walking, Scissors, Circles (NPCE Study Guide 2021, pp. 67–68) (see Chapter 5, Trier)
Intent	• Lumbopelvic femoral relative movement
	• Increase torso proprioception during LE movement
	• Unilateral variations to ease pelvic pain
Gait reasoning	• Pelvifemoral motions for leg swing
	• Increase hip joint articulation and medial glide
	• Improve hip joint flexion and control

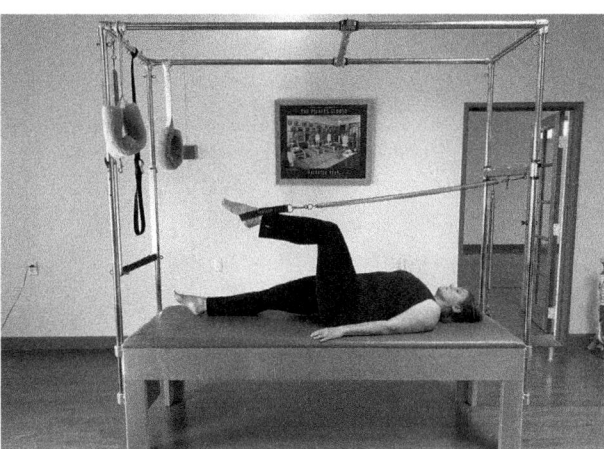

Figure 12.1

Set-up	• Medium leg spring sprung from slider bar lateral eye bolt

Starting position
- Supine on Trapeze Table
- One foot in strap, hip joint flexion, knee extended, foot plantar flexed
- Unsprung side: knee flexion, foot resting on mat

Editor note

The variety of Trapeze Tables have multiple eye bolts on the slider bar. The choice of placement of the leg spring will determine the angle of the variable resistance. The angle affects the dynamic pelvifemoral relationship. The training effect will vary according to the angle of the spring chosen.

Movement description
- Pull spring with hip extension
- Maintain resistance as femur returns to flexion
- Repeat 8 times
- Stay in flexion, flex, and extend the knee, preventing the femur from adducting or abducting
- Repeat 8 times
- Hip joint rotation: continuous arcing motion of flexion to abduction, pulling down toward table, adduction to midline/flexion
  - LE external rotation, 5 times
  - LE internal rotation, 5 times

3. Bridges with sling on Trapeze Table

Intent
- Improve hip joint extension
- Lumbopelvic femoral relative movement
- Use sling to support the pelvis

Gait reasoning
- Improve extension for push-off phase
- Pre-load torso

Set-up
- Sling sprung from above with 2 medium long springs

Starting position
- Supine on mat with knee flexion, heels in line with ischial tuberosities
- Place sling under pelvis for support
- UE at sides or resting on springs
- After the first few sessions, added placing the feet on an arc to increase hip joint ROM and activation of extensors

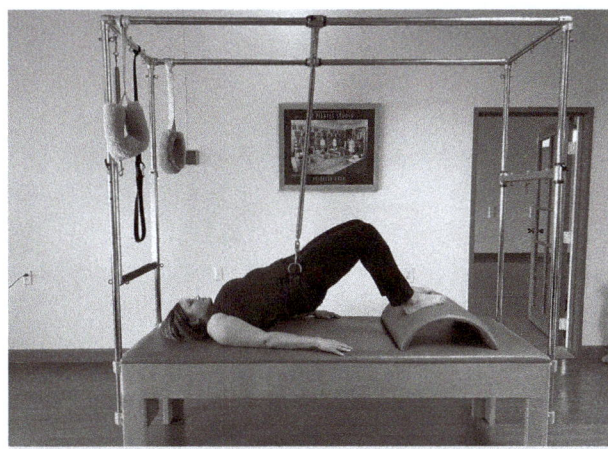

Figure 12.2

Movement description	● Press feet into mat or arc
	● Extend acetabular-femoral joints as torso lifts
	● Lower slowly returning to starting position

4. Hip joint extension with push-through bar on Trapeze Table

Intent	● Increase hip joint extension
	● Differentiate pelvifemoral motions
	● Pre-loading of LE
Gait reasoning	● Improve extension in the push-off phase
	● Improve timing of extension from feet to torso more efficiently
Set-up	● Push-through bar sprung from below with a very light or light push-through spring
	● Long box placed with one edge near push-through bar
Starting position	● Prone on long box with pelvis and superior aspect of femur at the edge
	● Place one heel underneath bar in contact with push-through bar

231

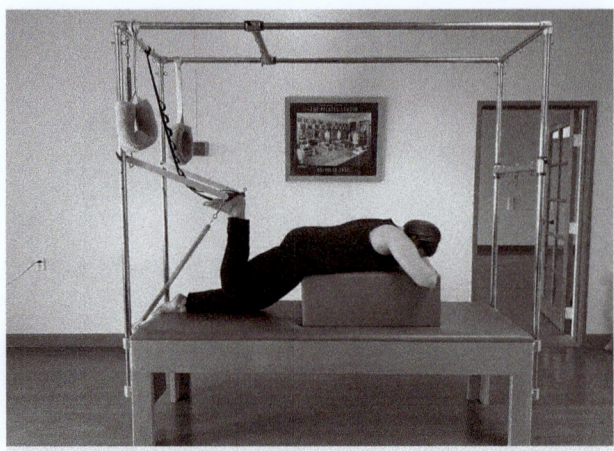

Figure 12.3

Movement description	• Press bar up with heel, extending hip joint • Knee remains flexed • Weight distribution of anterior pelvis on box remains constant

5. Nod and curl with push-through bar on Trapeze Table

Derivative of J. H. Pilates Push-Through Bar, Springs from Above, Upper Arms on Trapeze Table (NPCE Study Guide 2021, p. 63)

Intent	• Improve head and neck relationship for ease of cervical ROM
Gait reasoning	• Improve cervical and thoracic rotation for arm swing • Reduce lack of shoulder girdle glide to ease arm swing
Set-up	• Push-through bar loaded with 1 medium spring from above
Starting position	• Supine on Trapeze Table with head underneath bar • Both hands hold bar • Shoulders at 90 degrees flexion, hands in line with shoulders
Movement description	• Flex at the atlanto-occipital joint, focusing on rocking the occipital condyles • Lift head 1 in. (2.5 cm) off mat maintaining chin relationship to sternum • Articulate into flexion from head • Bar assists in pulling torso into flexion

6. Footwork on Universal Reformer

J. H. Pilates Footwork on Universal Reformer (NPCE Study Guide 2021, p. 52)

Intent
- Articulate pelvifemoral motions
- Pre-loading LE
- Improve timing and control of LE

Gait reasoning
- Articulation of LE for swing
- Initiating from hip joint extension rather than knee extension strategy for more efficient distribution of ground forces

Set-up
- Medium spring

Starting position
- Supine on Universal Reformer
- Arches of feet on footbar

Movement description
- Press into feet to activate LE
- Initiate from hip joint extension, pressing carriage away
- Extend knees
- Return carriage home, initiating from femoral glide into flexion
- Repeat 10 times

7. UE Press on Universal Reformer

Intent
- Proximal activation from torso to hand
- Maintain torso in frontal plane as UE extends

Gait reasoning
- Improve shoulder girdle and UE organization for arm swing
- Improve tissue resiliency and glide for ease in arm swing and reduction of pain

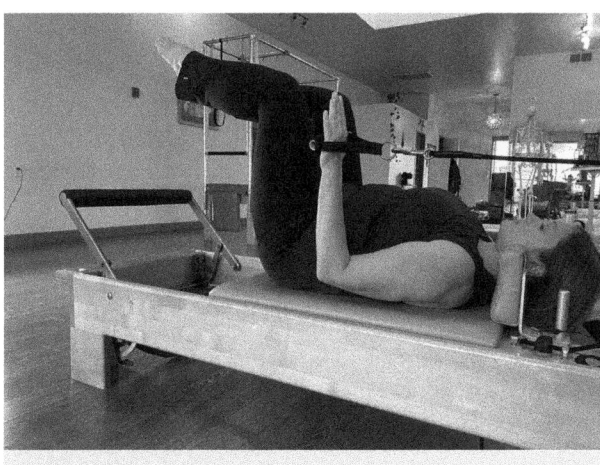

Figure 12.4

Starting position	● Supine on Universal Reformer
	● Hip and knee flexion at 90 degrees
	● One or both hands in straps or handles
	● Elbow flexion to 90 degrees
Movement description	● Keep elbows hovering slightly off mat
	● Pull handle into elbow extension with one or both arms down
	● Flex elbows
	● Return to starting position
	● Repeat 10 times

8. Modified Single Leg Stretch on Universal Reformer

Derivative of J. H. Pilates Single Leg Stretch on mat (NPCE Study Guide 2021, p. 46)

Intent	● Challenge flexion movement
	● Coordination of UE and LE movement
Gait reasoning	● Alternating LE flexion and extension
	● UE and LE coordination
Starting position	● Supine on Universal Reformer
	● Hip and knee flexion at 90 degrees
	● Elbows at 90 degree flexion with elbows at sides
	● Head remains on headrest
Movement description	● Exhale, extend right LE to 45 degrees, extending elbows at the same time
	● Flex right LE and elbows returning to starting position
	● Change to left LE
	● Repeat alternating right and left 5 times

9. Single leg ankle unilateral plantar and dorsiflexion on Universal Reformer

Derivative of J.H. Pilates Running on Universal Reformer Running (NPCE Study Guide 2021, p. 60)

Intent	● Articulate the foot through plantar flexion and dorsiflexion
	● Improve stamina of LE (prior history of LE issues may contribute to poor stamina)
	● Pre-load unilateral stance
Gait reasoning	● Articulate the foot to adapt to ground surfaces
	● Activate LE for push-off phase of gait
	● Pre-load for stance phase
	● Increase stride length

Set-up
- Springs: 1 or 2 medium

Starting position
- Supine on Universal Reformer
- Place right metatarsal arch on footbar with LE extended
- Left LE in 90 degrees hip joint and knee flexion

Movement description
- Press metatarsal arch on footbar to plantar flex ankle
- Dorsiflex ankle allowing the calcaneus to move under footbar
- Maintain LE extension
- Repeat 10 times

10. Modified Knee Stretch on forearms on Universal Reformer

Derivative of J. H. Pilates Knee Stretch Series on Universal Reformer (NPCE Study Guide 2021, p. 60)

Intent
- Increase awareness of femoral glide in flexion and extension
- Challenge torso organization during LE flexion and extension
- Challenge lumbopelvic femoral rhythm and coordination
- Initiate hip joint flexion without pelvic lateral elevation

Gait reasoning
- Three-dimensional movement of hip joint for swing
- Lessen innominate elevation during LE flexion

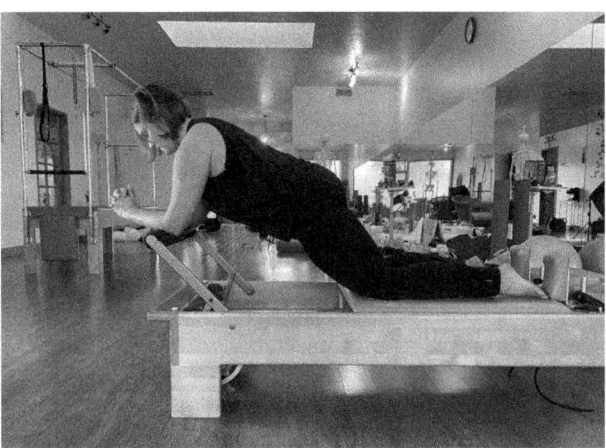

Figure 12.5

Starting position
- Quadruped on Universal Reformer with forearms on footbar
- Torso in optimal organization for movement task
- Plantar surface of feet in contact with shoulder stops
- Metatarsals extended in contact with carriage

Movement description
- Press into feet to move carriage away from footbar extending hip joints
- Flex hip joints, returning carriage home
- Maintain torso in starting position
- UE and shoulder girdle remain in starting position

11. Plantar flexion and dorsiflexion on Wunda Chair

Derivative of J. H. Pilates Achilles Stretch on Wunda Chair (NPCE Study Guide 2021, p. 79)

Intent
- Increase foot mobility
- Improve talar glide

Gait reasoning
- Increase potential for acceleration and deceleration
- Improve push-off phase
- Force absorption of heel strike
- Plantar flexion for force production and propulsion forward

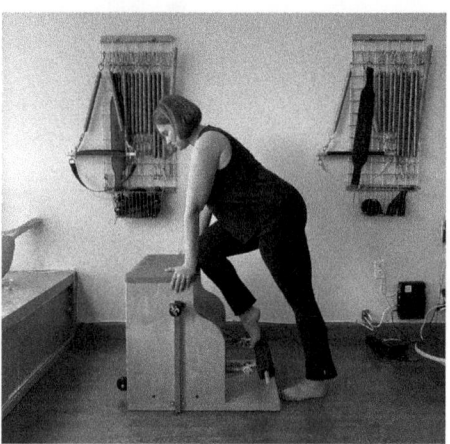

Figure 12.6

Starting position
- Standing facing Wunda Chair
- Place right metatarsal arch on foot pedal with ankle in dorsiflexion
- Right knee rests against edge of seat of chair
- Hands placed on either side of seat
- Torso in optimal organization for the task

Movement description
- Beginning in dorsiflexion, slowly plantar flex the foot
- Return to dorsiflexion

12. Respiration practice: Bellows breathing with knee folds with sling on Trapeze Table

(See Chapter 5, Gentry, Bellows breathing and knee folds)

Intent
- Proprioception of TLJ
- Improve breathing capacity, awareness, thoracic articulation, lung resiliency, and motility
- Train hip joint glide posteriorly and inferiorly in flexion

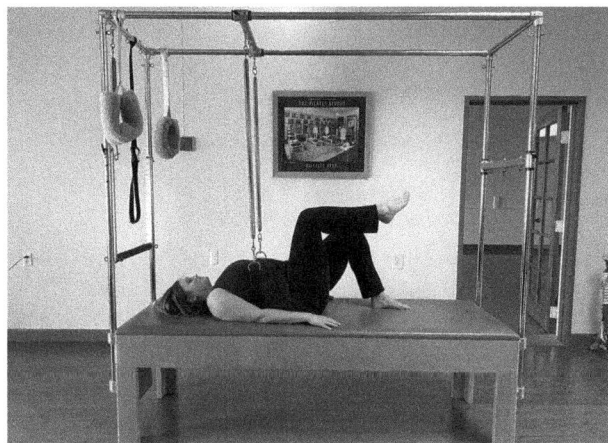

Figure 12.7

Editor note

Neuromyofascial organization affects organ mobility. When the connective tissue is dehydrated, lacking the ability to glide between levels, the biotensegrity balance between tension and compression is disrupted. During breathing, the lungs have an excursion that moves through all dimensions, a spherical-like motion.

Organ motility is the normal intrinsic rhythm of an organ. This movement is inherent to organ function. Motility can be reduced by an issue within the organ itself (such as inflammation), emotional concerns, or an issue related to medication. Motility reduction may also be due to surrounding structures that have been binding an organ and impinging on its cellular motion (Barral and Mercier 2006).

Gait reasoning
- Reinforce efficient standing organization by decreasing the tendency to extend the TLJ

Set-up	• Sling sprung from above on Trapeze Table with 2 medium long (leg) springs
Starting position	• Supine on table, sling at T11–T12/L1 • Feet flat on table, hip and knee flexion
Movement description	• Inhale into the back and sides of the sling, expanding the ribcage for increased flexion at the TLJ • Exhale, keeping sling in contact with table • Right hip and knee flexion, lifting foot off table • Pause at 90 degrees flexion • Lower LE to table • Repeat 10–20 times • Change to left LE and repeat

13. Pelvis level/unlevel on Wunda Chair	Derivative of J. H. Pilates Standing Leg Pump: Side on Wunda Chair (NPCE Study Guide 2021, p. 79)
Intent	• Lumbopelvic femoral movement in lateral plane • Challenge stance LE • Oscillate medial and lateral glide of hip joint with lumbopelvic adaptation in lateral flexion
Gait reasoning	• Improve weight transfer • Challenge supporting leg • Improve pelvic translation • Balance • Improve reciprocal motion in lumbar and thoracic lateral flexion

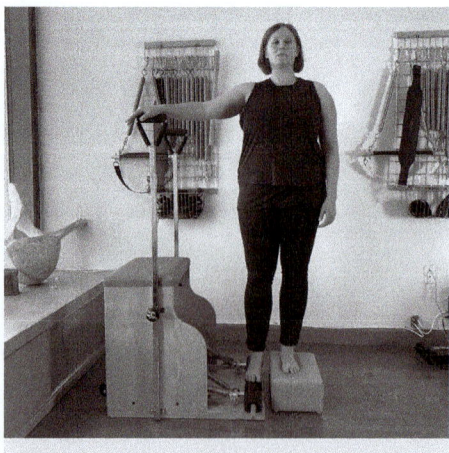

Figure 12.8

Set-up
- Wunda Chair sprung with 2 medium springs
- Place small box on floor on pedal side of chair

Starting position
- Stand perpendicular to chair
- Place left foot on small box and right foot on pedal
- Feet are parallel with each other
- Pedal is aligned with small box
- Inner hand holds handle on chair

Movement description
- Press pedal down slightly unleveling pelvis inferiorly and allowing supporting femoral joint to laterally glide
- Rise pedal upward unleveling pelvis superiorly in the other direction and allowing supporting femoral joint to medially glide
- Once a client feels confident, challenge balance by decreasing dependence of supporting hand on handle
- Repeat until fatigued on supporting LE

Session 11/12: Studio session

Fatigue scale 3

Pain scale 6–7

Client self-report
- Pain in right thoracic and lumbar area as a result of demonstrating an advanced Pilates movement without proper warm-up

Author note
The effects of multiple health-related issues (the combination of both Cushing's disease and COVID) and high levels of pain and fatigue challenged the progression of building a program. Scaling the movement back to basics, especially breathing practice, and the client's consistency of personal practice were a huge boost to her positive outcome.

Key changes observed by author at end of Session 11/12
- Improved ROM of torso
- Perceived back "spasm" was significantly reduced
- Able to breathe better, was less dizzy
- Easier time with movement transitions (sit to stand, supine to seated, etc.)

Reason behind choice of sequencing	• Balance dynamic motions for both gait and associated back pain in all dimensions • Practice breathing to help with dizziness and overall sense of instability • Improve rotation and translation motions to assist with easier weight transfer and transitions

Session movement sequence

1. Standing awareness (See Chapter 5, Kryzanowska: derivative of Wall Series)

Intent	• Bring awareness to distribution of weight while standing
Gait reasoning	• Facilitate verticality and midline orientation especially head and neck relationship • Improve proprioception of head and neck organization • Improve connective tissue glide of thoracolumbar region to reduce discomfort
Set-up	• Unobstructed wall space
Starting position	• Standing with back against wall • Feet are roughly 2 in. (5 cm) away from wall • The back of the head may or may not touch wall, depending on client's body structure
Movement description	• Sense the contact areas, especially TLJ on wall • Inhale, elevate sternum without moving TLJ away from wall • Exhale, allow anterior abdominal connective tissue to draw inward without pulling sternum inferiorly • Hold position for 1–5 breaths • Pause, repeat sequence 5 times

CUES
 • Maintain the lift of the sternum while TLJ remains in contact with wall
 • Head position: keep zygomatic arches level to the floor

Author note

This is a deceptively challenging exercise that allows the client to feel supported vertically. This activates whole-body support minimizing the flexion that occurs when supine. It requires a synergistic activation of the neuromyofascial system to connect the volumes of the pelvis, thorax, and cranium. Performing it against the wall provides increased proprioception. We returned to this exercise regularly to build stamina and awareness in all standing work.

2. Rolling with small ball for posterior-lateral pelvifemoral region

Intent	● Stimulate glide and circulation ● Improve ability for translational movement
Gait reasoning	● Improve ability in hemipelvis superior motion and lower innominates for lateral movement ● Balance medial and lateral hip glide
Set-up	● 3 in. (8 cm) small ball ● 4 in. (10 cm) yoga block ● Mat
Starting position	● Side lying on mat with ball directly under lateral pelvis above greater trochanter ● Knees flexed and slightly elevated on yoga block
Movement description	● Allow body weight to sink into ball ● Hold the place of tenderness until the sensation dissipates ● Move to another spot around the lateral pelvis

CUES
◆ Breathe to allow the tissue to ease
◆ Allow one spot to "ease" up before moving to another spot

Author note
It was necessary to create access to more supple movement in an area that was lacking connective tissue glide.

3. Supine hip adduction

Intent	● Activate continuity of LE to pelvic myofascia ● Bilateral LE adduction
Gait reasoning	● Facilitate midline orientation in sagittal plane motion ● Improve standing balance
Set-up	● 9 in. (23 cm) ball ● Mat
Starting position	● Supine, feet flat on mat, hip and knee flexion ● Feet in line with ischial tuberosities ● Ball between the femurs
Movement description	● Adduct femurs placing pressure on ball ● Hold for 5 seconds ● Release pressure but do not let ball go

CUES
+ Adduct without over activation of hip flexors
+ Avoid posterior tilt when adducting

Author note
Initially, it was challenging to uncouple the over-activation of the hip flexors with posterior pelvic tilt. Over time, the practice of this exercise improved the multi-dimensional activation sequencing of the LE.

4. Pelvic Clocks (Black 2022; Feldenkrais 1985)

Intent
- Articulation of lumbopelvic femoral joints
- Increase proprioception and awareness of lumbopelvic femoral rhythm, particularly tendency to hemipelvis superior motion
- Improve tissue glide

Gait reasoning
- Balance right and left LE movement and appropriate pelvic translation and rotation
- Facilitate figure 8 motion of the lumbopelvic femoral area

Editor note
Efficient gait involves coordinated motions in figure 8 patterns from the feet through to the head. Improving the capacity for movement in all planes is essential for gait patterning.

Set-up
- Partially deflated 9 in. (23 cm) ball
- Mat

Editor note
Placing the sacrum on top of a deflated ball provides the potential advantages of increasing proprioception to the posterior pelvis and elevating the pelvis relative to the thorax. It may also assist in facilitating thoracolumbar fascial glide. Consider also how this dynamic instability contributes to increasing chaos in the vectors of lumbopelvic ground forces.

Starting position
- Supine on mat
- Hip and knee flexion, feet flat on mat in line with ischial tuberosities
- Partially deflated ball placed under sacrum

Movement description	● Imagine wearing a clock
	● Navel is at 12 o'clock, pubis is at 6 o'clock
	● Allow the pelvis to move through all of the numbers on a clock face, from 1 to 12
	● Reverse the circle, pausing wherever there is a feeling of restriction

CUES

- ◆ Try to pause and breathe into areas that feel restricted
- ◆ Make sure to allow bones to drive the movement
- ◆ Try to imagine rolling around the perimeter of the sacrum
- ◆ As the pelvis tips to 3 or 9 o'clock, try to maintain parallel knees so that the pelvis is rotating on the femurs

Author note

The use of a partially deflated 9 in. (23 cm) ball instead of lying flat on the mat decreased the pressure that the client felt on L5/S1 due to stenosis. It provides an easier ability to move from pelvifemoral motion through the feedback of the ball. It increases the proprioception of the pelvis as it moves with a small bit of "assistance" from the ball. In addition, the slight elevation reduced the tension and pain in the thoracic region and allowed more attention to be placed on the lumbopelvic femoral area.

5. Knee folds and femoral abduction with pelvis elevated on partially deflated ball	Derivative of Eve Gentry knee folds and leg slide (see Chapter 5, Gentry)
Intent	● Facilitate femur on pelvis movement
	● Activate LE to torso in flexion/extension and abduction/adduction
	● Improve glide of the connective tissues that are continuous with LE to torso
Gait reasoning	● Improve ease of leg swing
Set-up	● Partially deflated 9 in (23 cm) ball
	● Mat
Starting position	● Supine on mat with pelvis slightly elevated on partially deflated ball
	● Knee flexion, feet flat on mat in line with ischial tuberosities
	● Hands resting on anterior pelvis for proprioception

Movement description
- Knee folds
  - Press into left foot on mat as right LE lifts off mat
  - Right lower limb is dangling, full knee flexion
  - Place right LE on mat 5 times
  - Repeat on other side 5 times
  - Progress to bilateral hip and knee flexion 90/90, lowering one leg toward floor without significant pelvic movement 5 times
  - Repeat on other side 5 times
- Hip joint abduction
  - Press into left foot on mat as right LE abducts
  - Counter the weight of the right LE by placing weight into left posterior pelvis
  - Adduct right LE and return to midline 5 times
  - Repeat on other side 5 times

CUES
- During hip flexion the femoral head glides posteriorly and inferiorly
- Initiate movement with the sensation of the head of the femur sinking prior to lifting foot
- During femoral abduction, feel the weight on the opposite posterior side of the pelvis weighted
- Sense the pelvis weight equally distributed on the ball throughout both movements

Author note
In the attempt of training pelvic awareness with a blood pressure cuff, it was apparent that proprioception was lacking. Supine position on the mat was uncomfortable and triggered pain. Elevating the pelvis slightly eased the stress and allowed for activation of the torso. With a history of inguinal hernias, training the torso on the partially deflated ball allowed for change in movement patterning and reduced pain.

6. Isometric knee folds (See Chapter 5, Gentry, knee folds)
(Black 2022)

Intent
- Facilitate LE to torso activation of flexors
- Enhance posterior femoral glide to improve positioning of femoral head on acetabulum

Gait reasoning
- Improve pelvifemoral glide for leg swing and stance
- Improve femoral head positioning for stance

Starting position
- Supine with feet flat on mat, hip and knee flexion
- Knee flexion, feet in line with ischial tuberosities

Movement description
- Unilateral hip flexion
- Place the ipsilateral hand against femur
- Hold isometrically
- Press femur into hand and hand into femur
- Hold for 5 seconds, release
- Repeat 5 times

CUES
- The amount of pressure on the femur is to activate the head of the femur and to match the amount of pressure with the outcome of activation
- Monitor pelvis motion, no rotation
- Allow the lower leg to dangle so the activation is proximal

Author note
Working on activation patterns from LE to pelvis helped the client to be aware of excess pelvic movement and hip joint congruence. It is useful for people who have had abdominal surgeries to experience the activation and awareness of LE to pelvic diaphragm and torso continuity. The synergy of movement plays a role in both centering the femoral head in the acetabulum and stimulating coactivations throughout the torso when moving the limbs.

7. Double-leg knee folds (See Chapter 5, Gentry, knee folds)

Intent
- Increase challenge progressing from unilateral knee fold to bilateral knee folds
- Facilitate synergistic patterning of LE flexion and torso adaptation
- Coordination of pelvifemoral movement

Gait reasoning
- Increase ease in leg swing
- Improve adaptability of torso to LE motion

Set-up
- Partially deflated 9 in. (23 cm) ball
- Mat

Starting position
- Supine on mat with partially deflated ball under sacrum
- Bilateral hip flexion to 90 degrees
- Lower limb dangling
- UE resting at sides

Movement description
- Lower both LE toward extension as far as possible maintaining TLJ anchor and anterior abdominal control, without abdominal doming
- Feet may or may not touch the floor
- Return LE to 90 degrees hip flexion without posterior rotation of pelvis

CUES
- Keep TLJ in contact with mat
- Monitor the loss of TLJ anchor with flexion or extension
- Watch for doming of anterior abdominals

Author note

Initially, the client excessively activated the anterior abdominals by doming rather than integrating the activation. She also had difficulty maintaining the TLJ anchor and moved into extension without any sort of leg lowering. Eventually, she achieved the ability to be fully integrated with the activation pattern of the torso while flexing and extending the LE. The client found this decreased pain levels that she was experiencing in the abdominal area due to two bilateral inguinal hernias.

8. Breathing with a ball

Intent
- Improve tissue glide in thorax to allow for improved elasticity in thorax
- Calm the nervous system to counter overactive cortisol production from Cushing's disease
- Improve organization of abdominal region during breathing
- Improve reduced lung capacity due to lingering effects of COVID-19
- Help mitigate COVID-19-related tachycardia symptoms

Gait reasoning
- Improve connective tissue glide and articulation of thorax for rotation and arm swing
- Lessen dizziness and improve balance
- Facilitate breathing pattern to support better endurance

Set-up
- Band or partially deflated 9 in. (23 cm) ball
- Mat

Starting position
- Supine on mat with mostly deflated ball underneath one side of torso between pelvis and lower ribs

Movement description
- Breathe in through nose with mouth closed
- Send the breath toward partially deflated ball imagining a spherical expansion
- Widen the inferior lateral angle (ILA) of the anterior ribcage
- Exhale, maintaining the widening of the ILA
- Inhale, increasing the width of the ILA
- Exhale and return to relaxed state of breathing
- Take a few natural breaths before repeating
- Repeat at least 5 times
- Move ball to other side of body and repeat progression

CUES
- Allow the torso to sink into the ball during inhale as the thorax expands
- Try to maintain that contact when exhaling
- Focus on the breath creating buoyancy and elasticity in the thorax
- Inhale and exhale through the nose with the mouth closed
- Do not try to extend the breath more than feels natural
- Find a slow but easy pace

Author note
The idea of using the deflated 9 in. (23 cm) ball is to provide proprioception of the expansion sensation to the connective tissues around the area of the respiratory diaphragm. This exercise became a staple of our sessions and home program. While improved breathing did not eliminate the COVID-19-related tachycardia, it reduced some of the panic associated with the symptoms, which may have also been exacerbated by living in a high-altitude environment.

9. Side lying Footwork on Universal Reformer

Intent
- Using closed kinematic chain for activation of LE to torso
- Improve medial hip glide
- Improve hip flexion and extension

Gait reasoning
- Client's gait is predominantly driven from UE rather than torso and LE
- Facilitate glide with weight shift
- Improve balance in one-leg stance

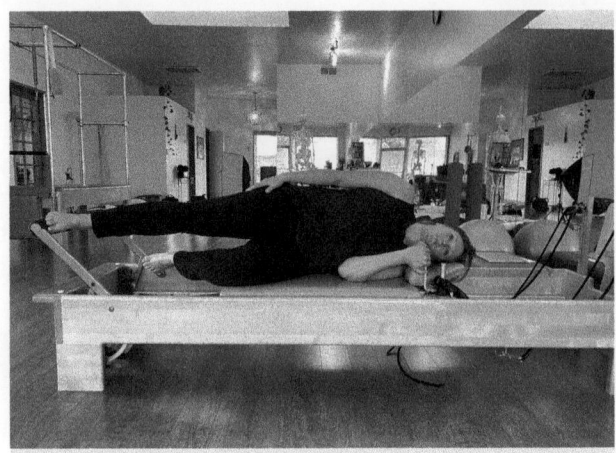

Figure 12.9

Set-up	● Springs: 1 medium or 1 medium and 1 light
Starting position	● Side lying on Universal Reformer
	● Bottom knee in flexion
	● Top LE extended in line with body, foot on footbar in parallel
	● Head resting on headrest
	● Hold shoulder stops
Movement description	● Press foot into footbar as if to reach leg away from torso
	● Feel activation of lateral torso without lateral flexion
	● Flex hip and knee moving carriage to footbar
	● Press again
	● Repeat 10 times

CUES

- Try to maintain activation on the lateral torso equally with no lateral flexion
- Monitor the pattern of joint activations from foot to pelvis
- Do not allow the LE to adduct during flexion

The journey to Session 11

Session 4/12
Client self-report

- Had less discomfort in the upper thorax, neck, and shoulders due to a combination of our work and dry needling performed by a physical therapist
- Pain scale 2–3
- Fatigue scale 2

Key changes observed

- Improved cervical ROM in transverse plane
- Scapula glides on thorax

Reasoning behind choice of movements

- Improve thoracic rotation for increased ease with arm swing
- Increase breathing capacity
- Facilitate oppositional thorax and pelvis in gait
- Improve hip centration for stance and glide for swing

Session movement sequence
1. Breathing

2. Pelvic Clocks

3. Bridging

4. Knee folds

5. Trapeze Table

- Mermaid
- Push-Through Bar Springs from Above: Upper Arms (derivative of J. H. Pilates Push-Through Bar Springs from Above: Upper Arms; NPCE Study Guide 2021, p. 63)
- Supine UE only, feet on table, knee flexion

- Leg Springs
  - Unilateral
  - Bilateral

6. Sling

- Bridging
- Bridging with unilateral plantar flexion with metatarsals on table, knee folds, LE abduction in knee flexion

7. Partially deflated 9 in. (23 cm) ball

- Pelvic Clocks
- Breathing
- Knee folds
  - Unilateral
  - Bilateral

8. Universal Reformer

- UE Press

9. Additional movement

- Ball rolling along medial edge of scapula in all directions for connective tissue glide of scapulohumeral motion

Session 5/12
Client self-report

- Ease in shoulder pain and less pain when sleeping
- Fatigue scale 3
- Pain scale 4

Key changes observed

- Improved cervical ROM in transverse plane
- Improved scapula glide on thorax
- Improved torso ROM in all dimensions

- Less overall pain in movement
- Increased the level of activity in our session
- Less pain in standing activities

Reasoning behind choice of movements

- Address structure and movement strategies that are affecting an increase in client's pain and discomfort stemming from degenerative disc changes and COVID-related numbness and tingling in right LE
- Increase capability to access breathing techniques to deal with dizziness and anxiety

Session movement sequence
1. Sling

- Breathing

2. Partially deflated 9 in. (23 cm) ball

- Pelvic Clocks
- Breathing
- Knee folds
  - Unilateral
  - Bilateral

3. Trapeze Table

- Mermaid
- Push-Through Bar Springs from Above: Upper Arms

4. Partially deflated 9 in. (23 cm) ball

- Pelvic Clocks and Nose Clocks
- Knee fall-outs
- Knee folds
- Modified Single Leg Stretch

5. Sling

- Breathing
- Knee fall-outs
- Knee folds
- Leg slides
- Bridges

6. Universal Reformer

- Leg Springs

Session 6/12
Client self-report

- Client's pain has increased recently, particularly around the SIJs and L5/S1, where degenerative changes as well as some stenosis are present
- Client had canceled the previous session due to issues with tachycardia and increased pain
- Pain scale 6–7
- Fatigue scale 5–6

Key changes observed

- ROM of hemipelvis inferior motion decreased from initial assessment
- ROM of left rotation decreased from initial assessment
- Improved extension of torso and LE for the first time in our sessions

Reasoning behind choice of movements

- Activating extensors for orientation of midline
- Increase articulation of torso especially scapulae glide
- Continue activation of torso for support and balance

Session movement sequence
1. Breathing

2. Partially deflated 9 in. (23 cm) ball

- Pelvic Clocks and Nose Clocks
- LE abduction
- Knee folds
- Modified Single Leg Stretch

3. Trapeze Table

- Modified Swan with long box

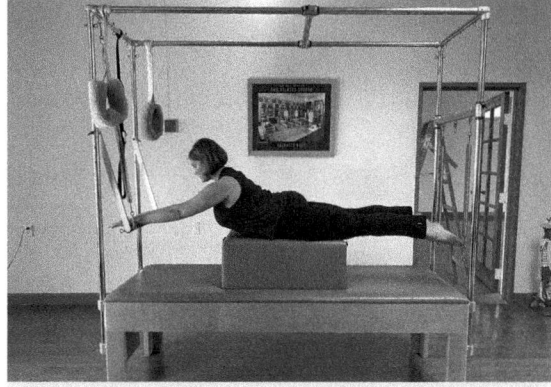

Figure 12.10

- Push-Through Bar Springs from Above: Upper Arms with LE abducted, dangling off table
- Teaser preparation
- Knee folds, supine holding on to push-through bar
- Leg Springs
  - Unilateral
  - Bilateral

4. Partially deflated 9 in. (23 cm) ball

- Pelvic Clocks
- Breathing
- Knee folds

5. Sling

- Bridging with feet also on the Pilates Arc
- Knee folds
- LE abduction
- Breathing with sling

6. Magic Circle breathing (Black 2022)

- Seated on box placed on floor near table
- Place one end of the Magic Circle on sternum, other end against edge of table

- UE resting on the table
- Facilitate flexion and extension initiating from sternum/Magic Circle
- Press into Magic Circle to facilitate extension
- Allow recoil of Magic Circle, press into sternum for flexion
- Alternate inhale and exhale, trying each breath with the movement and choosing optimal breath pattern that best facilitates desired movement

Editor note

Fascia facilitates movement by allowing gliding between the structures it surrounds (Pilat 2022). In a body region, a large number of neurovascular, visceral, and muscular structures can be found. These structures have free dynamic behavior during movement (Chaitow 2014).

7. Pilates Arc

- Bridging with feet on top of arc

8. Additional movements

- Nerve gliding
  - Brachial nerve gliding
    - Supine
    - UE at 90 degrees flexion
    - Abduct UE with extended wrists with phalanges extended
    - Adduct UE with flexed wrists with phalanges flexed
  - Sciatic nerve gliding
    - Seated on chair, both LE hanging freely
    - Extend right knee with ankle dorsiflexion while extending torso
    - Flex knee, plantar flexion while flexing torso

Author note

The client appeared to have high sensitivity to nerve stimulation. The range and amplitude of movement was kept to the simplest and less aggravating movement to stimulate nerve glide.

Session 7/12
Client self-report

- Client has been experiencing extreme COVID-related POTS and is now wearing compression socks
- Client has also had multiple emergency room visits
- Pain scale 7
- Fatigue scale 5–6

Key changes observed

- Feels more anxious than in past sessions
- Increased pain in her mid-thorax
- Client self-reporting less about LE symptoms

Reasoning behind choice of movements

- Increase ability to move torso in all dimensions
- Increase capacity of breathing
- Improve movement organization for torso support

Session movement sequence
1. Breathing

2. Partially deflated 9 in. (23 cm) ball

- Pelvic Clocks
- Supine nose circles (see Chapter 5, Gentry)
- Knee folds

- LE abduction
- Modified Single Leg Stretch

3. Trapeze Table

- Mermaid
  - Seated sideways to top-loaded bar
  - Hold bar with lower limb, pronated palm away
  - Pull bar increasing elbow flexion, extended elbow pressing bar away
  - Hold extended UE, laterally flex torso, while other UE abducts bringing hand overhead
  - Reverse the path to go back to starting position
- Teaser preparation
  - Supine head under push-through bar
  - Hold bar with extended elbows
  - Hip joint and knee flexion, feet on table
  - Flex torso from head to sit up pressing the bar overhead
  - Roll down to starting position
- Leg Springs
  - Unilateral
  - Bilateral

4. Sling

- Bridging
- Knee folds, marches
- Nerve gliding

5. Partially deflated 9 in. (23 cm) ball

- Pelvic Clocks
- Supine nose circles (see Chapter 5, Gentry)
- Knee fall-outs
- Knee folds
- Modified Single Leg Stretch

6. Side lying abduction

7. Additional movement

- Small 3 in. (8 cm) ball rolling plantar surface of feet

Session 8/12
Client self-report

- Improved articulation of torso; however, still has pain in lumbar area
- Fatigue scale 2
- Pain scale 4

Key changes observed

- Significant improvement of lateral flexion
- Significant improvement of rotation but limited left rotation

Reasoning behind choice of movements

- Increase ability to move torso in all dimensions
- Increase capacity and suppleness of breathing
- Improve organization of torso to increase support

Session movement sequence
1. Bridging

2. Pelvic Clocks

3. Breathing

4. Partially deflated 9 in. (23 cm) ball exercises

5. Trapeze Table

- Push-through modified Swan with long box
- Teaser preparation
- Leg Springs
  - Unilateral
  - Bilateral

6. Partially deflated 9 in. (23 cm) ball exercises

- Pelvic Clocks
- Breathing
- Knee folds
- Marching

7. Sling with Pilates Arc

- Breathing with sling
- Knee folds and fall-outs, marches
- Bridging with feet on Pilates Arc

8. Magic Circle breathing

9. Seated nerve gliding for brachial plexus and sciatic nerve

10. Additional movement

- Side lying in flexion, both hands behind head, small rotation with slight extension

---

Author note

Side lying in flexion is similar to a fetal position. Beginning a rotation from the flexed position facilitates moving into extension, eliminating the potential of hyperextension of the TLJ.

Session 9/12
Client self-report

- More ease in movement, less pain when walking and standing
- Fatigue scale 2
- Pain scale 3

Key changes observed

- The client was able to increase the amount of movement during this session, including adding Universal Reformer side lying Footwork without immediately fatiguing

Reasoning behind choice of movements

- Improve organization of torso to increase support for movement
- Facilitate thoracic and shoulder girdle glide to improve arm swing and find ease in head and neck relationship
- Activate and load hip joints

Session movement sequence
1. Bridging

2. Pelvic Clocks

3. Breathing

4. Partially deflated 9 in. (23 cm) ball exercises

5. Universal Reformer

- Side lying Footwork
  - Legs parallel
  - Legs externally rotated
- Straps: feet in loops, bilateral
- Lower and lift heels

6. Trapeze Table

- Mermaid
- Push-Through Bar Springs from Above: Upper Arms
- Teaser preparation including shoulder shrugs and UE overhead with push-through bar
- Modified Swan on long box

7. Partially deflated 9 in. (23 cm) ball exercises

- Pelvic Clocks
- Knee folds
- Swan

8. Sling

- Bridges with sling under pelvis
- Knee folds, knee fall-outs with sling under thoracic region
- Cervical nod and curl holding on to springs, breathing, legs in tabletop

Session 10/12
Client self-report

- Experiencing a headache from lying on her stomach at physical therapy
- Was able to sleep without a lumbar support pillow for over 2 weeks
- Fatigue scale 2
- Pain scale 4

Key changes observed

- Increased endurance and holding positions for longer periods of time
- ROM in general has improved
- Breathing has improved
- Felt emotional at one point in the session, because she was moving without pain for the first time in years

Reasoning behind choice of movements

- Improve organization of torso to increase support for movement
- Facilitate thoracic and shoulder girdle glide to improve arm swing and find ease in head and neck relationship
- Activate and load hip joints

Session movement sequence
1. Breathing: added a band around the ribs for increased proprioception

2. Partially deflated 9 in. (23 cm) ball exercises

3. Magic Circle breathing

4. Trapeze Table

- Mermaid
- Push-Through Bar Springs from Above: Upper Arms
- Teaser UE preparation with legs in 90/90 hip and knee flexion
- Modified Swan with long box
- Extension with Push-Through Bar: unilateral LE

5. Partially deflated 9 in. (23 cm) ball exercises

- Knee folds, knee fall-outs

- Pelvic Clocks
- Modified straight leg stretch
- Teaser preparation

6. Breathing with band

7. Pilates Arc bridging

8. Wall standing exercise

References

Barral, J.-P. and Mercier, P. (2006) *Visceral Manipulation.* Revised edition. Seattle, WA: Eastland Press, pp. 32–38.

Black, M. (2022) *Centered: Organizing the Body through Kinesiology, Movement Theory and Pilates Techniques.* 2nd Ed. Edinburgh: Handspring Publishing, pp. 83, 123–125, 194–195.

Chaitow, L. (2014) "Somatic dysfunction and fascia's gliding-potential." *Journal of Bodywork and Movement Therapies, 18,* 1, 1–3.

Feldenkrais, M. (1985 [2002]) *The Potent Self: A Study of Spontaneity and Compulsion.* Berkeley, CA: Somatic Resources/Frog Ltd., pp. 189–214.

Lee, D. (2018) *The Thorax: An Integrated Approach.* Edinburgh: Handspring Publishing, pp. 58–59.

Mayo Clinic Staff (2023a) Cushing Syndrome. Mayo Clinic. www.mayoclinic.org/diseases-conditions/cushing-syndrome/symptoms-causes/syc-20351310. [October 1, 2023].

Mayo Clinic Staff (2023b) Tachycardia. Mayo Clinic. www.mayoclinic.org/diseases-conditions/tachycardia/symptoms-causes/syc-20355127. [October 1, 2023].

NPCE Study Guide (National Pilates Certification Exam Study Guide) (2021) Miami, FL: National Pilates Certification Program, Inc.

Pilat, A. (2022) *Myofascial Induction: An Anatomical Approach to the Treatment of Fascial Dysfunction—Volume 1 The Upper Body.* Edinburgh: Handspring Publishing, pp.165, 166, 199.

Shah, N., Ruiz, H. H., Zafar, U., Post, K. D., Buettner, C., and Geer, E. B. (2017) "Proinflammatory cytokines remain elevated despite long-term remission in Cushing's disease: A prospective study." *Clinical Endocrinology, 86,* 68–74.

Walker, A. (2021) *The Trifecta Passport: Tools for Mast Cell Activation Syndrome, Postural Orthostatic Tachycardia Syndrome and Ehlers-Danlos Syndrome.* Kindle Direct Publishing.

Pilates for Long COVID: Effect on Gait

Elizabeth Larkam

Editor note

Long COVID was described, recognized, and named during the spring and summer of 2020 (Callard and Perego 2021). During the three years since the emergence of "post COVID-19 complex," social media discussions contributed to the acceleration of research publications (Davis *et al.* 2023), online education programming (DrTalks Summit 2023), medical conferences (FLCCC Alliance 2022, 2023), and media reporting. Differing—and at times controversial—opinions are still expressed regarding criteria for diagnosis, case-counting, economic costs to the labor force, and funding priorities for treatment trials (Cohrs and Ladyzhets 2023). Pilates professionals with clients who report a constellation of symptoms associated with long COVID must be informed about standards of care for this multi-systemic health condition. It is imperative that Pilates teachers understand post-exertional malaise (PEM) (Twomey *et al.* 2022), post-exertional symptom exacerbation (PESE) (Long COVID Physio 2023a), and pacing (Long COVID Physio 2023b) (see boxes).

Myalgic encephalomyelitis/chronic fatigue syndrome (ME/CFS)

Persistent (chronic) fatigue is consistently reported to be the most prevalent symptom of long COVID. Reports of chronic fatigue alongside fluctuating symptoms that worsen unpredictably or in response to exertion have led to comparisons between long COVID and other post-viral conditions, including ME/CFS. Chronic fatigue is a distressing, persistent feeling of weariness, tiredness, or exhaustion that is not alleviated by rest and is not proportional to recent activity levels (Cairns and Hotopf 2005). Chronic fatigue is a hallmark of multiple conditions, where it interferes with usual functioning and negatively impacts quality of life (Wong and Weitzer 2021).

Post-exertional malaise (PEM)

A hallmark symptom of ME/CFS and some cases of "post COVID-19 complex" is PEM. It is a worsening of symptoms and a reduction in function after physical, cognitive, social, or emotional exertions that would not have caused a problem before illness. The worsening of symptoms (for example, exacerbation of breathlessness or tachycardia) may occur immediately or lag in onset 24–72 hours after exertion. The recovery period may be days, weeks, or months. PEM can be mitigated by activity management known as "pacing" (see box: Pacing) and heart rate monitoring. Some forms of exercise such as aerobic conditioning and strength training may be harmful for patients with long COVID who have ME/CFS or PEM and should not be used as a treatment (Wright, Astill, and Sivan 2022).

Long COVID, also known as post-acute sequelae of COVID-19 (PASC) and "post-COVID conditions or syndrome," refers to the constellation of long-term symptoms experienced by people suffering persistent symptoms for one or more months after SARS-CoV-2 infection. A clinical case definition developed by the World Health Organization states: post COVID-19 conditions occur in individuals with a history of probable or confirmed SARS-CoV-2 infection, usually three months from the onset of COVID-19 with symptoms that last for at least two months and cannot be explained by an alternative diagnosis (Twomey *et al.* 2022). Long COVID is a major public health concern associated with all ages and acute-phase disease severities. The highest percentage of diagnoses are between the ages of 36 and 50 years. Long COVID impacts children of all ages (Kompaniyets *et al.* 2022).

The scale of the COVID-19 pandemic means that even if a small proportion of people infected with SARS-CoV-2 have prolonged symptoms, this translates to millions of people worldwide. The estimate that at least 65 million people worldwide have long COVID is based on a conservative estimated incidence of 10 percent of infected people and more than 651 million documented COVID-19 cases worldwide; the number is likely much higher due to many undocumented cases (Davis *et al.* 2023).

In March 2020, people with unresolved, mysterious symptoms after acute COVID infection turned to social media discussions for support. Long COVID was not identified initially by doctors who encountered similar sets of symptoms in their patients. The term "long-haulers" came from a patient convener of "long haul Covid fighters," who derived it from a trucker hat she was wearing when getting a test. "Long hauler" was shortened to "long haul" and led to the name "long COVID" (Callard and Perego 2021).

Although COVID-19 was initially recognized as a respiratory illness, SARS-CoV-2 has the capability to damage many organ systems (Slate 2023). The narrative that COVID-19 had only respiratory sequelae led to a delayed realization of the multi-system impacts of this mild-to-debilitating disease. More than 200 symptoms have been attributed to this complex infection that affects the neurologic, cardiovascular, pulmonary, hematologic, and endocrine systems. Many long COVID clinics and providers still disproportionately focus on respiratory rehabilitation, which results in skewed electronic health record data (Davis *et al.* 2023).

The damage across diverse tissues has predominantly been attributed to immune-mediated response and inflammation, rather than direct infection of cells by the virus. There is evidence that viral reservoirs are one leading driver of long COVID. The "viral persistence" theory posits that some people never fully eliminate the infection, that viral reservoirs are subsisting in the body, altering people's immune responses after the infection, and possibly triggering the symptoms of long COVID. Other mechanisms driving long COVID include autoimmunity, immune system dysregulation, inflammation of the endothelium that lines blood vessels, tiny blood clots, the reactivation of dormant viruses, and signaling problems with the brainstem and the vagus nerve (Stone 2023).

Researchers and clinicians have noted the similarity between ME/CFS (see box: Myalgic encephalomyelitis/chronic fatigue syndrome) and long COVID (Wong and Weitzer 2021); around half of individuals with long COVID are estimated to meet the criteria for ME/CFS (Haffke *et al.* 2022). The gut microbiota composition is significantly altered in patients with COVID-19 and gut microbiota dysbiosis is also a key component of ME/CFS. In studies where the cardinal ME/CFS symptom of post-exertional malaise is measured, the majority of individuals with long COVID report experiencing post-exertional malaise (see box: Post-exertional symptom exacerbation) (Twomey *et al.* 2022). Not all patients with long COVID experience PEM. Slow, deliberately paced movement integrated with controlled breath practices may help manage energy, tissue oxygenation, efficiency of movement, and stress (see box: Exhale-focused cyclic sighing).

The onset and time course of symptoms differ across individuals and by symptom type. Neurological and cognitive symptoms are a major feature of long COVID, including sensorimotor symptoms, memory loss, cognitive impairment, paresthesia, dizziness and balance issues, sensitivity to light and noise, loss of (or phantom) smell or taste, and autonomic dysfunction, often impacting activities of daily living (Davis *et al.* 2021). Audio-vestibular manifestations of long COVID include tinnitus, hearing loss, and vertigo (Almufarrij and Munro 2021).

The natural history and subtypes of neurologic post-acute sequelae of COVID-19 or neuro-PASC are being defined in the second half of 2023 (Mina *et al.* 2023).

Few people with long COVID demonstrate full recovery, with one study finding that 85 percent of patients who had symptoms two months after the initial infection reported symptoms one year after symptom onset (Tran *et al.* 2022). Future prognosis is uncertain, although diagnoses of ME/CFS and dysautonomia are generally lifelong (Ceban 2022).

The Brookings Institution estimated that long COVID is keeping the equivalent of 2 to 4 million full-time workers out of the American labor force, resulting in about $170 billion of lost earnings per year (Bach 2022). Economist David Cutler drew similar conclusions and estimated the US health costs of long COVID to be in the order of $100 billion per year. These combined estimates imply a real cost of more than $1 trillion over a five-year period, even before accounting for lost quality of life, increased disability costs, and the burden on caregivers and the health care system (Cutler 2022).

Client description: 46-year-old biological female, identifies as female; professional Pilates teacher in the lineage of Romana Kryzanowska (see Chapter 5)

Dates of case report: Session 1: February 8, 2022; Session 12: March 17, 2022; two one-hour online sessions per week for 6 weeks

Author note

The federal COVID-19 public health emergency declaration ended on May 11, 2023. More than 65 million worldwide have the condition called long COVID. The spike protein changes soluble clotting protein to insoluble microclots. Acute COVID activates platelets causing vascular damage, endothelial damage, and microclotting in some individuals. The clots caused by long COVID are made of unique proteins that contain an abnormal type of fibrin. When the body does not break down the insoluble microclots blood vessel damage and blocked blood flow to organs occur. Vasculature and oxygen transfer are compromised. The high level of microclots in long COVID patients might be the blood biomarker that could help explain long COVID's wide-ranging symptoms (Oza *et al.* 2023).

Post-exertional symptom exacerbation (PESE)

PESE is a physiological inability to provide sufficient energy on demand. Exercise intolerance observed in long COVID is not physical deconditioning. Managing PESE must be individualized by identifying specific symptoms, noting the duration and level of activity that provoke PESE, observing how long symptoms last, and how they change over time. It is imperative to appreciate physiological complexities when attempting to unravel post-COVID-19 syndrome exercise intolerance mechanisms (Long COVID Physio 2023a).

Postural orthostatic tachycardia syndrome (POTS)

POTS is a common heart condition of people with long COVID. When a person stands or sits up after lying down their heart rate accelerates by 30 beats per minute or more. This may be experienced as palpitations, chest pain, shortness of breath, and exercise intolerance. Neurological and other symptoms include exhaustion, lightheadedness, headaches, and mental clouding or "brain fog." In addition, muscle weakness, sleep disturbances, and gastrointestinal distress may result. In POTS, the brain, nervous system, and heart lack congruent communication which is normally managed automatically and unconsciously. The virus may infect and damage nerves that set heart rhythms and signal blood vessel contraction. Another explanation is that immune system overreaction harms nerves as it attacks the virus. The damaged nerves lose capacity for effective heartbeat control (Sutherland 2023).

Pacing

Pacing is a self-management strategy employed during physical and mental activity to avoid PESE. Activity management and heart rate monitoring are likely to be safe, effective interventions for living with fatigue. Prioritize tasks, then parse them into intervals of activity with intermissions for rest and rejuvenation. Develop symptom pattern recognition and familiarity with energy reservoir and baseline. Avoid the temptation to do just a little more. Finish each activity interval with some energy in the reservoir.

Skilled Pilates teachers will become realistic, flexible experts in pacing, recognizing early signs of client PESE and immediately initiating rejuvenating intermissions. Keep the focus on client accomplishments instead of on symptoms or what was not achieved. Rests from physical and mental exertion may include the client's preferred breathing practices, integrating humming (Chaitow 2018) resting the eyes, and "non-sleep deep rest" (NSDR) (Hutchinson 2022). Rests do not involve conversation, social media, mental stimulation, or physical activity. As client symptoms improve, gradually increase activities that align with short-term and long-term goals (Long COVID Physio 2023b).

Studio apparatus and props
Pilates equipment

- Ladder Barrel
- Wunda Chair with single pedal
- Ped-o-Pull with long, light springs attached to Stability Sling
- Trapeze Table with long springs attached to Stability Sling

---

Author note

In the prop list below, the Balansit, designed by osteopath Daniel Vladeta, is a dynamic, active sitting, posture-correcting tool made of proprietary foam. The patented two-curve design allows for forward and backward balance as well as side-to-side stability. The Balansit saddle provides support for the sitting bones, holding the pelvis in an optimal position for sitting (Vladeta 2022). Many cushions intend to improve sitting. I chose the Balansit for this program because it supports specificity of lumbopelvic-hip motion relevant to gait. Balance of the lumbopelvic region improves movement relationships of the thorax and diaphragm for efficient breathing. I placed the small Balansit on a 9 in. (23 cm) rotator disc without resistance. The client sat on the Balansit–rotator disc, both of which were on the Wunda Chair seat.

Props used with equipment

- Pinwheel
- Foot Corrector
- 2 dense foam yoga blocks
- 2 rotator discs, 9 in. (23 cm) in diameter, no resistance
- 2 non-skid rubberized pads to secure rotator discs
- Balansit®, small size
- Stability Sling

- Small Pilates box for foot support
- Magic Circle
- Non-skid rubberized mat

Home program props
The home program includes equipment because the client teaches Pilates and has access to equipment.

- Ladder Barrel
- Small Pilates box for foot support
- Paper
- Pen or pencil
- Outdoor walking shoes

Methods and materials

Session 1/12
1. Health history interview

- COVID-19 infection began in November 17, 2020
- Positive COVID-19 test in November 23, 2020

2. Symptoms

- Dysautonomia (chest pressure, palpitations, sound sensitivity, dizziness)
- Tachycardia (heart rate irregularities continue to present)
- Insomnia
- Hot flashes daily
- Loss of smell
- Hair loss
- Herpes outbreak (once or twice a month)
- Bronchial restriction
- Lung constriction concentrated on left side and in center of chest
- Ribcage tenderness and pain behind sternum continued for 6 months
- Sore, hoarse throat and vocal cords continued for 6 months
- Swollen neck
- Head pressure

- Sinus inflammation
- Right nostril bleeding
- Ear popping, ringing
- Balance compromised; single-leg balance not possible
- Unable to exercise for 3 months following diagnosis
- Panic attacks, fear of relapse and of never getting well
- Inability to work resulted in loss of income, financial anxiety
- Depression, loss of interest in life
- Cognition severely impaired; unable to read, follow directions, remember thoughts
- Improvement in cognitive clarity began in January 2022, 14 months after diagnosis

3. Medical examinations

- Chest X-ray in November 2020
- EKG during emergency room visit for severe tachycardia in December 2020
- Cardiac CT scan
- Lung CT scan in December 2020 showed "ground-glass opacities"
- Lung scan in June 2021 showed clear lungs
- Pulmonary function test
- Treadmill test
- Bloodwork

4. Medical treatment

- Sent home from the emergency room with pulse oximeter in December 2020
- Prescribed an albuterol inhaler 2 weeks later
- Prednisone, two five-day courses—February 2021 and April 2021
- Ivermectin, two rounds—March 2021 and May 2021
- Steroid inhaler—April 2021
- Vaccine—April and May 2021
- March–May 2021 breathing techniques using incentive spirometer for inhalation (up to 3000 on force, 1500–1800 in sustaining) and a straw for exhalation up to 21 seconds
- Implemented pacing and drinking 32–64 fl oz (0.94–1.89 L) of electrolytes to control PESE
- Took supplements to support health and well-being

5. Movement aids

- None

Final result of case report

Client gait demonstrates improved counter rotation of thorax and pelvis.

She stands with improved bilateral weight distribution and improved forefoot - rear foot weight distribution.

Client has resumed full schedule of teaching, podcasting and daily practice of Classical Pilates Intermediate program.

Irregular heart beat rhythms occur if she does not incorporate rests, electrolytes and supportive health practices.

Emotional distress triggers restricted breathing.

Somato-cognitive action network (SCAN)

The recently discovered brain structure named the somato (body)-cognitive (mind) action network, or SCAN, may be significant for individuals living with long COVID who integrate controlled breathing practices with movement of appropriate intensity to manage energy levels, reactions to stress, and cognitive clarity. A study published in April 2023 shows that brain regions controlling movement also control involuntary functions such as blood pressure and heart rate. These same brain areas are plugged into networks involved in thinking and planning. The SCAN reveals that the body-mind connection is embedded in the structure of the brain and expressed in physiology, movements, behavior, and thinking (Gordon *et al.* 2023).

Exhale-focused cyclic sighing

Exhale-focused cyclic sighing ("physiological sigh") is a controlled breathwork practice. The COVID-19 pandemic highlighted the importance of simple, fast-acting, and cost-effective techniques to address widespread physical and mental health challenges. The pattern and depth of breathing have direct physiological impact on oxygenation level, heart rate, ventilation, and blood pressure. Controlled breathwork practices have emerged as potential tools for stress management and well-being.

Daily 5-minute cyclic sighing has promise as an effective stress management exercise. Exhale-focused cyclic sighing produces greater improvement in mood and reduction in respiratory rate compared with mindfulness meditation. The tendency when feeling stress is to under-breathe, which can elevate the level of carbon dioxide in the blood and cause the alveoli to collapse. Alveoli are tiny sacs that inflate to increase the surface area of the lungs for gaseous exchange. The physiological sigh, which was discovered by physiologists in the 1930s, reduces anxiety. Inhale deeply through the nose and, when you feel your lungs are full, sniff in a little bit more air. This "double inhale" inflates the alveoli. Then sigh, exhaling slowly through the mouth to expel the carbon dioxide that is causing stress (Balban *et al.* 2023).

Session 2/12: Initial assessment

1. General observations of gait

◆ Extension at thoracolumbar junction prevalent throughout gait cycle

◆ Bilateral heavy heel strikes with right heel strike more pronounced than left

◆ Weight concentrated in right posterior region of the kinesphere

◆ Thoracic rotation not discernible

◆ Lumbar curve reduced

◆ Cervical curve reduced

◆ Retraction of head on neck

◆ Gaze fixed directly forward at horizon level throughout gait cycle

◆ Right leg external rotation more pronounced than left leg external rotation

◆ Asymmetrical gait rhythm with more time spent weight bearing on right leg than left leg

◆ Author note: Client began gymnastics training in preschool and continued at an elite level until young adulhood. She augmented gymnastics competitions with dance performances. Her right leg was her lead leg in 'take-off', or 'vaulting' into movement sequences. These training patterns throughout the first half of life may contribute to current gait strategies

Session 12/12: Post-assessment

1. General observations of gait

◆ Extension at thoracolumbar junction less pronounced throughout gait cycle

◆ Bilateral heel strikes less heavy; right heel strike still more pronounced than left

◆ Thorax and pelvis organized to middle region of kinesphere in all three planes

◆ Thoracic rotation observable with left thoracic rotation more pronounced than right

◆ Lumbar curve discernable

◆ Cervical curve discernable

◆ Retraction of head on neck less pronounced

◆ Gaze scans the horizon during gait cycle

◆ Right leg external rotation still greater than left leg external rotation, although, less pronounced

◆ Gait rhythm less asymmetrical, although more time still spent weight bearing on right leg than left leg

◆ Author note: Client remarks that her daily walking practice is more comfortable for her feet, pelvis and breathing. Prior to this gait-focused Pilates program she did not realize that walking strategies could contribute to whole body discomfort and restricted breathing

2. Standing tests

◆ Full torso rotation

● Observations of inefficient side:
  ■ Left rotation
  ■ Rotation of pelvis on femurs is not discernible
  ■ Thoracic rotation initiates from thoracolumbar junction
  ■ Segmental thoracic rotation is not discernible
  ■ Right foot and ankle supinated
  ■ Left foot and ankle did not adapt

◆ Hemipelvis inferior motion

● Observations of inefficient side: left

◆ Hemipelvis superior motion

● Observations of inefficient side: both
  ■ Right hemipelvis superior motion restricted
  ■ Right thoracic translation interferes with ability to transfer pelvis onto left leg
  ■ Left hemipelvis superior motion restricted since it is already near end range
  ■ Right thoracic translation contributes to left innominate elevation

◆ Lateral pelvic shift

● Observations of inefficient side: left
  ■ Attempts to shift pelvis left result in right thoracic translation
  ■ Restricted femoral-pelvic motion of right femoral abduction and left femoral adduction
  ■ Right foot and ankle supinate
  ■ Left foot and ankle do not adapt

2. Standing tests

◆ Full torso rotation

● Observations of inefficient side: left
  ■ Left rotation
  ■ Motion of pelvis on femurs supports left rotation of pelvic-lumbar region
  ■ Segmental thoracic rotation observable
  ■ Thoracic rotation does not accentuate extension at thoracolumbar junction
  ■ Right foot and ankle pronated
  ■ Left foot and ankle supinated

◆ Hemipelvis inferior motion

● Observations of inefficient side: left
  ■ Improved ability of left innominate to lower
  ■ Thoracic organization to the midline in the coronal plane improved during lowering of left innominate

◆ Hemipelvis superior motion

● Observations of inefficient side: both
  ■ Right hemipelvis superior motion less restricted
  ■ Reduction in right thoracic translation makes weight transfer of pelvis onto left leg more accessible
  ■ Left hemipelvis superior motion less restricted
  ■ Improved organization of thoracolumbar junction and S-2 to midline in all three planes supports left hemipelvis superior motion

◆ Lateral pelvic shift

● Observations of inefficient side: both

- Improved ability to shift pelvis left
- Reduced restriction of femoral-pelvic motion of right femoral abduction and left femoral adduction
- Right foot and ankle pronate
- Left foot and ankle adapt

3. Seated tests

◆ Thoracic rotation

● Observations of inefficient side: right
  - Improved ability to organize to the midline, bearing weight on both ischial tuberosities
  - Right thoracic translation is reduced
  - Right thoracic rotation is more accessible

◆ Hip joint and knee flexion

● Observations of inefficient side: both
  - Improvement in balanced weight distribution on right and left ischial tuberosities
  - Improvement in thoracic organization to the midline in the coronal plane
  - Right thoracic rotation is accessible
  - Improved ability to weight left ischial tuberosity and translate thorax left

4. Sit and stand

◆ Lateral view

● Improved bilateral pelvifemoral motion in hip flexion and extension

● Flexion of lumbar region less pronounced

● Extension at thoracolumbar junction less pronounced

3. Seated tests

◆ Thoracic rotation

● Observations of inefficient side: right
  - Right ischial tuberosity more weighted than left
  - Thorax is translated right
  - Right thoracic rotation is restricted

◆ Hip joint and knee flexion

● Observations of inefficient side: both
  - Right ischial tuberosity is more weighted than left
  - Thorax is translated right
  - Right thoracic rotation is restricted
  - Unable to weight left ischial tuberosity and translate thorax left

4. Sit and stand

◆ Lateral view

● Restricted bilateral pelvifemoral motion in hip flexion and extension

● Maintains lumbar region in flexion

● Maintains extension at thoracolumbar junction

- ◆ Anterior view
- ● Right hip abduction
- ● Pelvis translates right, reinforcing right leg dominance in weight bearing

5. Standing balance

- ◆ Two-leg stance, eyes open, 60 seconds
- ● Two-leg stance eyes closed, 40 seconds
- ◆ One-leg stance, eyes open
- ● Right leg eyes open 60 seconds
- ● Left leg eyes open 15 seconds
- ● Right leg eyes closed 35 seconds
- ● Left leg eyes closed 0 seconds

- ◆ Anterior view
- ● Improved bilateral hip-knee-ankle-foot tracking
- ● Reduced right translation of pelvis, accommodating left leg contribution to weight bearing

5. Standing balance

- ◆ Two-leg stance, eyes open 60 seconds
- ● Two-leg stance eyes closed, 60 seconds
- ◆ One-leg stance, eyes open
- ● Right leg eyes open 60 seconds
- ● Left leg eyes open 50 seconds
- ● Right leg eyes closed 45 seconds
- ● Left leg eyes closed 20 seconds

Session 3/12: Home program

Fatigue scale	6
Pain scale	4
Client self-report	● Hopeful, curious

Key changes observed by author at end of Session 3/12
- Initial organization in standing
  - On rear feet, plantar surface of toes has light or no contact with floor
  - Weight bearing biased toward right hemipelvis and right lower extremity (LE)
  - Right thoracic rotation
  - Thoracolumbar junction (TLJ) hyperextension
- Organization in standing following home program practice
  - More toward mid-foot, including both forefoot and rear foot, plantar surface of toes has contact with floor
  - Less pronounced weight bearing toward right hemipelvis and right lower extremity, more to midline
  - Decreased right thoracic rotation, more to midline
  - TLJ hyperextension, no discernible change

Reason behind choice of sequencing
- Respect client's need for pacing
- Avoid PESE
- Encourage efficient breath practices that reduce stress and support a calm state
- Encourage efficient breath practices that enhance tissue oxygenation (Nestor 2020)
- Encourage safe, easy-to-implement practices that support circulation (Chaitow 2002)
- Reduce TLJ hyperextension and right rotation
- Midline organization of pelvis, thorax, cranium over foundation of mid-feet and ankles in all three planes supports efficient gait

Session movement sequence

1. Ladder Barrel prone supported torso flexion with coherent breathing

Derivative of J. H. Pilates Ladder Barrel Stomach Jumps (NPCE Study Guide 2021, p. 86)
(See Figure 13.1 in Session 11, exercise 1)

Intent
- Facilitate efficient breathing
- Support calm physiological state

Gait reasoning ● Decrease TLJ hyperextension and right thoracic rotation

Starting position ● Prone over Ladder Barrel
● Hands hold ladder rung
● Feet on small box with ground force through heels
● Forehead supported on barrel

Movement description ● Coherent breathing through nose
● Inhale for 6 seconds, exhale for 6 seconds or longer according to comfort
● Hum during exhalation on a pleasing tone or tune of choice
● As comfort dictates, hands let go of ladder rung, cross arms, hands hold elbows
● Rest tongue on hard palate of roof of mouth to open airways
● Direct breathing movement toward posterior-lateral regions of thorax. Emphasize rib excursion of right side of thorax towards the right
● After 5 breath cycles or approximately 1 minute of coherent breathing leave the Ladder Barrel
● Stand upright
● Walk around the area, continuing nose breathing
● Practice at least twice a day, more if useful

Author note
– Nose breathing is preferred to mouth breathing for efficient tissue oxygenation (Nestor 2020)
– Humming stimulates the release of nitric oxide from the parasinuses, benefiting the endothelium to increase circulation (Chaitow 2018)
– Hyperextension at the TLJ may impede posterior and lateral excursion of the thorax and diaphragm, necessary for efficient breathing
– Excursion of the thoracic volume in the posterior and lateral dimensions may make more surface area of the lungs available for gaseous exchange (Lee 2018).

2. Forefoot and rear foot standing organization in sagittal plane

Intent ● Encourage whole-body standing strategy over mid-feet rather than rear feet

Gait reasoning	● Organizing entire body in adaptation to ankle plantar flexion/dorsiflexion supports efficient weight transfer
Starting position	● Stand, heels aligned with ischia ● Organize to midline in all planes ● Balance the volumes of pelvis, thorax, and cranium along vertical axis above foundation of feet
Movement description	● Dorsiflex at metatarsophalangeal (MTP) joints, minimizing posterior shift ● Metatarsal heads sustain contact with floor ● Tension lower abdominal region, creating a current that draws pubis in direction of xiphoid process ● Center volume of pelvis above mid-feet ● Return toes to contact floor ● Minimizing posterior weight shift, hover heels off floor ● Ankle plantar flexion requires balance on forefeet ● Translate entire central axis forward and up ● Lower heels to floor minimizing posterior weight shift ● Continue nose breathing, rhythmically alternating toes lift and lower with heels lift and lower ● Practice foot and ankle plantar flexon and dorsiflexion articulations for 1 minute sustaining whole-body organization around central axis ● Coherent breathing is optional ● Hum during exhalation unless it interferes with your rhythm and concentration. Practice at least twice a day; more if useful ● Avoid duration or frequency that causes fatigue, exaggerates symptoms, or compromises tissue comfort

Author note

Subtle, specific, whole-body reorganization to midline, primarily in the sagittal plane, is required to sustain rhythmic alternation between dorsiflexion at the MTP joints and ankle plantar flexion.

3. Drawing figure 8 mandalas in preparation for movement of lumbopelvic-hip complex in figure 8 patterns

Intent	● Drawing the infinity sign figure 8 pattern may prepare for coordinated movement of the lumbopelvic-hip complex in efficient gait

Gait reasoning	● Efficient gait involves movement of the lumbopelvic-hip complex in figure 8 patterns in three planes
Starting position	● Stand at a drawing table facing a blank piece of paper ● Hold a pencil or pen in dominant hand
Movement description	● Draw figure 8s with a horizontal axis, a vertical axis, and two diagonal axes ● Repeat drawing exercises holding pencil or pen in non-dominant hand ● Move pelvis in the same directions while drawing the figure 8s

4. Outdoor walking practice

● Once a day as stamina allows, walk outside along the neighborhood country road practicing nose breathing
● Include awareness of foot-ankle articulation

Intent	● Walking outdoors benefits exposure of eyes and skin to natural light ● Visual system benefits of scanning landscape and sky in the distance ● Decrease depression, reduce anxiety ● Support client awareness of subtle changes in physical capabilities and mood fluctuations
Gait reasoning	● Walking practice integrates home program coordination exercises into whole-body movement ● Walking practice develops cardiovascular and myofascial endurance
Starting position	● Note the beginning and end times of the walk ● Record the time spent walking outdoors ● Record physical, emotional, and cognitive responses
Movement description	● Once a day as stamina allows, walk outside along the neighborhood country road ● Practice nose breathing ● Include awareness of foot-ankle articulation ● Note the beginning and end times of the walk ● Record the time spent walking outdoors ● Record physical, emotional, and cognitive responses

Session 11/12: Studio session

Fatigue scale 3

Pain scale 2

Client self-report
- Walks neighborhood hill with no fatigue, no foot pain, no back pain, no exacerbation of symptoms
- Feels confident and secure about progress in health improvement
- Enjoys teaching her clients the new Wunda Chair exercises that have been helpful to her own progress

Key changes observed by author at end of Session 11/12
- Client appears animated, suffused with vitality
- Client seems confident and optimistic
- Movement transitions seem graceful rather than tentative

Reason behind choice of sequencing
- Experience all 10 exercises in a continuous sequence
- Acknowledge accomplishment of mastering a new movement program in 6 weeks
- Acknowledge improvements in motor control, endurance, strength, cognitive clarity

Session movement sequence

1. Ladder Barrel prone supported torso flexion with coherent breathing

Derivative of J. H. Pilates Ladder Barrel Stomach Jumps (NPCE Study Guide 2021, p. 86)

Author note
This exercise was introduced in Session 3, home program. It was practiced in Sessions 4 to 11. The orientation of partially upright, prone supported flexion may be preferable to supine or seated breathing practices. Supported, partially upright flexion on the Ladder Barrel minimizes a POTS response. The orientation minimizes sacroiliac joint (SIJ) irritation that may result from compression in sitting.

Intent
- Supported mild flexion may facilitate calm physiological state through ventral vagus nerve tone
- Posterior-lateral thoracic excursion may facilitate efficient breathing
- Decrease hyperextension of TLJ
- Decrease compression in right lumbar-pelvic region
- Stimulate release of nitric oxide from the parasinuses

Gait reasoning
- Client's current strategy of right rotation and hyperextension at TLJ may contribute to inefficient gait
- Orientation of supported flexion may decrease client's inefficient gait strategies
- Coherent breathing in supported mild flexion may prepare tissues and nervous system for new movement practices that develop efficient gait

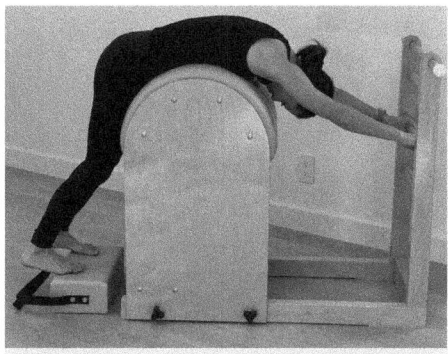

Figure 13.1

Set-up
- Position barrel a distance from ladder to support client structure and comfort
- Small box supports client's feet
- Towel or cushion supports client's forehead against barrel

Starting position
- Prone over barrel
- Hands hold ladder rung at comfortable level
- Forehead supported on a folded towel or cushion resting against the barrel facilitates ease of neck and jaw
- Knees in slight flexion
- Feet supported on small box, either forefoot or rear foot, according to comfort

Movement description
- Gently close lips
- Inhale through nose for 6 seconds
- Exhale through nose for 6 seconds
- During exhalation hum in register of preference
- Repeat for five breath cycles
- According to comfort and preference, let go of rungs, hold bent elbows
- Stand up from the barrel, walk, noticing changes in comfort or discomfort

CUES
- Direct inhalation movement excursion to right posterior-lateral thorax
- Direct inhalation movement to right lumbar region
- Aim ischial tuberosities toward heels
- During inhalation scroll the tongue up and back along the hard palate in the direction of the soft palate, as if to open airways for comfortable airflow
- During exhalation slide the tongue along the hard palate in the direction of the upper teeth, organizing the jaw

Coherent breathing

Coherent breathing and "resonant breathing" are names given to an efficient breathing rhythm in which a 5.5-second inhalation is followed by a 5.5-second exhalation. Nose breathing is recommended throughout inhalation and exhalation. This slow breathing pattern brings the body into a state of coherence when functions of heart, circulation, and nervous system are coordinated to peak efficiency. If the client prefers, start with an easier rhythm of 3-second inhales with at least the same length exhales (Nestor 2020).

Stimulating release of nitric oxide by humming during nose exhalation

Nitric oxide is a molecule made by the human body that nourishes muscle tissue. When you start to exercise and run out of oxygen (you feel your muscles ache), nitric oxide is released. Blood vessels dilate allowing more oxygen and nutrient delivery for muscle growth. Blood vessels only store about 90 seconds' worth of nitric oxide before they need to manufacture more. The body may regenerate nitric oxide every couple of hours, giving you the opportunity to release it multiple times a day. An effective way to increase your muscle function is to work out very briefly every few hours (Zachary Bush, MD). Clients experiencing long COVID symptoms may have blood vessels lined with impaired endothelium. This may affect circulation, contributing to fatigue during activities of daily living and movement. Respect pacing guidelines and avoid PEM. Hum during nose exhalation to stimulate release of nitric oxide from the parasinuses. This may improve circulation and support a calm state (Chaitow 2018).

2. Feet doming on foam yoga blocks

Derivative of J. H. Pilates Foot Corrector: Ball of Foot Over (Doming) (NPCE Study Guide 2021, p. 89)

Author note
- This exercise was introduced in Session 4 in sitting
- It was practiced in sitting and standing during Sessions 5 to 11
- This exercise prepares for standing doming exercises 4 and 6

Intent
- Stimulate synergistic activation of muscle tissue and connective tissue in support of efficient foot movement
- Prepare foundation of feet to support the volumes of pelvis, thorax, and cranium
- Decrease client's strategy to weight bear toward rear foot

Gait reasoning
- Improvement in foot-ankle movement coordination may improve gait efficiency
- Increase in foot-ankle tissue strength and endurance may improve gait efficiency
- Client's standing strategy to load rear foot may impede transfer of weight toward forefoot in preparation for push-off and swing phases of gait

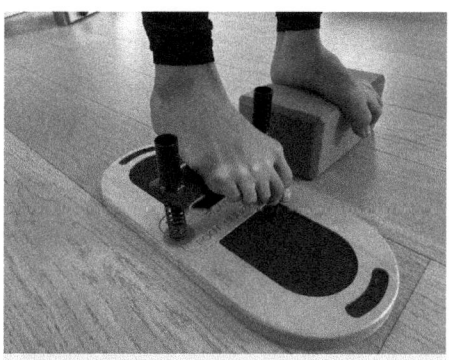

Figure 13.2

Set-up
- Place Foot Corrector with light spring on non-skid rubberized mat
- Place firm foam yoga block in most stable orientation on non-skid rubberized mat

Starting position
- Stand facing Foot Corrector and yoga block
- Right foot aligned with Foot Corrector
- Left foot aligned with yoga block
- Hands hold a stable surface to support balance
- If convenient, hold rungs of Ladder Barrel

Movement description
- Depress Foot Corrector pedal with right mid-foot just posterior to metatarsal heads
- Right forefoot creates a dome over and in front of pedal
- Shift pelvis forward over the right forefoot during pedal depression
- Repeat 8 times
- Return right foot to floor
- Front of left heel aligns over the back edge of yoga block
- Left metatarsal heads press onto the top facing of yoga block
- Left toes press against the front surface of yoga block that is perpendicular to floor
- Draw front of left heel forward toward left toes
- Press toes into yoga block back toward heel
- Sustain doming activity for 5 breath cycles
- Repeat on other side, aligning Foot Corrector with left foot and yoga block with right foot

CUES

- Intend to shorten the yoga block by doming foot
- Draw rear foot toward forefoot and forefoot toward rear foot
- As the foot domes, shift pelvis forward and up, centering the volume of the pelvis over the domed foot
- Activate doming during inhalation, then practice doming during exhalation, identifying preferred breath pairing

Foot doming (also known as the Janda short foot exercise)

The concept of "*the foot core*" was authored by McKeon *et al.* in 2014. The foot core consists of the plantar extrinsic and intrinsic foot muscles and connective tissue that control the amount and rate of strain with each foot strike. The foot core consists of 10 muscles in four groupings that have attachments only in the foot. These tissues function as stabilizers of the foot. The extrinsic foot muscle tissue and connective tissue attach in the foot and in the lower leg. They function as prime movers. Foot core training can develop foot and ankle articulation to support efficient function of the plantar fascia-Achilles tendon continuity. The "*short foot exercise,*" created by the late Czechoslovakian physiotherapist Vladimir Janda, is also called "*doming.*" This exercise develops coordination, strength, and endurance of the foot core structures (Davis 2021).

3. Wunda Chair seated thoracic lateral flexion with rotation toward sagittal flexion

Derivative of J. H. Pilates Wunda Chair Seated Mermaid/Side Arm Sit (NPCE Study Guide 2021, p. 73)

Author note
– This exercise was introduced in Session 3 and practiced in Sessions 4 to 11
– In recognition of the client's movement strategies:
  ♦ First exercise was practiced with left hand on pedal
  ♦ Next exercise was practiced with right hand on pedal
  ♦ Exercise was repeated with left hand on pedal

Intent
● Decrease compression that may result from right rotation and hyperextension at TLJ
● Counter client's strategy of loading right hemipelvis more than left
● Introduce client to novel uses of Pilates apparatus that were not included in her curriculum of study
● New movement patterns may stimulate dopamine release, elevate curiosity, and create optimism regarding improvement in health condition

Gait reasoning
● Balanced thoracic rotation on left and right supports efficient gait
● Encourage left thoracic rotation to counter current right thoracic rotation strategy
● Decrease hyperextension at TLJ

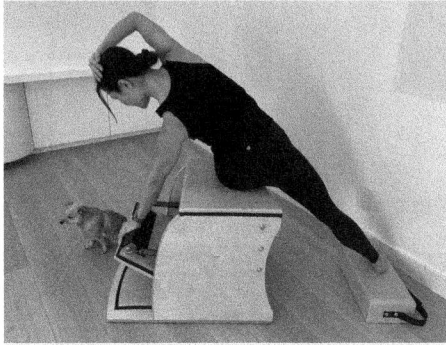

Figure 13.3

| Set-up | • Wunda Chair with single pedal attached to medium spring |
| | • Small box supports each foot |

Starting position	• Sit on chair, left side toward pedal
	• Small box supports left foot aligned forward of left hip
	• Small box supports right foot abducted from right hip
	• Left hand on pedal in plane of scaption
	• Bent right elbow palm on top of head, as if right palm could cover left ear

Movement description	• During inhalation depress pedal
	• During exhalation thoracic rotation left toward flexion
	• During inhalation derotate
	• During exhalation return to starting position
	• Repeat 8 times
	■ Variation 1: non-pedal arm elbow in flexion with hand on top of head, repeat 4 times
	■ Variation 2: non-pedal arm elbow in extension with upper arm alongside ear, continuing arc of thoracic lateral flexion, repeat 4 times
	• Repeat on other side

CUES

- ◆ Aim bent elbow away from pelvis
- ◆ Reach straight-elbow hand away from pelvis
- ◆ Arm reach encourages excursion of thorax in right lateral-posterior regions

4. Ladder Barrel standing whole-body rotation with feet doming on yoga blocks on rotator discs

Derivative of J. H. Pilates Trapeze Table Standing on Floor: Upper Arm Control Facing In (Vertical) and Standing on Floor: Twist (NPCE Study Guide 2021, p. 65)

Intent	• Develop endurance to sustain foot doming on dynamic surface
	• Encourage whole-body organization to midline in all planes
	• Stimulate integration of vestibular and proprioceptive systems to support balance
	• Stimulating coordination in standing full weight bearing may address brain fog

Gait reasoning	• Foot-ankle motor control, strength, and endurance provide a reliable foundation for gait
	• This exercise organizes the pelvis, thorax, and cranium over the mid-foot, preparing for efficient gait
	• Counter the client's strategy to stand toward rear foot

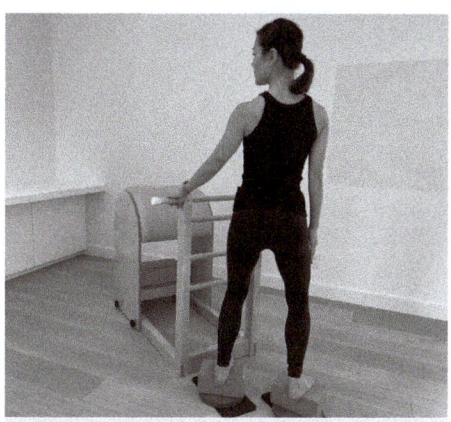

Figure 13.4

Set-up
- Place each yoga block in most stable orientation on a rotator disc adjacent to rungs of Ladder Barrel
- Position yoga blocks on discs apart, the width of greater trochanters

Starting position
- Stand on domed feet on yoga blocks
- Knees extended
- Hands hold rung of Ladder Barrel

Movement description
- Hand holds ladder rung, rotate whole body approximately 45 degrees to face right diagonally
- Hand holds ladder rung, rotate whole body approximately 45 degrees to face left diagonally
- Repeat 4 times knees extended. 4 times knees in flexion
- Variation 19: both eyes closed, neither hand holds rung, head and eyes track in the direction toes aim. Repeat 4 times right and left
  - Knees either in extension or flexion
- Variation 20: both eyes closed, neither hand holds rung, head and eyes track forward while thorax, pelvis, LE rotate right and left. Repeat 4 times right and left
  - Knees either in extension or flexion
- Variation 21: both eyes closed, neither hand holds rung, head and eyes track opposite the rotation of thorax, pelvis, LE. 4 times right and left
  - Knees either in extension or flexion

CUES

- ◆ Aim toes, navel, sternum, nose, eyes in the same direction at the same time
- ◆ Keep head and eyes steady while body and feet rotate right and left
- ◆ Turn head and eyes opposite the rotational aim of body and feet

Author note

- – This exercise was introduced in Session 5 and practiced in Sessions 5 to 11
- – Each session included more challenging variations culminating in the most challenging variations in Session 11

5. Wunda Chair: seated on Balansit on rotator disc facing pedals, ankle plantar flexion/dorsiflexion

Derivative of J. H. Pilates Wunda Chair Double Leg Pumps: Parallel (NPCE Study Guide 2021, p. 72)

Intent
- ● Refine alignment of hip joint with knee, ankle, 2nd toe
- ● Coordinate ankle plantar flexion/dorsiflexion with lumbo-sacral lateral flexion
- ● Coordinate rotation of pelvic-lumbar region with ankle plantar flexion/dorsiflexion

Gait reasoning
- ● Efficient gait includes aligned movement relationships of hip joint with knee, ankle, 2nd and 3rd toes
- ● Efficient gait includes coordination of lumbosacral lateral flexion with ankle plantar flexion/dorsiflexion
- ● Efficient gait includes coordination of lumbopelvic rotation with ankle plantar flexion/dorsiflexion

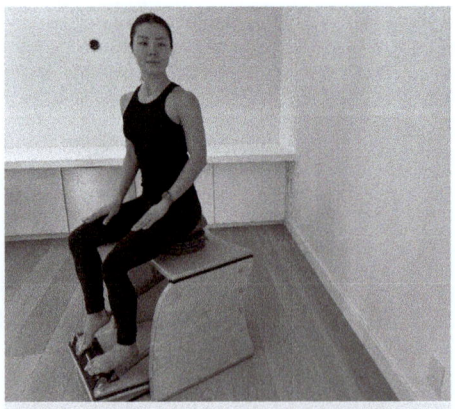

Figure 13.5

Set-up
- Place Balansit on rotator disc on chair seat
- Chair does not have split pedal
- Attach single pedal to 1 heavy spring

Starting position
- Sit on Balansit
- Each forefoot (soles of toes and metatarsal heads) on pedal
- Each palm on same side thigh

Movement description
- Variation 5: move pelvis and lumbar region in a figure 8 with a horizontal left-to-right axis integrating ankle plantar flexion with lumbosacral lateral flexion and rotation
  - Right ankle initiates plantar flexion
  - Left ischium depresses Balansit shifting weight forward left
  - Rotate pelvis to left
  - Left ankle initiates plantar flexion
  - Right ischium depresses Balansit shifting weight forward right
  - Rotate pelvis to right
  - Repeat pattern 12–16 times

CUES
- Steer pelvis in an infinity pattern, a figure 8 with a horizontal left-to-right axis
- Create a smooth movement flow

Author note
- This exercise was introduced in Session 6 and practiced in Sessions 6 to 11
- Each session included gait-relevant variations culminating in the most challenging variation 5 in Session

Soleus push-up (SPU)

The soleus is a posterior leg muscle that connects from just below the knee to the heel. Professor of Health and Human Performance at the University of Houston Marc Hamilton is pioneering the seated *soleus push-up* (SPU) which elevates muscle metabolism for hours. Hamilton's research suggests the SPU's ability to sustain an elevated oxidative metabolism to improve the regulation of blood glucose is more effective than any popular method including exercise, weight loss, and intermittent fasting. "When activated correctly, soleus muscle tissue can raise local oxidative metabolism to high levels for hours, not just minutes, and does so by using a different fuel mixture." The SPU activates the soleus muscle differently when standing or walking. The SPU performed while seated is the opposite of walking. When walking, the body is designed to minimize the amount of energy used. SPUs make the soleus use as much energy as possible for a long duration. Seated with feet flat on the floor and muscles relaxed, the heel rises while the front of the foot stays put. When the heel gets to the top of its range of motion, the foot is passively released to come back down. The aim is to simultaneously shorten the calf muscle while the soleus is naturally activated by its motor neurons. The SPU targets the soleus to increase oxygen consumption while also being resistant to fatigue (Hamilton, Hamilton, and Zderic 2022).

6. Ped-o-Pull standing facing pole, feet doming on yoga block on rotator disc with Stability Sling support TLJ

Derivative of J. H. Pilates Ped-o-Pull Deep Knee Bends: Facing In (NPCE Study Guide 2021, p. 91)

Intent	• Provide proprioceptive stimulation to TLJ region
	• Proprioceptive stimulation to TLJ region may decrease hyperextension at TLJ
	• Proprioceptive stimulation to TLJ region may decrease tendency toward right thoracic rotation
	• Standing rotation while doming on yoga blocks may refine proprioception supporting whole-body organization to midline
Gait reasoning	• Midline organization of the sacrum-TLJ-occiput during gait cycle supports efficient gait
	• Doming feet on dynamic surface of yoga blocks on rotator discs may encourage centering volume of pelvis above the mid-foot, improving weight transfer between forefoot and rear foot

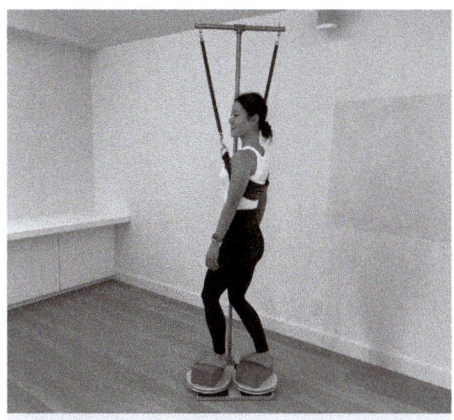

Figure 13.6

Set-up	● Attach Stability Sling to 2 light, long arm springs connected to crossbar
	● Place 2 rotator discs pelvis-width apart on non-skid rubberized mats
	● Place each yoga block in most stable orientation on a rotator disc
Starting position	● Stand facing the pole
	● Place Stability Sling around the back and sides of the lower thorax, supporting the TLJ
	● Dome one foot on yoga block
	● Dome other foot on yoga block
	● Hands hold central pole to assist balance and provide ground force for initiation of whole-body rotation
Movement description	● Knee flexion assists balance and contact of Stability Sling with TLJ
	● Rotate whole body approximately 45 degrees to face right diagonally
	● Rotate whole body approximately 45 degrees to face left diagonally
	● Simultaneously turn feet, pelvis, thorax, head in the same direction
	● Variation 5: thorax, neck, and head rotate in opposite direction to pelvis and LE

CUES

◆ Press soles of the big toes firmly onto the yoga blocks
◆ Create a force of adduction, drawing the tops of the inner thighs toward each other
◆ Aim the knees in the same direction as the 3rd toes
◆ Aim 3rd toes, navel, sternum, and nose in same direction
◆ Variation 5: feet and pelvis initiate right rotation as thorax, neck, and head rotate left

Author notes

– This exercise was introduced in Session 7
– New variations were introduced in Sessions 8 to 11

7. Wunda Chair: seated on Balansit on rotator disc, side to pedal, foot on forward pedal

Derivative of J. H. Pilates Wunda Chair Single Leg Pumps: Toes and Heels (NPCE Study Guide 2021, p. 72)

Intent
● Facilitate medial glide of hip joint
● Reinforce internal rotation of LE
● Coordinate torso rotation with LE sagittal movement

Gait reasoning
● Medial and lateral glides of the femur head in the acetabulum contribute to efficient gait
● Medial rotation of LE may contribute to efficient push-off phase of gait

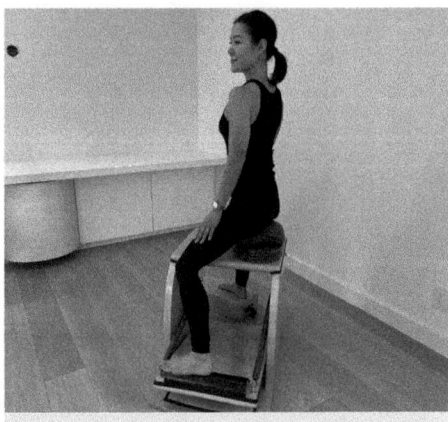

Figure 13.7

Set-up
- Place rotator disc at front corner of Wunda Chair seat
- Attach single pedal to 1 heavy spring

Starting position
- Sit on rotator disc with side to pedal
- Foot of LE closest to pedal contacts forward pedal in parallel
- Foot of LE furthest from pedal supported on small box

Movement description
- Variation 7
  - LE parallel, plantar surface of foot on forward pedal
  - Depress pedal with ankle plantar flexion rotating torso away from descending pedal
  - Rotate torso toward ascending pedal during ankle dorsiflexion
  - Repeat 12–16 times
- Variation 8
  - LE parallel, plantar surface of foot on forward pedal
  - Depress pedal with ankle plantar flexion rotating torso toward pedal
  - Rotate torso away from pedal ascending via ankle dorsiflexion
  - Repeat 12–16 times

CUES
- Inner thigh of pedal LE hugs toward the edge of the chair top
- Press sole of big toe/1st ray firmly on inner edge of pedal
- Steer ankle over 2nd toe
- Steer the rotator disc with ischial tuberosities
- Center thoracic region over pelvis, avoiding thoracic translation and lateral flexion

Author note
- This exercise was introduced in Session 8 and practiced in Sessions 9, 10, and 11
- Each session included new variations with the most challenging variations in Session 11
- The more advanced variations required sitting only on the rotator disc, not the Balansit

8. Ladder Barrel Horseback holding Magic Circle overhead — Derivative of J. H. Pilates Ladder Barrel Horseback (NPCE Study Guide 2021, p. 85) and Magic Circle Two Arm Press—Overhead (NPCE Study Guide 2021, p. 88)

Intent
- Integrate whole-body tension and compression network.
- Integrate proximal initiation of hip adduction with distal initiation of scapulohumeral movement.
- Organize volumes of pelvis, thorax and cranium to the midline in all three planes.
- Sustain synergistic activation of all structures required for pelvic lift off of Ladder Barrel.
- Sustain midline organization during differentiated rotation of pelvis, thorax, and cranium.

Gait reasoning
- Efficient gait requires both pelvi-femoral and femoral-pelvi motion.
- Efficient gait involves midline organization of pelvis, thorax and cranial volumes during counter rotation of pelvis and thorax.
- Open kinematic chain context of the plantar surfaces of the feet emphasizes proximal control of torso.

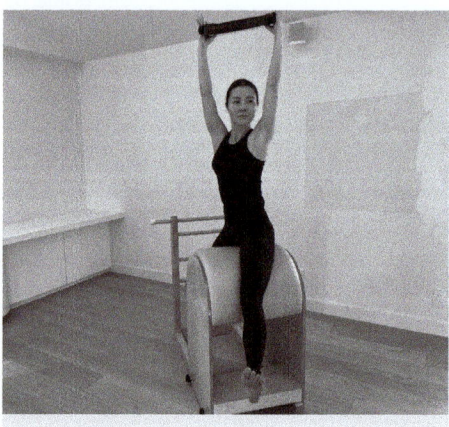

Figure 13.8

Set-up
- Adjust Ladder Barrel so that barrel is furthest away from the Ladder
- Hands hold Magic Circle

Starting position	• Straddle barrel
	• Knees extended
	• Ankles in dorsiflexion
	• LE slight flexion and internal rotation
	• Hands hold Magic Circle in front of lower thoracic area
	• Elbows extended

Movement description	• LE adduction and external rotation
	• Pelvic outlet region hovers off the barrel
	• Carry Magic Circle overhead
	• Thumbs pull outward on the Magic Circle handles
	▪ External rotation of upper extremity (UE) at glenohumeral joint (GHJ)
	• Rotate pelvis-torso-head right and left, 8 times
	• Repeat entire sequence holding Magic Circle with palms pressing handles outward
	▪ Internal rotation of UE

CUES

- ◆ Inner thighs hug the barrel
- ◆ Draw the pelvic outlet tissues up, away from the barrel
- ◆ Shoulders slide down away from the neck as thumbs pull the Magic Circle wide

Author note

- – This exercise was introduced in Session 9
- – Increasingly challenging variations were practiced in Sessions 10 and 11

9. Trapeze Table Stability Sling supported bridge with rotation	Derivative of J. H. Pilates Trapeze Table Roll-Down Bar: Breathing (NPCE Study Guide 2021, p. 66) and Hanging Half (NPCE Study Guide 2021, p. 70)
Intent	• Suspend thoracic area between supports of lumbopelvic and shoulder girdle regions
	• Facilitate ease of breathing by decreasing compression in areas of diaphragm attachments
Gait reasoning	• Decrease of thoracic compression may contribute to feelings of buoyancy during gait
	• Decrease of thoracic compression may encourage thoracic rotation during gait

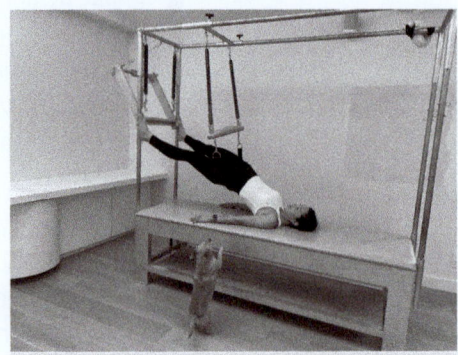

Figure 13.9

Set-up	• 2 heavy springs attach Stability Sling to overhead slider bar
	• Position overhead slider bar so that plantar surface of feet can press against the vertical frame bars when pelvis is supported by Stability Sling
Starting position	• Stand on Trapeze Table facing the upright frame bars at one end of table
	• Place Stability Sling behind lumbosacral area
	• Lower pelvis to table
	• Place feet on upright frame bars
	• Adjust position according to comfort
Movement description	• Press left foot against upright pole
	• Rotate lumbopelvic area right
	• Press right foot against upright pole
	• Rotate lumbopelvic area left
	• Repeat 8–12 times
	• Practice nose breathing
	• Practice coherent breathing
	• Hum at any register during exhalation
	• Relax and decompress as long as you like

CUES
- Imagine lungs resting in supportive rib basket hammock
- Imagine lungs puffing up with pillows of air

Author note
– This exercise was introduced in Session 10, variation 1, no rotation
– Variation 2 was practiced in Session 11

10. Trapeze Table supported Downward Facing Dog with thoracic rotation, hand reaches toward/holds opposite ankle

Derivative of J. H. Pilates Trapeze Table Spread Eagle (NPCE Study Guide 2021, p. 71) and Squirrel (NPCE Study Guide 2021, p. 71)

Intent
- Suspend torso from support of Stability Sling at front of upper thighs
- Decrease compression of diaphragm region
- Facilitate ease of breathing

Gait reasoning
- Sustained ankle dorsiflexion may improve posterior LE tissue glide
- Thoracic rotation in direction of flexion counters client's habitual strategy to rotate right in the direction of extension

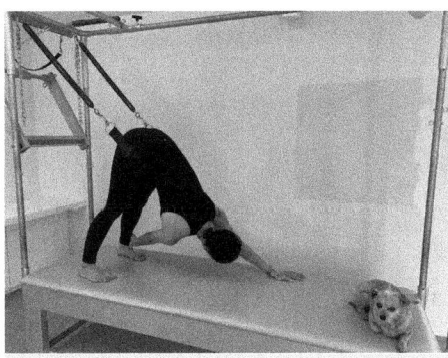

Figure 13.10

Set-up
- 2 heavy springs attach Stability Sling to upper crossbar frame at one end of the table
- Non-skid rubberized pads available for standing feet if needed

Starting position
- Stand with back to Stability Sling
- Place Stability Sling over head
- Secure Stability Sling at front of upper thighs
- Knee flexion to place palms on table
- Adjust distance between feet and hands
- Extend knees

Movement description
- When feeling secure, reach right hand across midline toward left lower leg or left ankle
- Sustain this arrangement as guided by comfort or for 5 breath cycles of coherent breathing
- Repeat other side
- Alternate sides as guided by comfort

CUES
- Press soles of feet and palms of hands into table
- Aim ischial tuberosities up, back, and wide
- During rotation wring out the contents of the rib basket making room for fresh circulation

Author note
Adjust the spring tension to provide optimal support for the client.

The journey to Session 11

Session 4/12
Client self-report

- Feels calmer when humming during nose exhalations
- Practices humming throughout the day
- Right SIJ irritated by figure 8 practice in Session 3
- Did not practice walking outdoors due to cold weather
- Prefers Ladder Barrel supported flexion holding elbows rather than rungs
- Fatigue scale 5
- Pain scale 3

Key changes observed

- Weight bearing less accentuated to rear feet
- Soles of toes contact the floor
- Speaking voice sounds more resonant, less anxious

Reasoning behind choice of movements

- Reinforce calm state with coherent breathing
- Reduce compression in right posterior-lateral lumbopelvic region

Session movement sequence
1. Remove standing pelvic figure 8s from home program

2. Ladder Barrel prone supported torso flexion with coherent breathing

- Each hand holds opposite elbow rather than rungs

3. Feet doming on foam yoga blocks

- Seated
- Standing

4. Wunda Chair seated thoracic lateral flexion with rotation toward sagittal flexion

- Non-pedal arm elbow in flexion with hand on top of head

Session 5/12
Client self-report

- Very happy with new Wunda Chair exercise of side bending and rotation, the "Pilates Mermaid"
- Right ear did not pop last night
- This is notable since she usually experiences tightness on right side of head accompanied by right ear popping
- Feels feet more in contact with floor
- Fatigue scale 4
- Pain scale 2

Key changes observed

- Thoracic rotation right less pronounced
- Thorax seems to be aligning with central axis of pelvis rather than posterior to it

Reasoning behind choice of movements

- Reinforce decompression of right posterior lateral torso region
- Develop awareness of midline organization in standing
- Challenge spatial organization in standing in hope that will contribute to cognitive clarity

Session movement sequence
1. Ladder Barrel prone supported torso flexion with coherent breathing

2. Feet doming on foam yoga blocks

- Omit Foot Corrector

3. Wunda Chair seated thoracic lateral flexion with rotation toward sagittal flexion

- Variation 1: non-pedal arm elbow in flexion with hand on top of head
- Variation 2: non-pedal arm elbow in extension with upper arm alongside ear, continuing arc of thoracic lateral flexion

4. Standing whole-body rotation, feet doming on yoga blocks on rotator discs

- Variation 1: hands hold Ladder Barrel rung
  - Both eyes open, head and eyes track in the direction toes aim
- Variation 2: hands hold Ladder Barrel rung
  - Both eyes open, head and eyes track forward during transverse plane rotation of thorax, pelvis, LE
- Variation 3: hands hold Ladder Barrel rung
  - Both eyes open, head and eyes rotate opposite the direction toes aim

Session 6/12
Client self-report

- Walked up neighborhood hill with improved power, speed, and less fatigue
- Aware of foot-to-pelvis connections during walking
- Increased fatigue attributed to excitement about improvement and decision to increase exertion rather than rest
- Fatigue scale 5
- Pain scale 3

Key changes observed

- TLJ seems to have sagittal alignment with sacrum rather than posterior to it
- Gait seems less rigid and brittle
- Heel strike seems less jarring

Reasoning behind choice of movements

- Reinforce midline organization in all planes
- Develop ankle articulation aligned with hip joint
- Challenge focus and concentration with motor control complexity

Session movement sequence

1. Ladder Barrel prone supported torso flexion with coherent breathing

2. Feet doming on foam yoga blocks

- Omit seated practice
- Standing only

3. Wunda Chair seated thoracic lateral flexion with rotation toward sagittal flexion

- Variation 2: non-pedal arm elbow in extension with upper arm alongside ear, continuing arc of thoracic lateral flexion

4. Standing whole-body rotation, feet doming on yoga blocks on rotator discs

- Variation 4: hands hold Ladder Barrel rung
  - Close one eye, head and eyes track in the direction toes aim
- Variation 5: hands hold Ladder Barrel rung
  - Close the other eye, head and eyes track in the direction toes aim
- Variation 6: hands hold Ladder Barrel rung
  - Close one eye, head and eyes track forward during transverse plane rotation of thorax, pelvis, LE
- Variation 7: hands hold Ladder Barrel rung
  - Close the other eye, head and eyes track forward during transverse rotation of thorax, pelvis, LE
- Variation 8: hands hold Ladder Barrel rung
  - Close one eye, head and eyes aim opposite during rotation of thorax, pelvis, LE
- Variation 9: hands hold Ladder Barrel rung
  - Close other eye, head and eyes aim opposite during rotation of thorax, pelvis, LE

5. Wunda Chair: seated on Balansit on rotator disc facing pedals, ankle plantar flexion/dorsiflexion

- Knees directly forward aligned with 2nd metatarsal and toe
- Do not rotate Balansit on disc
- Variation 1: keep pelvis steady as right ankle initiates plantar flexion and returns to dorsiflexion
  - Alternate right and left ankle initiation of plantar flexion/dorsiflexion
- Variation 2: as right ankle initiates plantar flexion press left ischial tuberosity into Balansit
  - Level pelvis as right ankle returns to dorsiflexion
- Variation 2: as left ankle initiates plantar flexion press right ischial tuberosity into Balansit
  - Alternate right and left ankle initiation of plantar flexion/dorsiflexion depressing opposite ischial tuberosity

Session 7/12
Client self-report

- Excited by new exercises she has learned that she can teach her clients
- Clients are responding enthusiastically to the rotation she is including in her own practice and her teaching clients
- No longer bothered by feeling stuck in right SI area
- Fatigue scale 3
- Pain scale 1

Key changes observed

- Decreased tendency to exaggerate right foot/ankle supination and left foot/ankle pronation

- Seems to enjoy new uses of familiar Pilates equipment, especially rotation and thoracic mobility

Reasoning behind choice of movements

- Focus on sensory stimulation at the TLJ in order to improve thoracic organization to midline in all planes
- Integrate domed feet with thorax using Stability Sling attached to Ped-o-Pull

Session movement sequence
1. Ladder Barrel prone supported torso flexion with coherent breathing

2. Feet doming on foam yoga blocks

3. Wunda Chair seated thoracic lateral flexion with rotation toward sagittal flexion

- Variation 2: non pedal arm elbow in extension with upper arm alongside ear, continuing arc of thoracic lateral flexion

4. Standing whole-body rotation, feet doming on yoga blocks on rotator discs

- Variation 10: hands hold Ladder Barrel rung
  - Close both eyes, head and eyes track in the direction toes aim
- Variation 11: hands hold Ladder Barrel rung
  - Close both eyes, head and eyes track forward
- Variation 12: hands hold Ladder Barrel rung
  - Close both eyes, head and eyes track opposite thorax, pelvis, toes

5. Wunda Chair: seated on Balansit on rotator disc facing pedals, ankle plantar flexion/dorsiflexion

- Variation 2: rotate pelvis, thorax, head away from the foot that depresses the pedal with ankle plantar flexion

- During right ankle plantar flexion rotate Balansit on disc to left
- During left ankle plantar flexion rotate Balansit on disc to right

6. Ped-o-Pull stand facing in, doming each foot on yoga block on rotator disc

- Stability Sling supports TLJ
  - Variation: knee flexion
  - Whole-body rotation approximately 45 degrees diagonally right and 45 degrees diagonally left

Session 8/12
Client self-report

- Walking felt lighter, easier after the Ped-o-Pull with Stability Sling last session
- Cannot explain why she did not sleep well
- Fatigue scale 5
- Pain scale 2

Key changes observed

- Decreased hyperextension at TLJ
- Voice sounds strained

Reasoning behind choice of movements

- Address medial and lateral glide of femoral head in the acetabulum to refine gait movement
- Refine TLJ movement relationship with feet and pelvis

Session movement sequence
1. Ladder Barrel prone supported torso flexion with coherent breathing

2. Feet doming on foam yoga blocks

3. Wunda Chair seated thoracic lateral flexion with rotation toward sagittal flexion

- Variation 1: non-pedal arm elbow in flexion with hand on top of head
- Variation 2: non-pedal arm elbow in extension with upper arm alongside ear, continuing arc of thoracic lateral flexion

4. Standing whole-body rotation, feet doming on yoga blocks on rotator discs

- Variation 11: both eyes open, one hand holds rung, head and eyes aim in the direction toes aim
- Variation 11: both eyes open, other hand holds rung, head and eyes aim in the direction toes aim
- Variation 12: both eyes open, one hand holds rung, head and eye aim forward while thorax, pelvis, LE rotate
- Variation 13: both eyes open, other hand holds rung, head and eyes aim in opposite direction of thorax, pelvis, toes

5. Wunda Chair: seated on Balansit on rotator disc facing pedals, ankle plantar flexion/dorsiflexion

- Variation 3: rotate pelvis, thorax, head toward the foot that depresses the pedal with ankle plantar flexion. During right ankle plantar flexion rotate Balansit on disc to right. During left ankle plantar flexion rotate Balansit on disc to left

6. Ped-o-Pull standing facing in, doming each foot on yoga block on rotator disc, Stability Sling supports TLJ

- Variation 2: knees in flexion, whole-body rotation approximately 45 degrees diagonally right and 45 degrees diagonally left

7. Wunda Chair: seated on Balansit on rotator disc, side to pedal, foot on forward pedal

- Variation 1: LE external rotation, heel on forward pedal, rotate torso away from pedal descending, rotate torso toward pedal ascending
- Variation 2: LE external rotation, heel on forward pedal, rotate torso toward pedal descending, rotate torso away from pedal ascending

Session 9/12
Client self-report

- Thrilled that she successfully performed her entire Universal Reformer workout in her home studio that she used to practice before contracting COVID
- This is an indication that strength, endurance, motor control, and focus are improving
- Fatigue scale 3
- Pain scale 1

Key changes observed

- Movement quality seems smoother, more graceful, more flow, less brittle
- Comments seem optimistic, less self-critical

Reasoning behind choice of movements

- Challenge whole-body control and endurance with Horseback on Ladder Barrel
- Focus on strength and endurance of pelvic outlet tissues to sustain activation

Session movement sequence
1. Ladder Barrel prone supported torso flexion with coherent breathing

2. Feet doming on foam yoga blocks

3. Wunda Chair seated thoracic lateral flexion with rotation toward sagittal flexion

- Variation 2: non-pedal arm elbow in extension with upper arm alongside ear, continuing arc of thoracic lateral flexion

4. Standing whole-body rotation, feet doming on yoga blocks on rotator discs

- Variation 14: both eyes open, neither hand holds rung, head and eyes aim in the direction toes aim
- Variation 15: both eyes open, neither hand holds rung, head and eyes aim forward while thorax, pelvis, LE rotate
- Variation 16: both eyes open, neither hand holds rung, head and eyes track opposite the rotation of thorax, pelvis, LE

5. Wunda Chair: seated on Balansit on rotator disc facing pedals, ankle plantar flexion/dorsiflexion

- Seated on Balansit on rotator disc facing pedals, knees directly forward aligned with 2nd meta-tarsal and toe
- Variation 4: aim head and eyes forward as torso rotates away from the ankle that initiates pedal depression with ankle plantar flexion
- Variation 5: aim head and eyes forward as tor-so rotates toward the ankle that initiates pedal depression with ankle plantar flexion

6. Ped-o-Pull standing facing in, doming each foot on yoga block on rotator disc, Stability Sling supports TLJ

- Variation 3: alternate 4 rotations knees in exten-sion with 4 rotations knees in flexion

7. Seated on Wunda Chair, on rotator disc, side to pedal, foot on forward pedal

- Variation 3: LE parallel, plantar surface of foot on forward pedal, rotate torso away from pedal descending, rotate torso toward pedal ascending
- Variation 4: LE parallel, plantar surface of foot on forward pedal, rotate torso toward ped-al descending, rotate torso away from pedal ascending

8. Ladder Barrel Horseback holding Magic Circle overhead

- Variation 1: LE adduction with Magic Circle over-head, thumbs inside of handles, creating a force of external rotation and abduction at the GHJ

Session 10/12
Client self-report

- Struggling with pacing
- Optimistic about improved strength and endurance
- Tries to accomplish more during the day—more physical practice, more clients
- Then experiences an energy crash so she can only rest to recover
- Fatigue scale 5
- Pain scale 1

Key changes observed

- Standing with weight balanced at mid-foot rath-er than rear foot
- Decreased tendency to supinate right foot in standing
- Decreased tendency to pronate left foot in standing

Reasoning behind choice of movements

- Comprehensive review of program to date
- Prepare for final movement session and post-assessment
- Refine movement relationships of LE alignment in sagittal plane and torso rotation in transverse plane
- Develop cognitive clarity by challenging concentration and focus in coordination and motor control

Session movement sequence

1. Ladder Barrel prone supported torso flexion with coherent breathing

2. Feet doming on foam yoga blocks

3. Wunda Chair seated thoracic lateral flexion with rotation toward sagittal flexion

- Variation 2: non-pedal arm elbow in extension with upper arm alongside ear, continuing arc of thoracic lateral flexion

4. Standing whole-body rotation, feet doming on yoga blocks on rotator discs

- Variation 17: one eye closed, neither hand holds rung, head and eyes aim in the direction of toes
- Variation 17: other eye closed, neither hand holds rung, head and eyes aim forward while thorax, pelvis, LE rotate
- Variation 18: one eye closed, neither hand holds rung, head and eyes aim opposite rotation of thorax, pelvis, LE
- Variation 18: other eye closed, neither hand holds rung, head and eyes aim opposite rotation of thorax, pelvis, LE

5. Wunda Chair: seated on Balansit on rotator disc facing pedals, ankle plantar flexion/dorsiflexion

- Variation 6: rotate thorax and head opposite rotation of pelvis on Balansit–disc
    - Pelvis rotates away from the ankle that initiates plantar flexion to depress pedal
- Variation 7: rotate thorax and head opposite rotation of pelvis on Balansit–rotator disc
    - Pelvis rotates toward the ankle that initiates plantar flexion to depress pedal
- Repeat Variations 6 and 7: opposite rotation of thorax and pelvis
    - Aim head and eyes forward

6. Ped-o-Pull standing facing in, doming each foot on yoga block on rotator disc, Stability Sling supports TLJ

- Variation 4: thorax, neck, head aim forward while pelvis and LE rotate right and left, 4 times knees in extension, 4 times knees in flexion

7. Seated on Wunda Chair, on rotator disc, side to pedal, foot on forward pedal

- Variation 5: LE external rotation forefoot on forward pedal
    - Rotate torso away from pedal descending via ankle plantar flexion
    - Rotate torso toward pedal ascending via ankle dorsiflexion
- Variation 6: LE external rotation forefoot on forward pedal
    - Rotate torso toward pedal descending via ankle plantar flexion
    - Rotate torso away from pedal ascending via ankle dorsiflexion

8. Ladder Barrel Horseback holding Magic Circle overhead

● Variation 2: LE adduction with Magic Circle overhead, palms press outward from inside handles creating a force of internal rotation and abduction at the GHJ

9. Trapeze Table Stability Sling supported bridge with rotation

● Variation 1: supported bridge with no torso rotation

References

Almufarrij, I. and Munro, K. J. (2021) "One year on: An updated systematic review of SARS-CoV-2, COVID-19 and audio-vestibular symptoms." *International Journal of Audiology, 60,* 12, 935–945.

Bach, K. (2022) Is "long Covid" worsening the labor shortage? Brookings. January 11, 2022. www.brookings.edu/research/is-long-covid-worsening-the-labor-shortage. [Accessed October 27, 2023].

Balban, M. Y., Neri, E., Kogon, M. M., Weed, L. *et al.* (2023) "Brief structured respiration practices enhance mood and reduce physiological arousal." *Cell Reports Medicine, 4,* 1. DOI: 10.1016/j.xcrm.2022.100895.

Bush, Z. (2017) *4 Minute Workout YouTube.* September 5, 6:36.

Cairns, R. and Hotopf, M. (2005) "A systematic review describing the prognosis of chronic fatigue syndrome." *Occupational Medicine (London), 55,* 1, 20–31.

Callard, F. and Perego, E. (2021) "How and why patients made Long Covid." *Social Science & Medicine, 268.* DOI: 10.1016/j.socscimed.2020.113426.

Ceban, F., Ling, S., Lui, L. M. W., Lee, Y. *et al.* (2022) "Fatigue and cognitive impairment in post-COVID-19 syndrome: A systematic review and meta-analysis." *Brain, Behavior and Immunity, 101,* 93–135.

Chaitow, L. (2018) *Fascial Dysfunction: Manual Therapy Approaches.* 2nd Ed. Edinburgh: Handspring Publishing, pp. 220–221.

Chaitow, L, et al. (2002) *Multidisciplinary Approaches to Breathing Pattern Disorders.* Churchill Livingstone Elsevier Science, UK.

Cohrs, R. and Ladyzhets, B. (2023) The NIH has poured $1 billion into long Covid research—with little to show for it. STAT. March 31, 2023. www.statnews.com/2023/04/20/long-covid-nih-billion. [Accessed October 27, 2023].

Cutler, D. (2022) The economic cost of Long COVID: An update—David Cutler. Harvard Kennedy School. www.hks.harvard.edu/centers/mrcbg/programs/growthpolicy/economic-cost-long-covid-update-david-cutler. [Accessed October 27, 2023].

Davis, H. E., Assaf, G. S., McCorkell, L., Wei, H. *et al.* (2021) "Characterizing long COVID in an international cohort: 7 months of symptoms and their impact." *eClinicalMedicine, 38.* DOI: 10.1016/j.eclinm.2021.101019.

Davis, H. E., McCorkell, L., Vogel, J. M., and Topol, E. J. (2023) "Long COVID: Major findings, mechanisms and recommendations." *Nature Reviews. Microbiology, 21,* 3, 133–146.

Davis, I. S. (2021) The Achilles tendon and plantar fascia: One functional unit. CONNECT 2021 Conference. Munich, Germany, March. [Online conference lecture].

Dennis, A., Cuthbertson, D. J., Wootton, D., Crooks, M. *et al.* (2023) "Multi-organ impairment and Long COVID: a 1-year prospective, longitudinal cohort study." *Journal of the Royal Society of Medicine, 116,* 3, 97–112.

DrTalks Summit (2023) Overcoming Long Haul & Chronic Fatigue Syndrome Summit. February 7–14, 2023. https://drtalks.com/calendar. [Accessed October 27, 2023].

FLCCC Alliance (Front Line COVID-19 Critical Care Alliance) (2022) Fall 2022 Conference: Understanding & treating spike protein-induced diseases. October 14–16, 2022. https://covid19criticalcare.com/conference-fall-2022. [Accessed October 27, 2023].

FLCCC Alliance (Front Line COVID-19 Critical Care Alliance) (2023) Spring 2023 Conference: Emerging approaches to treating spike protein-induced diseases. April 28–29, 2023. https://covid19criticalcare.com/conference-spring-2023. [Accessed October 27, 2023].

Gordon, E. M., Chauvin, R. J., Van, A. N., Rajesh, A. *et al.* (2023) "A somato-cognitive action network alternates with effector regions in motor cortex." *Nature, 617,* 7960, 351–359.

Haffke, M., Freitag, H., Rudolf, G., Seifert, M. *et al.* (2022) "Endothelial dysfunction and altered endothelial biomarkers in patients with post-COVID-19 syndrome and chronic fatigue syndrome (ME/CFS)." *Journal of Translational Medicine, 20,* 1, 138.

Hamilton, M. T., Hamilton, D. G., and Zderic, T. W. (2022) "A potent physiological method to magnify and sustain soleus oxidative metabolism improves glucose and lipid regulation." *iScience, 25,* 9. DOI: 10.1016/j.isci.2022.104869.

Hutchinson, B. (2022) Andrew Huberman's NSDR (non-sleep deep rest) protocol. BrainFlow. November 26, 2022. https://brainflow.co/2022/11/06/andrew-hubermans-non-sleep-deep-rest-protocol. [Accessed October 27, 2023].

Kompaniyets, L., Bull-Otterson, L., Boehmer, T. K., Baca, S. *et al.* (2022) "Post–COVID-19 symptoms and conditions among children and adolescents—United States, March 1, 2020–January 31, 2022." *Morbidity and Mortality Weekly Report (MMWR), 71,* 31, 993–999.

Lee, D. (2018) *The Thorax an integrated approach.* Edinburgh: Handspring Publishing.

Long COVID Physio (2023a) Exercise. March 3, 2023. https://longcovid.physio/exercise. [Accessed October 27, 2023].

Long COVID Physio (2023b) Pacing. June 9, 2023. https://longcovid.physio/pacing. [Accessed October 27, 2023].

Mina, Y., Enose-Akahata, Y., Hammoud, D. A., Videckis, A. J. *et al.* (2023) "Deep phenotyping of neurological post-acute sequelae of SARS-CoV2 infection." *Neurology:*

Neuroimmunology and Neuroinflammation, 10, 4. DOI: 10.1212/nxi.0000000000200097.

McKeon, P, Hertel J, Bramble D, Davis I, The foot core system: a new paradigm for understanding intrinsic foot muscle function, British Journal of Sports Medicine 2015 Volume 49 Issue 5 .

Nestor, J. (2020) *Breath: The New Science of a Lost Art.* Riverhead Books, pp. 83–84. New York

NPCE Study Guide (National Pilates Certification Exam Study Guide) (2021) Miami, FL: National Pilates Certification Program, Inc.

Oza, A., Ramirez, R., Kwong, E., Spitzer, G., Cirino, M., and McCoy, B. (2023) Long COVID scientists try to unravel blood clot mystery. NPR. May 15, 2023. www.npr.org/2023/05/10/1175217130/long-covid-scientists-try-to-unravel-blood-clot-mystery. [Accessed October 27, 2023].

Stone, W. (2023) Why viral reservoirs are a prime suspect for long COVID sleuths. NPR. May 2, 2023. www.npr.org/sections/health-shots/2023/05/02/1172806898/why-viral-reservoirs-are-a-prime-suspect-for-long-covid-sleuths. [Accessed October 27, 2023].

Sutherland, S. (2023) Long COVID now looks like a neurological disease, helping doctors to focus treatments. Scientific American. March 21, 2023. www.scientificamerican.com/article/long-covid-now-looks-like-a-neurological-disease-helping-doctors-to-focus-treatments1. [Accessed October 27, 2023].

Tran, V.-T., Porcher, R., Pane, I. and Ravaud, P. (2022) "Course of post COVID-19 disease symptoms over time in the ComPaRe long COVID prospective e-cohort." *Nature Communications, 13,* 1, 1812.

Trewartha, J. (2023) Humming and nasal breathing – keys to efficient breathing, calm and improved immunity. The Fascia Hub. https://thefasciahub.com/blog/humming-and-nasal-breathing-keys-to-efficient-breathing-calm-and-improved-immunity. [Accessed October 27, 2023].

Twomey, R., DeMars, J., Franklin, K., Culos-Reed, S. N., Weatherald, J., and Wrightson, J. G. (2022) "Chronic fatigue and postexertional malaise in people living with Long COVID: An observational study." *Physical Therapy 102,* 4. DOI: 10.1093/ptj/pzac005.

Vladeta, D. (2022) www.balansit.com.au/about

Williamson, A. E., Tydeman, F., Miners, A., Pyper, K., and Martineau, A. R. (2022) "Short-term and long-term impacts of COVID-19 on economic vulnerability: A population-based longitudinal study (COVIDENCE UK)." *BMJ Open, 12.* DOI: 10.1136/bmjopen-2022-065083.

Wise, J. (2023) *Long COVID Comes Into the Light.* slate.com Technology Section, Medical Examiner.

Wong, T. L. and Weitzer, D. J. (2021) "Long COVID and myalgic encephalomyelitis/chronic fatigue syndrome (ME/CFS)—a systemic review and comparison of clinical presentation and symptomatology." *Medicina (Kaunas), 57,* 418.

Wright, J., Astill, S. L., and Sivan, M. (2022) "The relationship between physical activity and Long COVID: A cross-sectional study." *International Journal of Environmental Research and Public Health, 19,* 9. DOI: 10.3390/ijerph19095093.

Yeoh, Y. K., Zuo, T., Lui, G. C., Zhang, F. *et al.* (2021) "Gut microbiota composition reflects disease severity and dysfunctional immune responses in patients with COVID-19." *Gut, 70,* 698–706.

Pilates and Metabolic Syndrome and Weight Control: Effect on Gait

Su Yeon Roh

Prevalence of metabolic syndrome

Metabolic syndrome is a burgeoning global problem, with an increasing prevalence in urban populations of some developing countries (Wang *et al.* 2021). Approximately a quarter of the adult European population is estimated to have metabolic syndrome, with a similar prevalence in Latin America. It is also considered an emerging epidemic in developing East Asian countries, including China, Japan, and Korea. The prevalence of metabolic syndrome in East Asia may range from 8–13 percent in men and 2–18 percent in women (Wang *et al.* 2021). In the US about a quarter of the adult population has metabolic syndrome, and the prevalence increases with age, with racial and ethnic minorities being particularly affected.

Definition

Metabolic syndrome is a clustering of at least three of the five following medical conditions: central obesity, high blood pressure, high blood sugar, high serum triglycerides, and low serum high-density lipoprotein (HDL). Metabolic syndrome is associated with the risk of developing cardiovascular disease and type 2 diabetes.

Symptoms

Most of the disorders associated with metabolic syndrome do not have obvious signs or symptoms. One sign that is visible is a large waist circumference. And if your blood sugar is high, you might notice the signs and symptoms of diabetes—such as increased thirst and increased urination, fatigue, and blurred vision.

Causes

The cause of the syndrome is an area of ongoing medical research. The syndrome is thought to be caused by an underlying disorder of energy utilization and storage. Metabolic syndrome is closely linked to overweight or obesity and inactivity. It is also linked to a condition called insulin resistance. Insulin is a hormone made by the pancreas that helps sugar enter the cells to be used as fuel. In people with insulin resistance, cells do not respond normally to insulin and glucose cannot enter the cells as easily. As a result, blood sugar levels rise as the body churns out more and more insulin to try to lower the blood sugar.

Author note

A research study shows that a Pilates program is effective for weight control and hypertension. A single session of Pilates was shown to reduce blood pressure (BP) by about 5–8 mm Hg in adults with hypertension during the first 60 minutes of post-exercise recovery (Rocha *et al.* 2020). The findings are promising for the use of Pilates as an alternative exercise modality to lower BP. The Martins-Meneses *et al.* study showed that mat Pilates reduced clinical and ambulatory BP in hypertensive women using antihypertensive medications. These results support the recommendation of mat Pilates as a non-drug treatment for hypertension (Martins-Meneses *et al.* 2015). The Şavkin and Aslan 2017 study showed that eight weeks of Pilates exercises had positive effects on body composition in sedentary overweight and obese women. They suggested that Pilates exercises can be applied for improving body composition.

Client description: 69-year-old, identifies as female; mother of one son and two daughters

Dates of case report: Session 1: March 20, 2020; Session 12: May 19, 2020; virtual sessions

Studio apparatus and props
Pilates equipment

- Trapeze Table
- Universal Reformer
- Wunda Chair with split pedal
- CoreAlign®

Props used with equipment

- Pilates Arc
- Resistance band, medium
- Rotator disc, 12 in. (30.5 cm), no resistance
- 2 rotator discs, 9 in. (23 cm), no resistance, to attach to Universal Reformer footplate
- Foot Corrector

Home program props

- Pilates Arc
- Resistance band, medium
- Hand towel (for toe curl)
- Bed
- Chair
- Small ball, 2.5 in. (6.5 cm)

Methods and materials

Session 1/12
1. Health history interview

- Late 1987: broken left leg was immobilized with brace for 2 months
- 1997: concurrent myoma uteri and urinary incontinence surgery
- 1999: diagnosed with osteoporosis
- Prescribed medication for osteoporosis; subsequently medication replaced by vitamin D injection every 3 months
- 2011: prescribed angiotensin, a receptor blocker for hypertension
- 2012: microscopic surgery for rupture of left rotator cuff
- 2013: L4–L5 herniated nucleus pulposus ruptured requiring emergency surgery
- 2020: cataract surgery

2. Symptoms

- General fatigue amplified after 2 hours of walking
- Short gait stride
- Digestion deficiency
- Headaches of unknown origin at irregular intervals

- Right hallux valgus, cannot wear high heels; prefers customized shoes or flexible shoes
- Balance deficiency
- Awakened from sleep by right leg spasms

Author note
The client takes nutritional supplements for blood circulation.

---

3. Movement aids

- Flexible shoes accommodate hallux valgus
- Wore sneakers, with customized lateral edge for right heel

Final result of case report
The client was able to stand with balanced upright stance. She has improved torso rotation during gait. She is sleeping well without being awakened by right lower extremity spasms.

Session 2/12: Initial assessment

1. General observations of gait

◆ Limited thoracic rotation, leading with arm swing

◆ Gait stride short

◆ Not able to maintain the midline during walk

◆ Limited dorsiflexion

◆ Loads the right lateral foot

2. Standing tests

◆ Full torso rotation

● Observations of inefficient side: left
  ■ Limited torso rotation
  ■ Tends to rotate cervical region
  ■ Right foot inversion

◆ Hemipelvis inferior motion

● Observations of inefficient side: both
  ■ Hard to perform this assessment because of balance deficiency
  ■ Limited hemipelvis inferior motion bilaterally
  ■ Tends to thoracic rotation rather than lowering hemipelvis

◆ Hemipelvis superior motion

● Observations of inefficient side: both
  ■ Limited hemipelvis elevation bilaterally
  ■ Inability to maintain left lower extremity orientation anteriorly

◆ Lateral pelvic shift

Session 12/12: Post-assessment

1. General observations of gait

◆ Improved bilateral thoracic rotation

◆ Gait stride length increased

◆ Able to maintain midline orientation

◆ Limited dorsiflexion

◆ Improved loading throughout foot

2. Standing tests

◆ Full torso rotation

● Observations of inefficient side: left
  ■ Limited torso rotation
  ■ Tends to rotate cervical region
  ■ Right foot inversion

◆ Hemipelvis inferior motion

● Observations of inefficient side: both
  ■ Improved balance, able to perform assessment task
  ■ Hemipelvis lowers without anterior rotation
  ■ Decreased thoracic rotation

◆ Hemipelvis superior motion

● Observations of inefficient side: both
  ■ Improved hemipelvis elevation bilaterally
  ■ Left lower extremity orientation remains anterior

◆ Lateral pelvic shift

- Observations of inefficient side: both
  - Compensates with hip flexion
  - Pronounced bilateral translation of pelvis
  - Bilateral foot-ankle supination and pronation

3. Seated tests

- ◆ Thoracic rotation

- Observations of inefficient side: both
  - Limited rotation bilaterally
  - Compensates for limited thoracic rotation with rotation of cervical region

- ◆ Hip joint and knee flexion

- Observations of inefficient side: left
  - Translates torso away from midline during left hip joint flexion
  - Left lower extremity (LE) trembles during left knee flexion

4. Sit and stand

- ◆ Lateral view

- Slight lumbar flexion
- Generally performed well without evidence of knee pain

- ◆ Anterior view

- Shifts weight from left to right

5. Standing balance

- ◆ Two-leg stance, eyes open

- 60 seconds

- Observations of inefficient side: both
  - Less compensation of hip flexion
  - Excessive bilateral pelvic translation
  - Bilateral foot-ankle supination and pronation

3. Seated tests

- ◆ Thoracic rotation

- Observations of inefficient side: left
  - Improved bilateral rotation
  - Tends to rotate cervical region

- ◆ Hip joint and knee flexion

- Observations: both sides efficient
  - Ability to maintain midline orientation
  - Left leg does not tremble during movement

4. Sit and stand

- ◆ Lateral view

- Slight lumbar flexion
- Generally performed well without evidence of knee pain

- ◆ Anterior view

- Whole body organized to midline throughout movement

5. Standing balance

- ◆ Two-leg stance, eyes open

- 60 seconds

◆ One-leg stance, eyes open

◆ Information not recorded

◆ One-leg stance, eyes open

● Maintained balance with single stance on each side. Further information not recorded.
● Able to perform with eyes closed. Further information not recorded.

Session 3/12: Home program

Fatigue scale 4

Pain scale 2

Client self-report
- Encouraged, eager to learn

Key changes observed by author at end of Session 3/12
- Comfortable with exercise
- Improved awareness of her physical position during exercise with instructor's cueing
- Adapted well to movement tasks

Reason behind choice of sequencing
- Improve proprioception and midline orientation
- Awareness of hip, knee, and ankle articulations

Session movement sequence

1. Morning bed

Author note
The client's first experience with Pilates required time to become familiar with Pilates equipment. She needed to sip water often during the session. All exercises in this session began with slow tempo, light resistance, low intensity.

Intent
- Whole-body sensory stimulation
- Reduce whole-body rigidity
- Encourage joint articulations

Gait reasoning
- Stimulate proprioceptive acuity
- Preparation for gait prior to full weight bearing

Starting position
- Supine in a comfortable position on bed
- Relax whole body

Movement description
- 5 quiet breath cycles with closed eyes
- 5 quiet breath cycles with open eyes
- Slow flexion of hip joints and knee extension
- Hold for 20 seconds
- Ankle plantar flexion
- Ankle dorsiflexion
- Alternate 10 times
- Legs adduct with hip joints flexed and knees extended
- Move bilateral LE to right laterally 30 degrees
- Move bilateral LE to left laterally 30 degrees

- Repeat 5 times
- Bilateral knee flexion
- Bilateral femur circles in both directions
- Repeat 5 times
- Return to midline
- Slowly lower both legs
- Roll body to the side and sit

2. Rolling small ball on plantar surface of foot

Intent	• Sensory stimulation of feet • Reducing foot-ankle rigidity
Gait reasoning	• Stimulate proprioceptive acuity of feet and ankles • Prepare feet for efficient weight bearing • Foot stimulation prepares entire LE and torso for efficient weight bearing
Starting position	• Sit on bed in an optimal position • Equal weight on right and left ischial tuberosities • Plantar surfaces of feet in firm contact with floor
Movement description	• Place ball on the floor • Plantar surface of right foot in firm contact with ball • Roll smoothly for 10 seconds • Change to left foot • Hold ball in hand • Roll ball on dorsum of right foot for 10 seconds • Repeat on left foot

3. Lower limb with resistance band

Intent	• Increase range of motion (ROM) ankle plantar flexion and dorsiflexion • Improve circulation and tissue glide of LE
Gait reasoning	• Develop foot-ankle adaptability • Develop proprioceptive acuity of ankle dorsiflexion and plantar flexion
Starting position	• Sit on bed or chair in an optimal position • Even weight on right and left ischial tuberosities • Feet in firm contact with floor • Tie a loop at end of resistance band • Place right foot into loop and hold with left hand

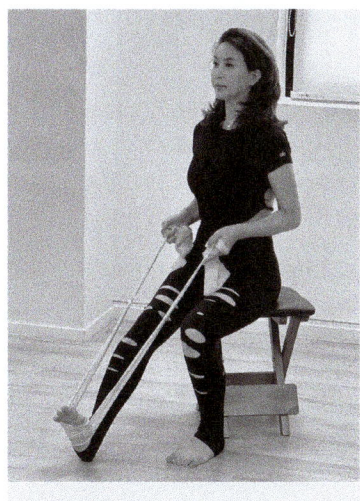

Figure 14.1

Movement description
- Plantar flex the foot slowly
- Dorsiflex the foot slowly
- Repeat 5 times
- Move loop to left foot
- Repeat
- Articulate forefoot and rear foot in ankle plantar flexion and dorsiflexion

4. Towel toe curls

Intent
- Improve toe flexion
- Activate metatarsophalangeal (MTP) regions of forefoot

Gait reasoning
- Improve foot loading
- Improve metatarsal and mid-foot articulation
- Develop control of intrinsic foot structures

Starting position
- Sit on bed or chair
- Place towel on floor
- Right foot on towel

Movement description
- Dome right foot and hold towel
- Pull towel taut for 10 seconds
- 1st phalange extends as 2nd to 5th flex pressing into floor
- Reverse 1st phalange flexes as 2nd to 5th extend
- Repeat 3–4 times
- Change to left foot
- Repeat

5. Seated torso flexion and extension

Intent
- Awareness of articulation of hip region
- Increased awareness of midline orientation during torso flexion and extension
- Preparation for a squat

Gait reasoning
- Awareness of organization to the midline in all planes
- Hip joint stimulation through torso on femurs

Starting position
- Sit on the edge of a chair
- Bilateral foot contact with floor
- Feet parallel, knees a hand's width apart

Movement description
- Place each hand on lateral hemipelvis
- Sustain upright orientation
- 3 slow breath cycles
- Flex the torso about 45 degrees
- Return to starting position
- Repeat 6–8 times

6. Seated thoracic extension

Intent
- Improve thoracic articulation
- Decrease lumbar lordosis

Gait reasoning
- Improve sagittal plane orientation
- Facilitate thoracic rotation
- Torso extension and rotation for push-off phase of gait

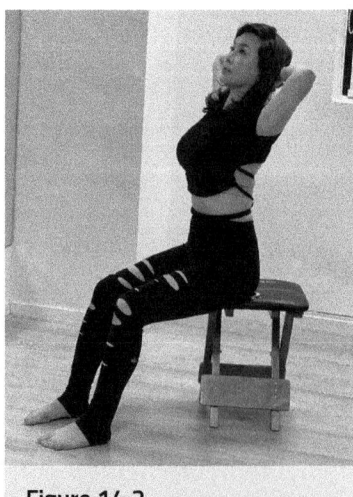

Figure 14.2

Starting position
- Sit on edge of chair, weight balanced on ischial tuberosities
- Feet in full contact with floor
- Feet parallel, a hand's width apart
- Hands on occiput supporting head

Movement description
- Inhale during preparation
- Exhale during thoracic extension
- Return to starting position
- Repeat 6–8 times
- Perform slowly
- Maintain elbows in peripheral vision
- Repeat 3 times
- Rotate and extend thorax to right
- Return to starting position
- Repeat on other side
- 3 times for each side

7. Standing squat on Pilates Arc (Larkam 2017)

Intent
- Training LE adaptability
- Develop ROM of ankle dorsiflexion
- Refine LE movement relationships from feet to torso
- Challenge balance

Gait reasoning
- Increase proprioception on uneven surface
- Sensory input for foot loading
- Improve dynamic control of ankle dorsiflexion

Starting position
- Stand on side of arc
- Carefully stand on step
- Place hands on hemipelvis

Movement description
- Slowly flex and extend LE
- Repeat 3–4 times
- Add torso leaning anteriorly from pelvifemoral movement
- Increase level of horizontal torso position
- Extend the knee avoiding hyperextension
- Repeat 3–4 times
- Return to starting position
- Step off slowly and carefully

8. Step-ups on step of Pilates Arc

Intent	<ul><li>Challenge balance</li><li>Awareness of LE weight distribution</li><li>Training LE adaptability</li></ul>
Gait reasoning	<ul><li>Increase proprioception on dynamic surface</li><li>Sensory input for foot loading</li><li>Improve ROM of dorsiflexion</li><li>Improve stair climbing</li></ul>
Starting position	<ul><li>Stand on the floor facing the step and convexity of Pilates Arc</li><li>Stand with feet parallel</li><li>Place hands on hemipelvis</li></ul>
Movement description	<ul><li>Right foot steps up on step</li><li>Left foot steps up on step</li><li>Right foot steps down to floor</li><li>Left foot steps down to floor</li><li>Repeat 6–8 sets</li><li>Change sides, stepping left foot first</li><li>Repeat 6–8 sets</li></ul>

9. Lunge on step of Pilates Arc

Intent	<ul><li>Challenge balance</li><li>Awareness of LE weight distribution</li><li>Training LE adaptability</li></ul>
Gait reasoning	<ul><li>Increase proprioception on dynamic surface</li><li>Sensory input for foot loading</li></ul>
Starting position	<ul><li>Stand facing step and convexity of body of Pilates Arc</li><li>Stand with feet parallel</li><li>Place hands on hemipelvis</li><li>Right foot on top of step</li></ul>
Movement description	<ul><li>Bilaterally flex knees</li><li>Slowly extend</li><li>Step down</li><li>Repeat on left side</li><li>Repeat 6–8 times</li></ul>

10. Lateral flexion and rotation on Pilates Arc — Derivative of J. H. Pilates Mermaid on Universal Reformer (NPCE Study Guide 2021, p. 58)

Intent
- Encourage thoracic rotation and lateral flexion

Gait reasoning
- Efficient gait includes bilateral thoracic rotation
- Bilateral thoracic rotation supports oppositional rotation of the lumbopelvic region

Starting position
- Sit on the step, left side toward convexity of arc
- Left hemipelvis at junction of step and body of arc
- Left hip joint in flexion/external rotation with knee flexion
- Right hip joint abducted in parallel, right knee extended
- Right LE in line with torso
- Support head with left hand

Movement description
- During inhalation, abduct and flex right upper extremity (UE) with elbow extended
- During exhalation, laterally flex torso over curve of Pilates Arc
- During inhalation direct movement toward right lateral thoracic region
- During exhalation reverse the arm movement and return to seated starting position
- Repeat 3 times
- Resume lateral flexion
- Thoracic rotation toward body of Pilates Arc
- Hold top of arc with both hands, elbows in flexion
- Sustain thoracic rotation during extension and flexion of elbows, extending torso
- Repeat 3 times
- Change to other side

11. Pilates Arc plank with ankle dorsiflexion — Derivative of J. H. Pilates Leg Pull: Front (NPCE Study Guide 2021, p. 50)

Intent
- Challenge whole-body organization to midline
- Whole-body motor control, challenging torso integration and LE extension

Gait reasoning
- Whole-body integration
- Activate ankle dorsiflexion and plantar flexion
- Improve articulation at 1st MPJ

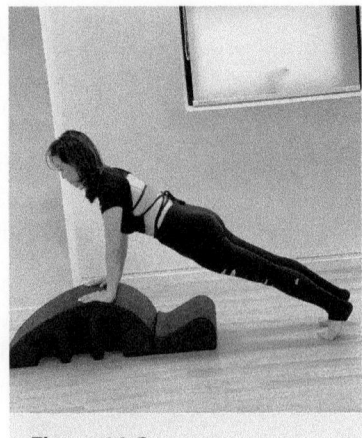

Figure 14.3

Starting position	● Place hands on convexity of Pilates Arc, front of body facing floor
	● Move into a plank position with 90 degrees arm flexion
	● LE adducted
	● Ankles in dorsiflexion
	● MTP joints extended
	● Phalanges on mat
Movement description	● Ankle dorsiflexion, moving torso back toward feet
	● Ankle plantar flexion propels the torso forward
	● Alternate ankle dorsiflexion and plantar flexion
	● Repeat 4–6 times

12. Walking on the Pilates Arc

Intent	● Lateral weight shift on unstable surface
	● Challenge balance
Gait reasoning	● Develop proprioception
	● Develop agility and balance
	● Develop foot/ankle adaptation on dynamic surface
Starting position	● Stand on front of the Pilates Arc
	● Feet parallel
Movement description	● Walk on step and convexity
	● Reverse, walk back backward on Pilates Arc
	● Walk around the arc
	● Walk on the side well of arc
	● Repeat 6–10 times with deliberate steps

Session 11/12: Studio session

Fatigue scale	2–3
Pain scale	1
Client self-report	● Excited, optimistic, high self-esteem
Key changes observed by author at end of Session 11/12	● Comfortable using exercise props ● Able to maintain balance during single stance ● Able to change gait pattern and decrease fatigue
Reason behind choice of sequencing	● Performed all exercises in order during last movement session ● Client now has no apprehension regarding exercises with Pilates equipment ● Improve awareness, self-adaptations for motor control

Session movement sequence

1. Trapeze Table Footwork: dorsiflexion

Intent	● Motor control coordinating articulation of ankle-knee-hip joints
Gait reasoning	● Increase foot and ankle articulations ● Increase ROM and control of LE
Set-up	● Push-through bar sprung from above with 2 medium springs
Starting position	● Supine with pelvis toward push-through bar end of Trapeze Table ● Place dorsum of right foot over push-through bar ● Right knee extended
Movement description	● Dorsiflexion of ankle to pull the bar down ● Return to starting position ● Repeat 6–8 times ● Change feet ● Repeat 6–8 times ● Flex knee of foot on bar ● Maintain knee flexion, dorsiflex foot to pull bar down ● Return to starting position ● Repeat 6–8 times ● Change feet ● Repeat 6–8 times

Movement description
- Variation: lying on side
  - External rotation of LE with foot on bar
  - Ankle dorsiflexion and knee flexion to pull bar down
  - Repeat
  - Change feet
  - Repeat 6–8 times

CUES
- Maintain centration of the hip, knee, and ankle joints
- Exhalation during ankle dorsiflexion

Author note
Ankle dorsiflexion with the dorsum of the foot on the push-through bar develops tissue glide of foot-ankle region, contributing to efficient gait.

2. Trapeze Table standing on rotator disc with long spring

Intent
- Develop motor control of hip joint in multiple vectors
- Challenge dynamic control of lumbopelvic to LE movement relationships

Gait reasoning
- Motor control of pelvifemoral movement
- Improve proprioception on dynamic surface

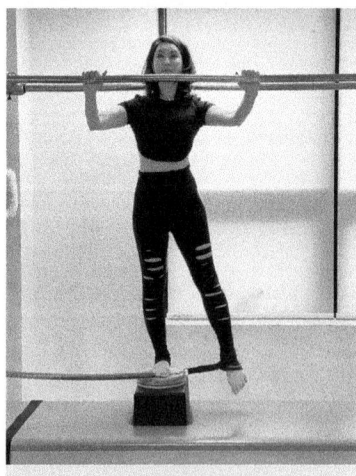

Figure 14.4

Set-up
- Light long spring
- Spring attached to eye bolt at level of hip joint
- Velcro® strap secures spring to ankle
- Rotator disc, 12 in. (30.5 cm) in diameter, placed on top of Trapeze Table

Starting position
- Stand with right foot on rotator disc
- Velcro strap around left ankle
- Organize the body to midline
- Hold upper bars of Trapeze Table frame
- Attach spring to eye bolt aligned to ankle midline

Movement description
- Hip flexion
  - Stand facing away from spring attachment
  - Hip flexion resisted by spring, maintaining standing organization
  - Return to starting position
  - Change sides
  - Repeat 5 times on each side
- Hip extension
  - Stand facing spring attachment
  - I lip extension resisted by spring, maintaining standing organization
  - Return to starting position
  - Change to left
  - Repeat 5 times on each side
- Hip adduction
  - Stand with right side toward spring
  - Pull spring across the midline
  - Return to starting position
  - Change sides
  - Repeat 5 times on each side
- Hip abduction
  - Stand with right side facing spring
  - Pull spring away from midline of the body
  - Return to starting position
  - Change sides
  - Repeat 5 times on each side

CUE
- Press the sole of the 1st ray onto the rotator disc to re-inforce the connection between the foot, LE, and pelvis regions

Author note
- Practice the exercise prior to standing on rotator disc, with resistance band tied to a door or chair
- Rotator disc provides awareness of preferred rotation movement pattern
- Client recognized her dominant direction of rotation, facilitating self-correction

3. Supine Footwork with rotator disc on Universal Reformer footplate

Derivative of J. H. Pilates Footwork on Universal Reformer (NPCE Study Guide 2021, p. 52)

Intent
- Activate pelvifemoral movements in low load, partial weight-bearing environment
- Improve lumbopelvic-femoral motor control
- Increase hip ROM

Gait reasoning
- Motor control of limbs on torso with unstable surface
- Activate and load LE in a variety of vectors

Set-up
- Springs: 2 medium and 1 light
- 2 rotator discs, 9 in. (23 cm), with no resistance
- Attach Velcro straps of rotator discs to jump board

Starting position
- Supine on carriage
- Entire plantar surface of each foot on rotator disc
- Heels hip-width apart
- LE parallel
- 90 degrees knee flexion

Movement description
- Extend hip and knee joints moving carriage away
- Flex hip and knee joints moving carriage in
- Repeat 3 times
- Plantar flex ankles with metatarsals on discs
- Extend hip and knee joints moving carriage away
- Flex the hip and knee joints moving carriage in
- Repeat 3 times
- Dorsiflex ankles with heels on the discs
- Extend hip and knee joints moving carriage away
- Flex the hip and knee joints moving carriage in
- Repeat 3 times
- Internally rotate LE
- Extend hip and knee joints moving carriage away
- Flex hip and knee joints moving carriage in
- Repeat 3 times

● Externally rotate LE
● Extend hip and knee joints moving carriage away
● Flex hip and knee joints moving carriage in
● Repeat 3 times

CUE
◆ Steer the disc with the rear-foot/heels to facilitate LE external and internal rotation

Author note
External rotation at the hip joint frequently encourages hyperextension at the thoracolumbar junction. Prior to and during LE rotation intensify tissue activation to reinforce organization to midline in all planes.

4. Side lying unilateral Footwork with rotator disc and Pilates Arc on Universal Reformer

Intent
● Assist in activation of pelvifemoral movements in a low load environment
● Improve lumbopelvic-femoral dynamic stability
● Refine hip ROM

Gait reasoning
● Integrated movement of LE with torso
● Single-leg partial weight bearing prepares for lateral weight shifts in full weight bearing

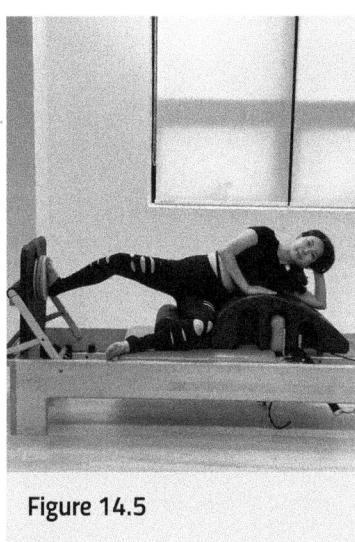

Figure 14.5

317

Set-up	● Medium spring
	● 9 in. (23 cm) rotator discs, with no resistance, attached with Velcro straps to jump board
	● Pilates Arc placed on Universal Reformer
	● Head support
Starting position	● Right side of torso supported by body of arc
	● Left foot on rotator disc
	● Parallel LE
Movement description	● Extend left hip and knee joints moving carriage away from footbar
	● Flex hip and knee joints moving carriage toward footbar
	● Repeat 5 times
	● Externally rotate left LE
	● Extend hip and knee joints moving carriage away from footbar
	● Flex hip and knee joints moving carriage toward footbar
	● Repeat 5 times
	● Maintain hip joint external rotation
	● Internal rotation of tibia on femur
	● Extend left hip and knee joints moving carriage away from footbar
	● Flex hip and knee joints moving carriage toward footbar
	● Repeat 5 times
	● Repeat on other side

CUE

◆ Prior to LE external rotation aim the same side ASIS forward, opposite the direction of LE rotation. Prior to LE internal rotation aim the same side ASIS back, opposite the direction of LE rotation. This facilitates proximal stability

Author note
The rotator disc may be attached to the footplate to facilitate flexion, neutral position, or extension of the hip joint.

5. Supine hip circumduction with knee flexion on Universal Reformer (See Chapter 5, Gentry: Knee stirs)

Intent	● Facilitate lumbopelvic-femoral motor control
	● Increase LE ROM in partial weight bearing
Gait reasoning	● Motor control in lumbopelvic region through multiple vectors of hip ROM support efficient gait

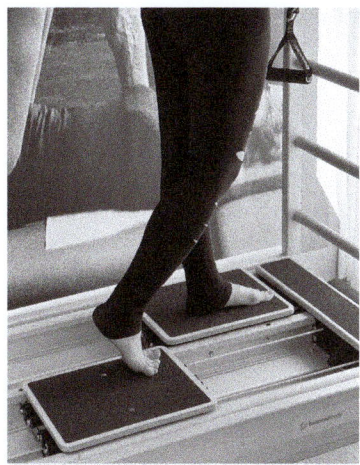

Figure 14.6

Set-up	● 3 medium springs
	● Y-loops
Starting position	● Supine
	● Place cushion under the head
	● Flex hip and knee joints to 90 degrees
	● Place Y-loops around knees
Movement description	● Abduct LE
	● Extend LE
	● Adduct LE
	● Flex LE
	● Repeat 3 times
	● Reverse
	● LE external rotation and internal rotation smoothly
	● Repeat 5 times
	● Cross the strap and place the loop to opposite knee
	● Abduction/external rotation bilaterally touching plantar surface of feet together
	● Adduction/internal rotation bilaterally touching knees in midline
	● Repeat 4 times
	● Bilateral LE adducted
	● Torso rotates to right
	● Torso rotates to left
	● Repeat 4 times

CUE
◆ Practice three variations: abduction/adduction; rhythmical movement of external rotation and internal rotation; smooth flow

Author note

Practice knee stirs on the mat prior to Universal Reformer.

6. Universal Reformer Splits: Side with squat variation

Derivative of J. H. Pilates Splits: Side on Universal Reformer (NPCE Study Guide 2021, p. 61)

Intent
● Increase whole-body activation to improve stance and gait
● Activate and increase load in lumbopelvic-hip region through a variety of vectors and ROM

Gait reasoning
● Improve stance on a dynamic surface
● Lateral transfer of weight from one side to the other

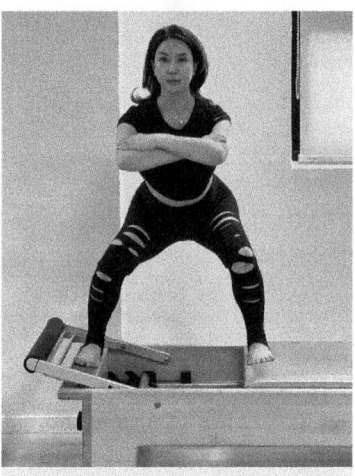

Figure 14.7

Set-up
● Light spring
● Footbar down

Starting position
● Stand on the Universal Reformer, one foot on the standing platform, one foot against the shoulder stop
● LE parallel, hip and knee joints extended

Movement description	● Abduct, slide the carriage away from footbar
	● Adduct, slide the carriage toward footbar
	● Repeat 5 times
	● Change sides
	● Repeat
	● Reposition feet, aiming toes to right diagonally
	● Slide carriage away from and toward footbar
	● Repeat 5 times
	● Reposition feet, aiming toes to left diagonally
	● Slide carriage away from and toward footbar
	● Repeat 5 times
	● Change to 1 medium spring or 1 light spring
	● Feet parallel
	● Squat position
	● Slide carriage away from and toward footbar
	● Sustain squat position
	● Repeat 3 times
	● Change sides

CUES

- ◆ Avoid knee hyperextension
- ◆ Maintain pelvis facing anterior in optimal position in sagittal plane

Author note

Safety is the priority. Assist the client's balance, holding their hand or providing a stick for ground support.

7. Wunda Chair dorsiflexion with various vectors	Derivative of J. H. Pilates Wunda Chair Achilles Stretch (NPCE Study Guide 2021, p. 79)
Intent	● Load lower limb during ankle dorsiflexion and plantar flexion
	● Lower limb compartment gliding
Gait reasoning	● Resiliency of lower limb to withstand ground forces
Set-up	● Heavy spring at medium setting
Starting position	● Stand facing Wunda Chair
	● Place right foot in front of platform
	● Place left knee on edge of chair with forefoot on foot pedal
	● Place hands on the seat
	● Torso leans forward

Movement description	
	● Ankle plantar flexion pressing foot pedal down without moving knee
	● Ankle dorsiflexion, return to starting position
	● Repeat 10 times slowly, with control
	● Change sides
	● Place hand on right edge of chair
	● Ankle plantar flexion pressing foot pedal down without moving knee
	● Ankle dorsiflexion, return to starting position
	● Repeat 10 times slowly, with control
	● Change sides
	● Place hand on left edge of chair
	● Ankle plantar flexion pressing foot pedal down without moving knee
	● Ankle dorsiflexion, return to starting position
	● Repeat 10 times slowly, with control
	● Change sides
	● Standing upright, hands off the chair
	● Ankle plantar flexion pressing foot pedal down without moving knee
	● Ankle dorsiflexion, return to starting position
	● Repeat 10 times slowly, with control

CUES

- ◆ Move smoothly throughout both phases of the exercise
- ◆ Press the pedal down quickly and release it slowly

Author note

- – Pad the patella tendon contact with the edge of the chair
- – Advance to add LE external and internal rotation
- – Advance to add ankle plantar flexion on standing leg

8. Standing Leg Pumps with rotator disc on Wunda Chair	Derivative of J. H. Pilates Standing Leg Pump: Front on Wunda Chair (NPCE Study Guide 2021, p. 79)
Intent	● Activate and load LE in different vectors
	● Improve single stance balance
Gait reasoning	● Fall prevention
	● Address lower limb motor control
	● Improve gait stance
Set-up	● Heavy spring at medium setting
	● Handles in place to support balance
	● Rotator disc placed in front of Wunda Chair platform

Starting position
- Stand facing Wunda Chair
- Place right foot on rotator disc
- Place left metatarsal arch on foot pedal
- LE parallel
- Hands hold handles

Movement description
- Plantar flex left foot pressing pedal down maintaining midline organization
- Return pedal to starting position
- Repeat 3–4 times
- Stand with left side facing Wunda Chair
- Externally rotate right LE turning the disc
- Externally rotate left LE placing metatarsal arch on foot pedal
- Press pedal down maintaining midline organization
- Return pedal to starting position
- Repeat 3–4 times
- Take foot off foot pedal
- Stand in external rotation with left side facing Wunda Chair
- Cross over right foot in front of left foot
- Press foot pedal down
- Stand on the leg closest to pedal and place outer leg on pedal by crossing in front of standing leg
- Return pedal to starting position
- Repeat 3–4 times

CUE
- Press the pedal down smoothly and evenly maintaining control

Author note
The client practiced Standing Leg Pumps several times without rotator discs, then added rotator discs as control improved and confidence developed.

9. CoreAlign ankle plantar flexion with dorsiflexion of metatarsophalangeal joints

(See Editor note, Volume 2 Chapter 6)

Intent
- Develop lower leg alignment in push-off phase of gait
- Develop coordination required for reciprocal leg movement
- Develop whole-body organization while moving on dynamic surface
- Refine upright standing posture
- Train coordination and balance

Gait reasoning
- The CoreAlign is a useful environment for addressing gait because it develops the ability to perform reciprocal leg movements with resistance from different directions
- Hands holding the ladder rung support balance while client adapts to the novel training environment
- Adjustable resistance provided by elastic cords supports progressive strength and endurance training

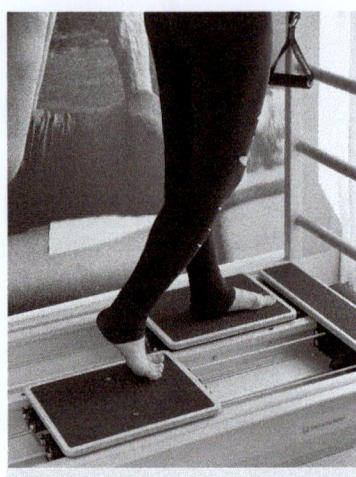

Figure 14.8

Set-up
- Facing the ladder, one cart aligned in the left lane, the other aligned in the right lane
- 1 or 2 light elastic tubes attach each cart to ladder end of frame
- Calibrate elastic resistance for client safety in upright stance
- If resistance is too light client is at risk for instability
- If resistance is too heavy shear forces will compromise tissue integrity

Starting position
- Stand facing the ladder
- One foot per cart
- Hands hold ladder at waist height
- Upright stance organized to midline in all planes
- Gaze at horizon level

Movement description
- Flex one knee and plantar flex same side ankle, raising heel to push cart backward as if showing bottom of foot to someone behind you
- Maintain thighs parallel to each other
- Maintain torso upright during LE articulation
- Return to starting position by lowering heel and returning carts to starting position beside ladder
- Alternate each leg during desired number of repetitions
- Return to starting position by lowering heel and returning cart to stoppers
- Repeat 6–8 times
- Repeat above and press cart back while bending both knees to 90 degrees
- The back knee should align with the torso and head
- Extend both knees, returning whole body to starting position
- Alternate sides
- Repeat 6–8 times

CUES
- Keep the head, torso, pelvis, and both knees in one vertical line as the lower leg moves
- As the heel lifts and lowers, articulate through the foot
- For the lunge, keep the front knee aligned with or behind the toes

Author note
The client tried chair lunge standing on the Wunda Chair but was afraid of the height. If there is no CoreAlign then we completed lunge on the Wunda Chair in this session. Place a small box under the pedal for safety and confidence.

The journey to Session 11

Session 4/12
Client self-report

- Fatigue scale 3
- Pain scale 2

Key changes observed

- Client follows instructor's direction well
- Feet articulation improved

Reasoning behind choice of movements

- Sensory stimulation of feet
- Increasing proprioception
- Developing coordination of LE
- Torso control

Session movement sequence

1. Morning bed

2. Lower limb with resistance band

3. Seated torso flexion and extension, added thoracic rotation

4. Trapeze Table

- Footwork
  - Dorsiflexion
- Leg spring work without rotator disc

5. Universal Reformer

- Supine Footwork without rotator disc
- Unilateral Footwork without rotator disc and arc
- Supine hip full ROM with knee flexion (see Chapter 5, Gentry: Knee stirs)

6. Additional movements

- Foot Corrector
- Trapeze Table with push-through bar loaded from below
  - Hip and knee flexion and extension
  - Reciprocal plantar flexion and dorsiflexion with knee flexion and extension

Session 5/12
Client self-report

- Fatigue scale 2
- Pain scale 2

Key changes observed

- Improved hip internal and external rotation
- Improved standing with midline organization

Reasoning behind choice of movements

- Sensory stimulation of feet
- Increasing proprioception
- Developing coordination work for LE
- Improve adaptability for dynamic stability

Session movement sequence

1. Pilates Arc

- Bridge and reach added

2. Trapeze Table

- Footwork
  - Dorsiflexion
- Leg spring work without rotator disc

3. Universal Reformer

- Supine Footwork without rotator disc
- Unilateral Footwork without rotator disc and arc
- Supine hip full ROM with knee flexion (see Chapter 5, Gentry: Knee stirs)

4. Additional movements

- Rotator disc
  - Standing on one disc
  - Standing on two discs

Session 6/12
Client self-report

- Fatigue scale 1
- Pain scale 1

Key changes observed

- Improved torso organization during LE movements

- Increased willingness to try challenging movements

Reasoning behind choice of movements

- Integration of UE and LE coordination
- Improve ankle proprioception for balance and stance
- Activate optimal foot loading

Session movement sequence
1. Universal Reformer

- Supine Footwork with rotator disc
- Unilateral Footwork with rotator disc and arc
- Supine hip full ROM with knee flexion (see Chapter 5, Gentry: Knee stirs)
- Splits: Side with squat variation

2. Wunda Chair

- Standing unilateral plantar flexion and dorsiflexion with knee on chair with various vectors

3. Additional movement

- Use towel sliding on the floor for squat variation to prepare for Universal Reformer Splits: Side with squat variation

Session 7/12
Client self-report

- Fatigue scale 3
- Pain scale 3
- Could not sleep well, body feels tight

Key changes observed

- Difficulty with smooth thoracic rotation
- Develop awareness of thorax movement

Reasoning behind choice of movements

- Improve thoracic rotation
- Footwork for improved foot loading
- Continue to develop a session progression

Session movement sequence
1. Half squat 10 times after seated torso flexion and extension

2. Universal Reformer

- Supine Footwork with rotator disc
- Unilateral Footwork with rotator disc and arc
- Supine hip full ROM with knee flexion (see Chapter 5, Gentry: Knee stirs)
- Splits: Side with squat variation

3. Wunda Chair

- Standing unilateral plantar flexion and dorsiflexion with knee on chair with various vectors

4. Additional movements

- Half squat on floor
- Trapeze Table
  - Thoracic rotation with push-through bar

Session 8/12
Client self-report

- Fatigue scale 1
- Pain scale 0
- Less night spasms, does not interrupt sleep
- Walking easily without fatigue

Key changes observed

- Able to increase light spring to medium spring for Universal Reformer Splits: Side

- Able to position self on Universal Reformer without assistance

Reasoning behind choice of movements

- Integrating exercises into whole-body movement
- Improve torso control

Session movement sequence

1. Pilates Arc
- Heel raise on slope of arc
- Side lunge on arc on step

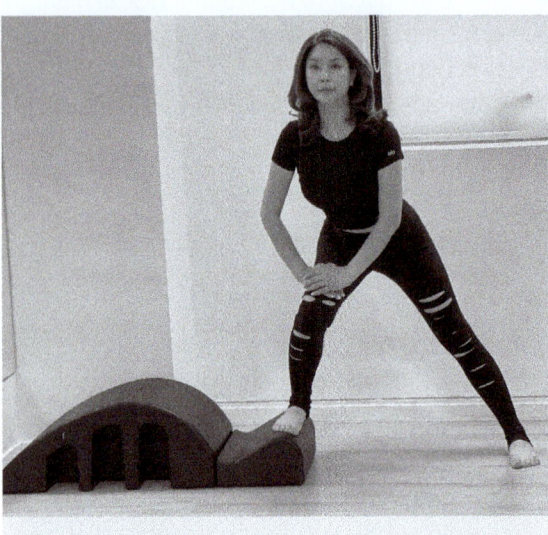

Figure 14.9

2. Trapeze Table

- Leg spring work
- Standing on rotator disc with long spring

3. Universal Reformer

- Supine Footwork with rotator disc
- Unilateral Footwork with rotator disc and arc

- Supine hip full ROM with knee flexion (see Chapter 5, Gentry: Knee stirs)
- Splits: Side with squat variation

4. Wunda Chair

- Standing unilateral plantar flexion and dorsiflexion with knee on chair with various vectors

5. Additional movements

- Universal Reformer
  - Jumping on footplate (with different vectors, foot positions)
- Wunda Chair
  - Standing unilateral plantar flexion and dorsiflexion with knee on chair with various vectors

Session 9/12
Client self-report

- Fatigue scale 2
- Pain scale 0
- Tried different shoes with low heel for a few hours

Key changes observed

- Improved left thoracic rotation
- Improved unilateral standing
- Exhibiting self-confidence

Reasoning behind choice of movements

- Continue progressions
- Integrate movement for whole body and gait
- Encouraging Pilates movement to continue even though the sessions were ending
- Reciprocal movement training

Session movement sequence
1. Pilates Arc

- Added standing on arc

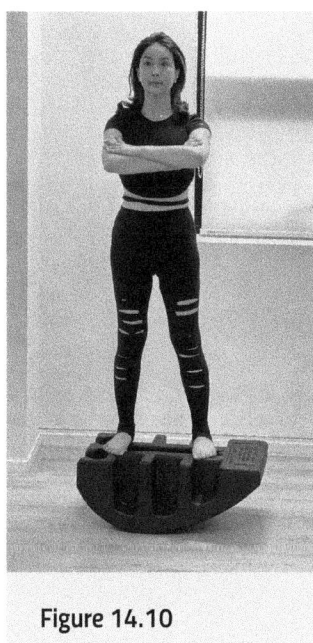

Figure 14.10

2. Universal Reformer

- Splits: Side with squat variation

3. Wunda Chair

- Standing unilateral plantar flexion and dorsiflexion with knee on chair with various vectors
- Standing leg pumps with rotator disc

4. CoreAlign

- Ankle plantar flexion with dorsiflexion of MTP joints
- Sagittal lunge (see Volume 2, Chapter 6, Session 11, exercise 5)

5. Additional movements

- Universal Reformer
  - Jumping on footplate (with different vectors, foot position)
- Wunda Chair
  - Standing unilateral plantar flexion and dorsiflexion with knee on chair with various vectors

Session 10/12
Client self-report

- Fatigue scale 1
- Pain scale 0
- Ability to control her mind not to have stress that exacerbates hypertension

Key changes observed

- Full body rotation improved
- Awareness of midline
- Balance improved

Reasoning behind choice of movements

- Fine-tune session movement sequences
- Integrate movement for whole body and gait
- Encourage Pilates movement to continue even though the sessions were ending
- Reciprocal movement training

Session movement sequence
1. Pilates Arc

- Added standing on arc

2. Universal Reformer

- Splits: Side with squat variation

3. Wunda Chair

- Standing unilateral plantar flexion and dorsiflexion with knee on chair with various vectors
- Standing leg pumps with rotator disc

4. CoreAlign

- Ankle plantar flexion with dorsiflexion of MTP joints
- Sagittal lunge

5. Additional movements

- Universal Reformer
  - Splits: Side with squat variation to standing hip abduction/adduction with torso rotation (Larkam 2017)
- CoreAlign
  - Ankle plantar flexion with dorsiflexion of MTP joints with torso rotation
  - Sagittal lunge with torso rotation

References

Larkam, E. (2017) *Fascia in Motion: Fascia-Focused Movement for Pilates.* Edinburgh: Handspring Publishing.

Martins-Meneses, D. T., Antunes, H. K., de Oliveira, N. R., and Medeiros, A. (2015) "Mat Pilates training reduced clinical and ambulatory blood pressure in hypertensive women using antihypertensive medications." *International Journal of Cardiology, 179,* 262–268.

NPCE Study Guide (National Pilates Certification Exam Study Guide) (2021) Miami, FL: National Pilates Certification Program, Inc.

Rocha, J., Cunha, F. A., Cordeiro, R., Monteiro, W., Pescatello, L. S., and Farinatti, P. (2020) "Acute effect of a single session of Pilates on blood pressure and cardiac autonomic control in middle-aged adults with hypertension." *Journal of Strength and Conditioning Research, 34,* 1, 114–123.

Şavkin, R. and Aslan, U. B. (2017) "The effect of Pilates exercise on body composition in sedentary overweight and obese women." *The Journal of Sports Medicine and Physical Fitness, 57,* 11, 1464–1470.

Wang, Y., Chen, Z., Wu, Z., Ye, X., and Xu, X. (2021) "Pilates for overweight or obesity: A meta-analysis." *Frontiers in Physiology, 12.* DOI: 10.3389/fphys.2021.643455.

Pilates and Type 2 Diabetes: Effect on Gait

Ji Hyun Koo and Eunju Lim

Type 2 diabetes is the most common type of diabetes, accounting for around 90 percent of all diabetes cases. Diabetes is a chronic, metabolic disease characterized by elevated levels of blood glucose (or blood sugar) which leads over time to serious damage to the heart, blood vessels, eyes, kidneys, and nerves (World Health Organization 2021a).

More than 420 million people are living with diabetes, a number that is expected to rise to 578 million by 2030 (World Health Organization 2021b). One in two adults living with type 2 diabetes are undiagnosed, because the symptoms can be so mild. As a result, the disease may be diagnosed several years after onset, and after complications have already arisen.

The symptoms of type 2 diabetes are similar to those of type 1 diabetes and include: excessive thirst and dry mouth, frequent urination, lack of energy, tiredness, slow-healing wounds, recurrent infections of the skin, blurred vision, and tingling or numbness in the hands and feet.

Several risk factors have been associated with type 2 diabetes and include: a family history of diabetes, being overweight, an unhealthy diet, physical inactivity, increasing age, high blood pressure, ethnicity, impaired glucose tolerance, a history of gestational diabetes, and poor nutrition during pregnancy.

The cornerstone of managing type 2 diabetes is a healthy lifestyle, which includes a healthy diet, regular physical activity, not smoking, and maintaining a healthy body weight. Over time, a healthy lifestyle may not be enough to keep blood glucose levels under control and people with type 2 diabetes may need to take oral medication. If treatment with a single medication is not sufficient, combination therapy options may be prescribed. When oral medication is not sufficient to control blood glucose levels, people with type 2 diabetes may require insulin injections.

The most commonly used oral medications for type 2 diabetes include:

- Metformin, which reduces insulin resistance and allows the body to use its own insulin more effectively. It is regarded as the first-line treatment for type 2 diabetes in most guidelines around the world.
- Sulfonylureas, which stimulate the pancreas to increase insulin production. Sulfonylureas include gliclazide, glipizide, glimepiride, tolbutamide, and glibenclamide.

There are several factors that influence the development of type 2 diabetes. The most influential are lifestyle behaviors commonly associated with urbanization. Research indicates that a majority of cases of type 2 diabetes could be prevented through healthy diet and regular physical activity. Regular physical activity is essential to help keep blood glucose levels under control. It is most effective when it includes a combination of both aerobic exercise (e.g., jogging, swimming, cycling) and resistance training, as well as reducing the amount of time spent being inactive (International Diabetes Federation 2021).

The American College of Sports Medicine (ACSM) confirms that exercise science research indicates physical activity can help prevent type 2 diabetes as well as help patients manage its effects. ACSM guidelines for managing type 2 diabetes (ACSM 2022) specify that regular aerobic exercise helps manage blood glucose. High-intensity resistance exercise benefits those with type 2 diabetes more than low- to moderate-intensity exercise.

Editor note

A Pilates program may prepare the client to safely sustain a medically guided regular practice of aerobic and resistance exercise of appropriate, effective intensity. Susceptibility to injury and overuse symptoms may be decreased by a customized Pilates practice that develops a well-organized structure, conscious body awareness, and accurate motor control.

Client description: 65-year-old biological female, identifies as female; retired teacher (2015)

Dates of case report: Session 1: March 20, 2020; Session 12: May 8, 2020; all in-person sessions

Studio apparatus and props
Pilates equipment

- Trapeze Table
- Universal Reformer
- Wunda Chair

Props used with equipment

- Spine Corrector
- Rotator disc, 12 in. (30.5 cm), no resistance and light resistance
- Toe Corrector
- Stability Sling

Home program props

- Wall space
- Spine Corrector/Pilates Arc
- Toe Corrector
- 2 rollers, 36 in. (92 cm) long, 6 in. (15 cm) in diameter
- Soft spikey ball, 4 in. (10 cm) in diameter

- Hard ball, 1 in. (2.5 cm) in diameter
- Towel

Methods and materials

Session 1/12
1. Health history interview

- 2003: high stress levels and fatigue from excessive work and caring for ill father-in-law
- 2004: diagnosed with type 2 diabetes
- 2004: due to menopause prescribed sleeping pills until 2007
- 2008: diagnosed herniated intervertebral disc (L4–L5)
- 2008: experienced side effects of the medication (steroid pill) for Cushing's syndrome
- 2012: epidural neuroplasty
- 2014: diagnosed with varicose veins in lower extremities
- Lower extremity edema with subsequent changes to feet, bunions

2. Symptoms

- Decreased sensory function of feet
- Leg edema
- Balance deficiency
- General fatigue due to a sleep disorder
- Low back pain after housework
- Digestion deficiency

3. Movement aids

- None

Final result of case report

The client was able to have arm swing naturally with thorax rotation. Her stance was wide and her balance upright. She has more power in her feet to push off the ground. After the program, the client felt less fatigue and enjoys line dancing more. She has lost 8 lb (3.6 kg) of weight.

Session 2/12: Initial assessment

1. General observations of gait

◆ Lacks thoracic rotation

◆ Lateral shift of torso

◆ Only right arm swing without thoracic rotation

◆ Gait stance is short

◆ Propulsion phase: plantar flexion was minimal, especially right foot

◆ Heel strike phase: right foot strikes toes first not heel due to a foot drop

2. Standing tests

◆ Full torso rotation

● Observations of inefficient side: left
  ■ Left rotation
    ○ Torso shifts and translates to right
    ○ Right foot pronates and right knee slightly bent, left foot slides slightly on lateral side
  ■ Tendency to rotation from the shoulders

◆ Hemipelvis inferior motion

● Observations of inefficient side: left
  ■ Small range of motion
  ■ Limited innominate lowering
  ■ Thorax translates to right

◆ Hemipelvis superior motion

● Observations of inefficient side: right
  ■ Right innominate not able to hike

Session 12/12: Post-assessment

1. General observations of gait

◆ Improved thoracic rotation

◆ Less lateral shifting, increased rotation

◆ Swing with arm and torso rotation coordinated

◆ Increased stride length

◆ Improved right foot push-off strength

◆ Minimal improved dorsiflexion on right foot

2. Standing tests

◆ Full torso rotation

● Observations of inefficient side: left
  ■ Left rotation
  ■ Less torso shift and translation, near to axis
  ■ Right knee straight and femur rotation improved
  ■ Rotates torso and shoulders together

◆ Hemipelvis inferior motion

● Observations of inefficient side: left
  ■ Left hemipelvis inferior motion improved due to hip joint gliding smoothly
  ■ Increased innominate lowering
  ■ Thorax was more centered

◆ Hemipelvis superior motion

● Observations: both sides efficient

- Thorax excessively translates to left
- Pelvis rotates to left

◆ Lateral pelvic shift

● Observations of inefficient side: right
  - Thorax translates to left
  - Pelvis rotates to left
  - Feet not adapting
  - Inability of left pronation and right supination

3. Seated tests

◆ Thoracic rotation

● Observations of inefficient side: right
  - Limited thoracic rotation to right
  - Thoracic flexion
  - Pelvis rotates right, left sitz bone slides anteriorly
  - More weight on right ischial tuberosity

◆ Hip joint and knee flexion

● Observations of inefficient side: right
  - Posterior pelvic tilt bilaterally
  - Thorax shifts to right

Author note
Included dorsiflexion and knee flexion test. Right was inefficient; limited range of motion in ankle dorsiflexion. Included hip abduction with external rotation. Right limited compared to left; right hemipelvis posteriorly rotated.

4. Sit and stand

◆ Lateral view

● Unable to stand without pushing on the chair

- Right innominate hikes
- No excessive translation of thorax to left
- Pelvis does not rotate to left

◆ Lateral pelvic shift

● Observations of inefficient side: right
  - Less thoracic translation to left
  - No left pelvic rotation
  - Feet adaptation slightly improved
  - Inability of right supination

3. Seated tests

◆ Thoracic rotation

● Observations of inefficient side: right
  - Increased right rotation
  - Small improvement of thoracic flexion
  - No pelvic rotation right
  - Equal weight on ischial tuberosities

◆ Hip joint and knee flexion

● Observations of inefficient side: right
  - Improved upright position
  - Slight thoracic shift to right

Author note
Included dorsiflexion and knee flexion test. Right dorsiflexion improved a small amount; limited range of motion in ankle dorsiflexion. Right external rotation and abduction: pelvic stability position improved.

4. Sit and stand

◆ Lateral view

● Good torso position throughout
● Hip hinge maintained

- Torso flexes forward
- Pelvis posteriorly rotates

◆ Anterior view

- To stand: weighted on left side
- Sways left to right to sit

5. Standing balance

◆ Two-leg stance, eyes open

- 60 seconds

◆ Two-leg stance, eyes closed

- 50 seconds

◆ One-leg stance, eyes open

- Left: 40 seconds
- Right: 35 seconds

◆ One-leg stance, eyes closed

- Could not perform

- Moves faster than before

◆ Anterior view

- To stand: still with more weight on left side
- Sitting position improved

5. Standing balance

◆ Two-leg stance, eyes open

- 60 seconds

◆ Two-leg stance, eyes closed

- 60 seconds

◆ One-leg stance, eyes open

- Left: 60 seconds
- Right: 50 seconds

◆ One-leg stance, eyes closed

- Left: 2 seconds
- Right: 2 seconds

Session 3/12: Home program

Fatigue scale	6
Pain scale	2
Client self-report	● Excited
Key changes observed by author at end of Session 3/12	● Better movement after exercise ● Good mind-body awareness ● Performs functional movement in daily activities
Reason behind choice of sequencing	● Foot training for awakening of foot sensory function ● Feel the whole connection from head to toe ● Counterbalance training for thoracic and lumbar area ● Hip activation and harmonious movement of joints of lower body through standing ● Upper body and lower body, whole-body integration

Session movement sequence

1. Spikey ball and hard ball plantar fascia release

Intent	● Awakening foot sensory function ● Releasing held tension
Gait reasoning	● Proprioception ● Foot sensory awakening to feel the ground with each step
Starting position	● Place spikey ball under right foot
Movement description	● Roll spikey ball from right heel to toe by shifting weight on right side ● Roll ball following right lateral arch ● Repeat 10 times with slow tempo ● Roll ball following right midline arch ● Repeat 10 times with slow tempo ● Roll the ball following medial arch line ● Repeat 10 times with slow tempo ● Lift left foot while pressing the ball ● Repeat 10 times slowly while standing on one leg ● Place superball under each metatarsal and roll ● Repeat on other side

2. Toe Corrector: Standing toe extension and flexion
Derivative of J. H. Pilates Toe Corrector: Pulling Down (NPCE Study Guide 2021, p. 89)

Intent
- Extension and flexion of toes
- Separate movement of 1st metatarsophalangeal (MTP) joint and 2nd to 5th MTP joints
- Increase mobility of the 1st MTP joint

Gait reasoning
- To improve the force for push-off from the ground

Starting position
- Place each loop of Toe Corrector around bilateral 1st MTP joints

Movement description
- Extend both 1st phalanges at MTP joint
- Flex other four MTP joints by pressing distal phalanges into the ground
- Flex both 1st phalanges and extend other four
- Repeat this movement slowly
- Maintain centralization of talus during all movement
- Repeat 6 times
- Be aware of the whole body, especially the pelvis, to avoid excess movement

3. Supine longitudinal rotation
(Larkam 2017)

Intent
- Encourage rotational motion of torso

Gait reasoning
- Counter-rotation training from feet through torso
- Connect shoulder girdle and upper extremity (UE) in counter-rotations

Starting position
- Supine, both legs extended
- Align right heel with right ischial tuberosity
- Place the left Achilles tendon between 1st and 2nd phalanges of right foot
- Interlace fingers and place hands above head, palms pressing away from head

Movement description
- Rotate pelvis, legs, and feet to right while the head, neck, and eyes turn to left
- Return to center
- Rotate pelvis, legs, and feet to left while the head, neck, and eyes turn to right
- Return to center
- Repeat 10 times
- Repeat on other side

4. Prone longitudinal rotation (Larkam 2017)

Intent	● Encourage rotational motion of torso
Gait reasoning	● Counter-rotation of pelvis and thorax from feet
Starting position	● Prone on mat ● Overlap hands and place forehead on back of hand ● Right foot dorsiflexion in line with right ischial tuberosity ● Place 1st and 2nd toes of left foot around right Achilles tendon
Movement description	● Rotate pelvis, legs, and toes to left ● Return to center ● Rotate pelvis, legs, and toes to right ● Return to center ● Repeat 10 times

5. Bridge with pelvic lateral translation

Intent	● Training torso articulation and activation ● Sensing the continuity from feet to torso ● Improve thoracic translational movement
Gait reasoning	● Activating torso with lower extremity (LE) for improved balance during stance phase ● Increase torso articulation ● Increase ability to extend hips and torso
Starting position	● Supine ● Feet parallel, hip-width apart ● Knees flexed ● Arms alongside body
Movement description	● Articulate from feet to extend hips and torso into bridge position ● Hold position ● Translate pelvis side to side, 5 times each side ● LE and shoulders remain on mat ● Articulate torso in flexion to starting position ● Repeat 5 times ● Repeat extending hips and torso articulating into bridge half way ● Translate pelvis side to side, 3 times each side ● Articulate torso in flexion to starting position ● Repeat 3 times

6. Side lying roller assisted counter-rotation of pelvis and thorax (Larkam 2017)

Intent	● Increase lateral articulation ● Improve rotation
Gait reasoning	● Improve torso rotation ● Training torso rotation with arm swing

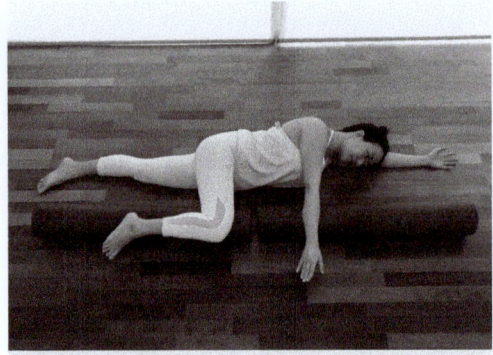

Figure 15.1

Starting position	● Place two rollers in front and parallel to the body in a vertical line ● Lie on side on mat, place top arm on roller above ● Flex hip and knee to 90 degrees and place top leg on roller
Movement description	● Top leg remains still as top arm rolls roller forward and back ● Allow thorax to follow arm and rotate ● Repeat 5 times ● Top arm remains still as top leg rolls roller forward and back ● Allow pelvis to follow leg and rotate ● Repeat 5 times ● Counter-rotation by rotating arm forward and leg back, and reverse ● Repeat 5 times ● Repeat on other side

7. Side leg lift with Pilates Arc

Intent	● Activation of posterior-lateral hip ● Stimulate posterior and lateral hip activation through hip internal and external rotation

Gait reasoning	• Balanced one-leg stance
	• Decrease unnecessary lateral shift during swing phase
	• Improve stance phase for both standing leg and swinging leg
Starting position	• Sit in well of Pilates Arc facing sideways
	• Side bend over arc, support with underneath elbow flexed on floor
	• Place the top arm in a comfortable position
	• Flex hips and knees
Movement description	• Extend hip and knees in alignment with the greater trochanter
	• Abduct and adduct the legs with feet together
	• Abduct top leg and hold
	• Internally rotate and adduct leg, knee to bottom knee
	• Externally rotate and abduct leg, top foot to bottom foot
	• Repeat 4 times slowly
	• Rest for 1 or 2 seconds
	• Repeat, abducting top leg
	• Internally rotate leg and extend leg posteriorly
	• Hold extended hip and knee
	• Abduct and adduct leg 10 times
	• Return to starting position
	• Repeat, abducting top leg
	• Externally rotate leg and extend posteriorly
	• Hold extended hip and knee
	• Abduct and adduct leg 10 times
	• Return to starting position
	• Repeat on other side

8. Swan on Spine Corrector

Derivative of J. H. Pilates Swan on Spine Corrector (NPCE Study Guide 2021, p. 82)

Intent	• Activate torso extensors
	• Increase articulation in extension for upright stance
Gait reasoning	• Extensor activation enhancing upright stance
	• Improve rotation
Starting position	• Lie on top of the arc, facing away from the step
	• Place hands on floor

Movement description
- Use hands to press up into Swan
- Extend torso feeling scapula set on thorax
- Minimize force of palm and arms
- Flex elbows
- Repeat 8 times slowly
- From the last repetition, pause at the top
- Hover both hands off floor
- Hold for 10 seconds
- Return to starting position

9. Wall assisted heel raise

Intent
- Improve ankle dorsiflexion and plantar flexion
- Challenge torso organization with dynamic feet

Gait reasoning
- Improve the force of push-off during gait
- Challenge torso adaptations during movement of the foot

Starting position
- Stand facing wall
- Feet parallel, hip-width apart
- Knees extended

Movement description
- Raise calcaneus slowly
- Lower calcaneus slowly
- Maintain the distance between wall and face
- Repeat 10 times
- Maintain central position of talus
- Distribute the force throughout metatarsal arch

10. Standing single lower leg push-off with towel

Intent
- Articulation of ankle dorsiflexion and plantar flexion
- Motor control of pressing through plantar flexion and hip extension with center of mass moving forward

Gait reasoning
- Practice push-off distributing force from foot to propel forward

Starting position
- Stand facing wall
- Legs parallel
- Place towel under right foot
- Place both hands on wall if it is hard to maintain midline organization

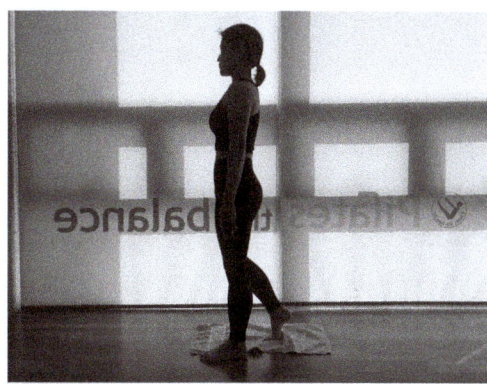

Figure 15.2

Movement description
- Stand with weight equally distributed on feet
- Sweep towel behind with right heel lifted and knee flexed
- Lower heel and return to starting position
- Repeat 10 times
- Repeat on other side

11. Standing on both feet, facing away from a corner

Intent
- Stimulate torso rotation
- Stimulate hip joint internal and external rotation

Gait reasoning
- Improve torso rotation
- Closed kinematic chain exercise stimulates femoral joint rotations that occur in gait

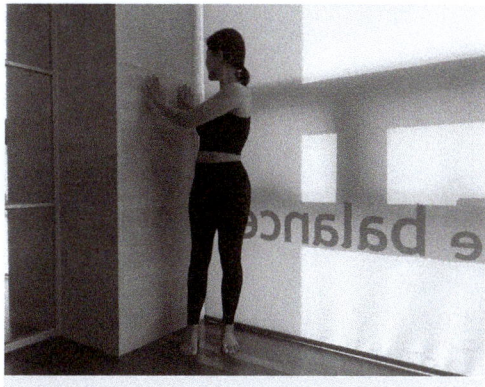

Figure 15.3

Starting position	● Standing facing away from corner of wall
	● Feet parallel, hip-width apart
Movement description	● Flex both elbows, and position both palms to face the front
	● Stand with both legs extended and rotate torso to right
	● Stop at the point where pelvis would rotate
	● Touch wall on right side
	● Keep axis of torso during rotation
	● Keep nose and sternum in one line
	● Return to center
	● Rotate torso to left
	● Touch wall on left side
	● Return to center
	● Repeat 10 times

12. Pilates Arc balance squat

Intent	● Motor control of hip and knee joint in flexion and in extension
	● Challenge balance
Gait reasoning	● Challenge adaption for balance during a squat on an unstable surface
	● Proprioception
	● Increase dorsiflexion
	● Training posterior-lateral hip activation in squat

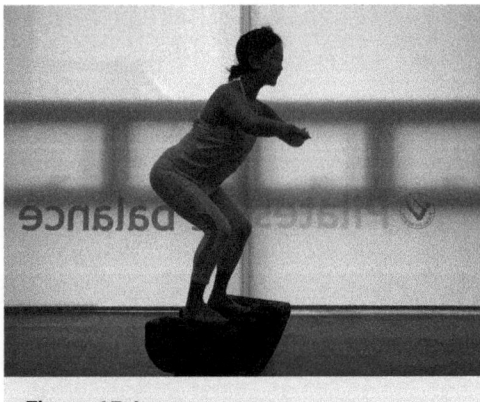

Figure 15.4

Starting position   ● Place Pilates Arc upside down
  ● Stand on underside of arc
  ● Step up on low slope first and place other foot on high slope
  ● Keep the feet parallel

Movement description   ● Find balance standing with both LE extended
  ● Flex hips and knees to client's optimal organization
  ● Extend hips and knees to stand
  ● Repeat 5 times
  ● Increase hip and knee flexion as possible
  ● Repeat 5 times
  ● Repeat on other side

Session 11/12: Studio session

Fatigue scale   3

Pain scale   0

Client self-report   ● During line dancing, feeling smooth movement and less edema

Key changes observed by author at end of Session 11/12   ● Client integrates whole-body movement
  ● Client applies new movement skills to gait

Reason behind choice of sequencing   ● Improved torso rotation with arm swing
  ● Improved feet articulation
  ● Less excessive lateral pelvic shift during heel strike

Session movement sequence

1. Trapeze Table supine to side lying assisted torso rotation with arm internal and external rotation   (Larkam 2017)

Intent   ● Full torso rotation
  ● Torso rotation coordination with UE

Gait reasoning   ● Rotation from foot articulating through torso and UE
  ● Working with and against resistance to load derotation of torso

Set-up   ● 2 light springs crossed, top-loaded on push-through bar
  ● Carabiners attach handles to eye bolts of push-through bar

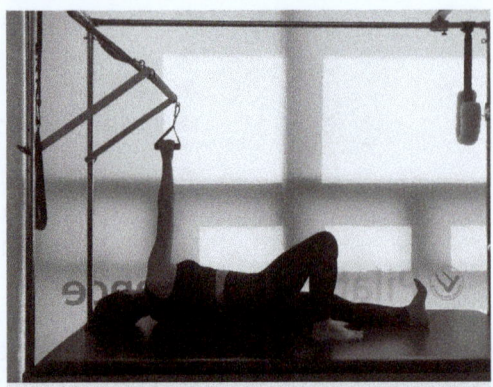

Figure 15.5

Starting position	● Supine, head toward tower end
	● Left knee flexion, left hand holding right-side handle
	● Right LE extended
Movement description	● Press left foot on Trapeze Table to rotate toward right side
	● Articulate rotation from foot through pelvis, torso, head, and eyes to right
	● Left UE follows the rotation bringing shoulder joint to lateral abduction
	● Reverse the rotation and return to starting position
	● Repeat 6 times
	● Repeat on other side

CUES
- Press the foot strongly and knee toward the ceiling
- Keep the torso's midline orientation
- Inhalation during rotation
- Exhalation during derotation

2. Lateral flexion with rotation on Wunda Chair	Derivative of J. H. Pilates Seated Mermaid/Side Arm Sit on Wunda Chair (NPCE Study Guide 2021, p. 73)
Intent	● Increase lateral body mobility
	● Torso rotation
	● Release tension held in torso
Gait reasoning	● Improve lateral flexion and rotation
Set-up	● Heavy spring in high position

Starting position	● Sit sideways on the chair with right side facing pedal
	● Right knee flexed over side of chair
	● Left leg extended with foot on floor
	● Laterally flex torso placing right UE extended on pedal
	● Left hand behind head, elbow flexed
Movement description	● Press pedal down with lateral flexion of torso
	● Return to starting position
	● Rotate torso to right and press pedal
	● Return to starting position
	● Rotate torso to left and press pedal
	● Return to starting position
	● Repeat in each direction 4 times
	● Repeat on other side

CUES

- ◆ Press the foot into the floor throughout the exercise
- ◆ Use a long exhale to increase the lateral flexion when lowering the pedal
- ◆ Rotate only the torso—do not swing the pelvis anterior

Author note

If it is difficult to reach the foot to the floor or maintain the foot in contact with the floor, place a box under the foot. The client's assessment showed limited rotation to the left. She repeated left lateral flexion using the breath. For this client, it was uncomfortable to hold the hand behind the head and she placed the back of the hand on the forehead. After a few repetitions, she changed the position of the hand to behind the head.

3. Footwork on Universal Reformer using jump board and rotator disc	Derivative of J. H. Pilates Footwork on Universal Reformer (NPCE Study Guide 2021, p. 52)
Intent	● Rotate LE femur moving pelvis
	● Dynamic activation of LE through rotation and sagittal plane motions
Gait reasoning	● Adaptability of LE in all planes of movement
	● LE control on an unstable surface
	● Dynamic continuity of LE with torso
Set-up	● Place rotator disc on jump board
	● 2 medium springs
	● Toe Corrector on both 1st phalanges

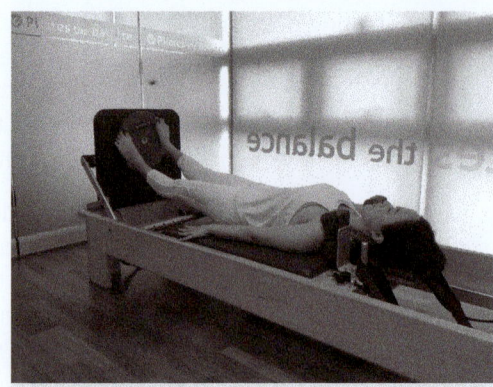

Figure 15.6

Starting position	● Supine on carriage
	● Place feet on disc, legs parallel
	● Extend Toe Corrector's spring and spread all toes
Movement description	● Press parallel feet into disc and extend hips and knees
	● With control, flex hips and knees returning the carriage home
	● Repeat 6 times
	● Extend both hips and knees, hold
	● Rotate disc to right activating right hip external rotation and left hip internal rotation with extended legs
	● Hold rotated position as hips and knees flex
	● Return carriage home
	● Stay in home position, in flexion, rotate both legs to left activating hip external rotation and right hip internal rotation
	● Press feet into disc and extend hips and knees
	● With extended legs rotate both feet to the right
	● Hold rotated position as hips and knees flex
	● Continuously repeat rotations with hip/knee flexion and extension
	● Repeat 6 times
	● Repeat the pattern starting with legs extended rotating left 6 times

CUES

- Maintain the pelvis facing front as the LE rotates especially on the internal rotation
- Keep the feet centralized with the femoral joint
- Maintain an equal distance between the legs

Author note

Use equal force of the 1st phalange when extending the spring. This will enhance the arch of the foot. Once accomplished try placing the 1st and 2nd phalanges into the Toe Corrector.

4. Footwork on Universal Reformer with jump board: metatarsal jumping

Derivative of J. H. Pilates Footwork on Universal Reformer (NPCE Study Guide 2021, p. 52)

Intent
- Proprioception of feet in jumping
- Training adaptability to ground forces
- Training feet articulation

Gait reasoning
- Improve feet articulation for distributing and adapting ground forces
- Improve force of push-off
- Torso adaptation to force generated from feet

Set-up
- Universal Reformer with jump board
- Medium spring

Starting position
- Supine on carriage
- Feet parallel on jump board
- Hip and knees extended

Movement description
- Lift the heels, plantar flex with metatarsals on jump board
- Press off the toes for a small jump
- Exhale on landing
- Repeat 10 times

CUES
- Inhale for a small jump
- Exhale on the landing
- Land softly and quietly
- Align the center of the feet with center of femoral joints
- Maintain the same placement of the feet on the jump board

Author note

To begin, the client first performed heel raise and lower before jumping. Then she began jumping continuously. Observe for how the feet land. Encourage the client to land with feet level on the jump board.

5. Side lying single-leg jumps with Pilates Arc on Universal Reformer

Intent
- Stimulating posterior lateral hip
- Activation of hip internal and external rotation
- Motor control of foot to torso in side lying orientation

Gait reasoning
- Training lateral orientation facilitating activation for improved stance phase
- Decrease excessive pelvic lateral shift during swing and stance phases

Set-up
- Place Pilates Arc on shoulder rest of Universal Reformer with step toward footbar
- Medium spring

Starting position
- Lie with right side over arc in lateral flexion
- Right hip and knee flexed resting on carriage
- Place right hand behind head and left hand on pelvis
- Place left foot on jump board
- Left knee flexed, foot dorsiflexed

Movement description
- Press foot into board to jump
- Extend left hip and knee, plantar flex the foot
- Landing quietly
- Repeat 10 times
- Change the leg position from external rotation, internal rotation, extension
- Repeat on other side

CUES
- Heel down in landing
- Maintain centralized foot and femoral joint
- On landing, the foot neither pronates nor supinates
- Keep the torso in lateral position without falling forward or back

Author note
Clients can be afraid of jumping and intend to look down to watch the landing. At first, allow them to watch, then guide the client's gaze.

6. Swan facing back on Universal Reformer

Derivative of J. H. Pilates Long Box: Swan and Long Box: Pulling Straps (NPCE Study Guide 2021, p. 54)

Intent
- Activate torso extensors
- Improve scapula mobility and awareness of UE connection
- Coordination of torso and UE in prone position

Gait reasoning
- Axial elongation for improved torso mobility
- Improve extension for push-off

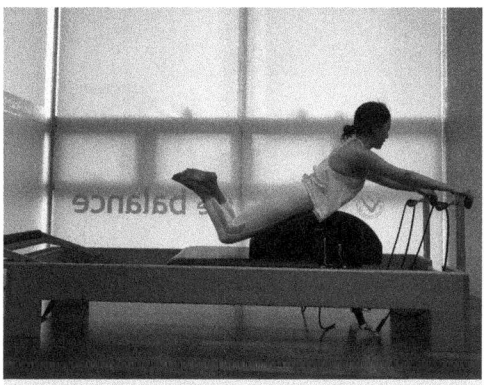

Figure 15.7

Set-up
- Separate the Pilates Arc from the seat
- Place the low slope toward footbar
- Middle arch over shoulder stops
- Very light spring

Starting position
- Prone on Pilates Arc
- Facing the risers
- Hold risers with shoulders flexed and elbows extended
- Head, torso, and LE active in a horizontal position

Movement description
- Pull and push risers to lower and elevate scapulae
- Maintain extended elbows
- Repeat 6 times
- Set the scapulae on the ribs with elbows extended
- Begin to articulate into extension from head through mid-torso moving the carriage toward risers
- Slowly lower down to starting position
- Repeat 6 times

351

CUES
- LE active in maintaining the horizontal body position
- Keep scapulae set on the ribs throughout the movement

Author note

If the client is uncomfortable with the prone position, place a suitable mat under the front of the pelvis. Place the sticky pad on the Pilates Arc to prevent slipping.

7. Standing ankle plantar flexion and dorsiflexion with Wunda Chair and light resistance disc

Intent
- Improve articulation of ankle
- Challenge balance

Gait reasoning
- Improve force of plantar flexion in push-off phase
- Increase hip glide
- Improve integration of foot to hip activation

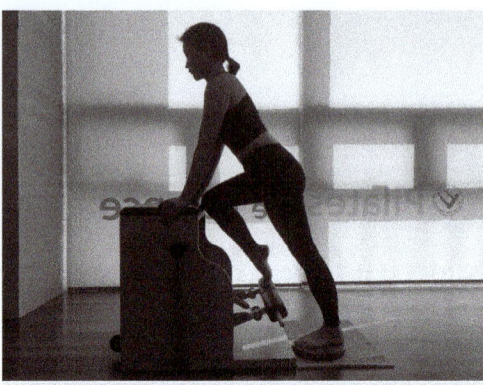

Figure 15.8

Set-up
- Heavy spring in high position
- Place light resistance disc under standing leg

Starting position
- Stand facing chair
- Stand with right foot on disc
- Place left knee on edge of chair and metatarsals on pedal
- Hold seat of chair

Movement description
- Right standing leg externally rotates
- Return right standing leg to front
- Repeat 8 times
- Plantar flex left foot and press pedal down
- Return to starting position
- Repeat 8 times
- Repeat on other side

CUES
- Move smoothly throughout the movement
- Observe how the foot to hip are organized in both the standing leg and pedal leg

Author note
Add a variation of internal rotation of standing leg.

8. Half squat with arm rotation on Trapeze Table

Intent
- Counter-rotation with torso and pelvis
- Coordination of arm and torso

Gait reasoning
- Improve arm swing with torso rotation
- Training rotational pattern for gait

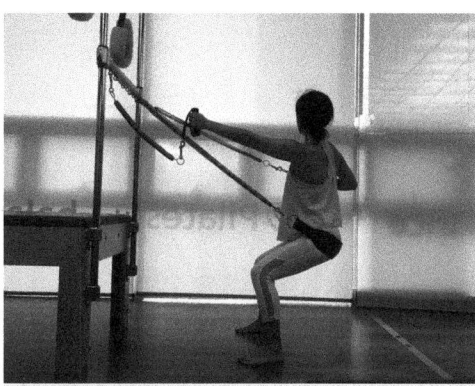

Figure 15.9

Set-up
- 2 medium long springs attached to a Stability Sling
- 2 very light springs attached to handles
- Springs attached to open end of table at appropriate height

Starting position
- Stand facing Trapeze Table
- Place Stability Sling at level of sacrum
- Hold handles

Movement description
- Extend the long springs and squat into sling
- Alternate pulling and pushing handles
- Keep pelvis still and rotate torso to pulling arm side
- Repeat 10 times

CUES
- The gaze follows the torso rotation
- Move smoothly and with control

Author note

At first, the client had difficulty with coordination of arm movement. Time was spent on the squat. With improved coordination of UE and squat, single-leg lift and lower was added.

9. Lunges and running with sling on Trapeze Table

Intent
- Coordination of walking forward with resistance
- Dynamic movement experience
- Motor control of moving forward and back working with and against resistance

Gait reasoning
- Resistance against forward momentum
- Practice arm swing with stepping forward

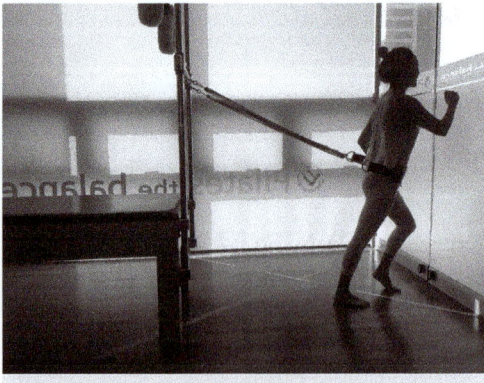

Figure 15.10

Set-up	● 2 light long springs attached to a Stability Sling ● Springs attached to open end of table at appropriate height
Starting position	● Place Stability Sling at level of anterior superior iliac spine (ASIS)
Movement description	● Right step forward into lunge position ● Pause for 2 seconds ● Step back ● Left step forward into lunge position ● Pause for 2 seconds ● Step back ● Repeat 5 times on each side ● Run toward the front with natural arm swing ● Run for 30 seconds, step back, finish

CUES

- Track knee over 3rd metatarsal in lunge
- Resist the spring when stepping back
- Even rhythm when running forward
- Contralateral arm swing to foot forward

Author note
There will be an increase in heart rate.

The journey to Session 11

Session 4/12
Client self-report

- Scapular glide difficult to feel
- Fatigue scale 6
- Pain scale 2

Key changes observed

- Improved orientation to midline

Reasoning behind choice of movements

- Proprioception of foot and adaptation of torso
- Motor control of LE

Session movement sequence
1. Bridge with pelvic lateral translation

2. Side lying roller assisted counter-rotation of pelvis and thorax

3. Supine longitudinal rotation

4. Trapeze Table

- Supine to side lying assisted torso rotation with arm internal and external rotation

5. Wunda Chair

- Lateral flexion with rotation

6. Universal Reformer

- Footwork
- Jump board with disc
- Pilates Arc Swan facing back

7. Additional movements

- Universal Reformer lunge
- Prone arms on roller, scapular elevation and depression

Session 5/12
Client self-report

- Fatigue scale 4
- Pain scale 2

Key changes observed

- Improved torso rotation from central axis

Reasoning behind choice of movements

- Improved proprioception and articulation of feet

Session movement sequence
1. Trapeze Table

- Supine to side lying assisted torso rotation with arm internal and external rotation

2. Wunda Chair

- Lateral flexion with rotation

3. Universal Reformer

- Footwork
- Supine ankle jumps with knees extended
- Pilates Arc Swan facing back

4. Additional movement

- Universal Reformer
  - Footwork with spikey ball under feet

Session 6/12
Client self-report

- Fatigue scale 3
- Pain scale 1

Key changes observed

- Less edema of lower legs
- Improved sensory function of the foot

Reasoning behind choice of movements

- Articulate feet and ankles
- Activate doming of foot
- Improve balance

Session movement sequence
1. Wunda Chair

- Seated lateral spine flexion with rotation

2. Universal Reformer

- Footwork
- Supine ankle jumps with knees extended
- Side lying single-leg jumps
- Pilates Arc Swan facing back

Session 7/12
Client self-report

- Could not sleep well
- Fatigue scale 5
- Pain scale 3

Key changes observed

- Using Toe Corrector induces a little pain

Reasoning behind choice of movements

- Improve force of push-off
- Improve articulation of feet
- Activate doming of feet

Session movement sequence
1. Standing single-leg heel push-off with towel

2. Wunda Chair

- Seated lateral spine flexion with rotation

3. Universal Reformer

- Footwork
- Supine ankle jumps with knees extended
- Side lying single-leg jumps
- Pilates Arc Swan facing back

4. Wunda Chair

- Standing ankle plantar and dorsiflexion

Session 8/12
Client self-report

- Seated for 2 hours playing the guitar causing increased edema of lower legs
- Fatigue scale 4
- Pain scale 3

Key changes observed

- Improve motor control of LE driven movements
- Decrease edema through LE exercises

Reasoning behind choice of movements

- Adapting a variety of pelvic and hip motions
- Improve walking by adapting to uneven surfaces

Session movement sequence
1. Supine longitudinal rotation

2. Wunda Chair

- Seated lateral spine flexion with rotation

3. Universal Reformer

- Supine ankle jumps with knees extended—single leg
- Side lying single-leg jumps, both external and internal rotation
- Pilates Arc Swan facing back

4. Wunda Chair

- Standing ankle plantar flexion and dorsiflexion

5. Additional movement

- Universal Reformer
  - Twist bridge

Session 9/12
Client self-report

- Walking without pain in big toe
- Fatigue scale 3
- Pain scale 1

Key changes observed

- Increased ease in gait through articulated hip joint movement without torso flexion

Reasoning behind choice of movements

- Torso mobility for better rotation
- Extensors for improved axial elongation
- Arm swing and LE coordination

Session movement sequence
1. Wunda Chair

- Seated lateral spine flexion with rotation

2. Universal Reformer

- Footwork
- Pilates Arc Swan facing back

3. Wunda Chair

- Standing ankle plantar flexion and dorsiflexion

4. Trapeze Table

- Half squat with arm rotation

5. Additional movement

- Universal Reformer
  - Double knee stretch

Session 10/12
Client self-report

- Fatigue scale 2
- Pain scale 0

Key changes observed

- Improve and balance torso rotation with arm swing

Reasoning behind choice of movements

- Coordination of torso rotation and arm swing
- Integrate whole-body movement

Session movement sequence
1. Roller

- Contralateral arm and leg lift

2. Trapeze Table

- Supine to side lying assisted torso rotation with arm internal and external rotation

3. Wunda Chair

- Standing ankle plantar flexion and dorsiflexion with light resistance disc

4. Trapeze Table

- Half squat with arm rotation
- Lunges and running with sling

References

ACSM (American College of Sports Medicine) (2022) ACSM publishes new recommendations on type 2 diabetes and exercise. February 9, 2022. www.acsm.org/news-detail/2022/02/09/acsm-publishes-new-recommendations-on-type-2-diabetes-and-exercise#:~:text=Small%20%E2%80%9Cdoses%E2%80%9D%20of%20physical%20activity,%2D%20to%20moderate%2Dintensity%20exercise. [Accessed October 23, 2023].

International Diabetes Federation (2021) Type 2 diabetes: Delaying or preventing type 2 diabetes. www.idf.org/aboutdiabetes/type-2-diabetes.html. [Accessed October 23, 2023].

Larkam, E. (2017) *Fascia in Motion: Fascia-Focused Movement for Pilates.* Edinburgh: Handspring Publishing, pp. 71, 77, 179, 189.

NPCE Study Guide (National Pilates Certification Exam Study Guide) (2021) Miami, FL: National Pilates Certification Program, Inc.

World Health Organization (2021a) Diabetes. April 5, 2023. www.who.int/news-room/fact-sheets/detail/diabetes. [Accessed October 23, 2023].

World Health Organization (2021b) New WHA Resolution to bring much needed boost to diabetes prevention and control efforts. May 27, 2021. www.who.int/news/item/27-05-2021-new-wha-resolution-to-bring-much-needed-boost-to-diabetes-prevention-and-control-efforts. [Accessed October 23, 2023].

Anatomical Illustrations References

Gait assessment

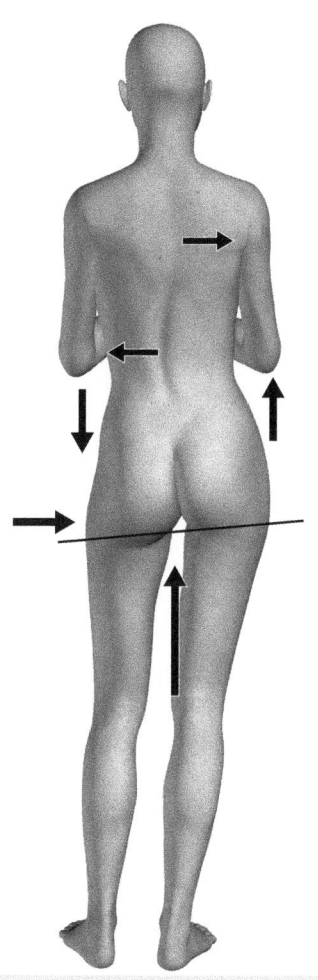

Figure A.1 Efficient gait.
(Black 2022, p. 75, Figure 3.9)

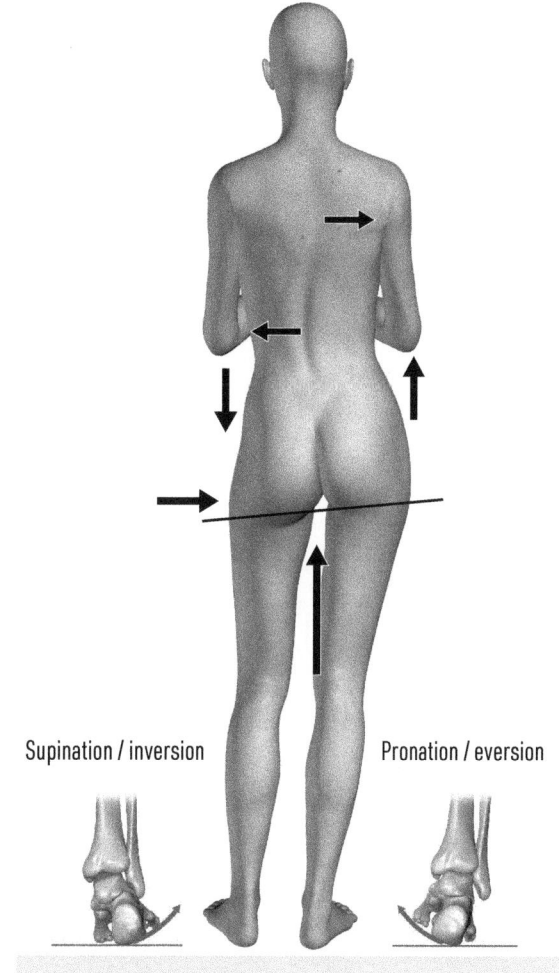

Supination / inversion   Pronation / eversion

Figure A.2 Efficient lateral shift.
(Black 2022, p. 75, Figure 3.9 and p. 14, Figure 1.10)

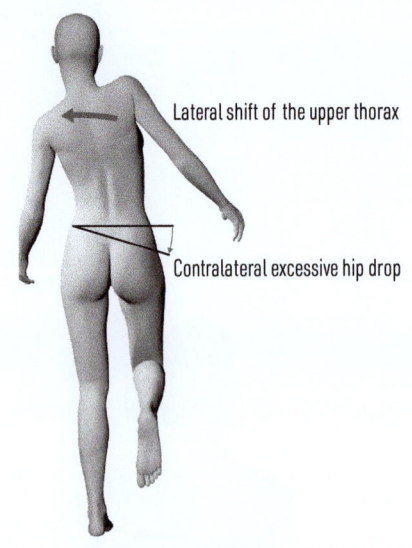

Lateral shift of the upper thorax

Contralateral excessive hip drop

Figure A.3 Inefficient gait.
(Black 2022, p. 68, Figure 3.2)

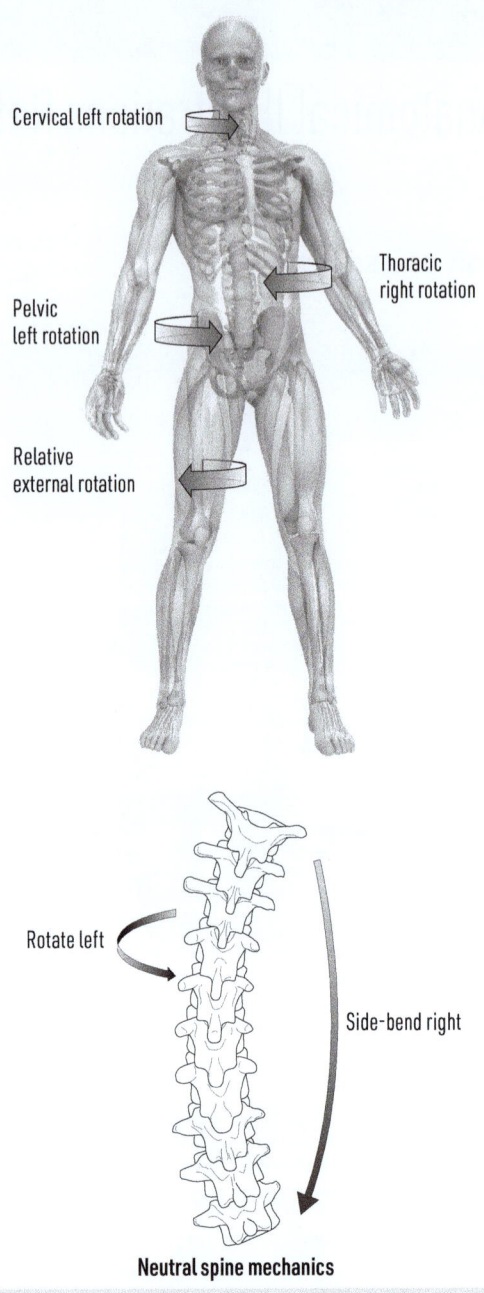

Cervical left rotation

Thoracic right rotation

Pelvic left rotation

Relative external rotation

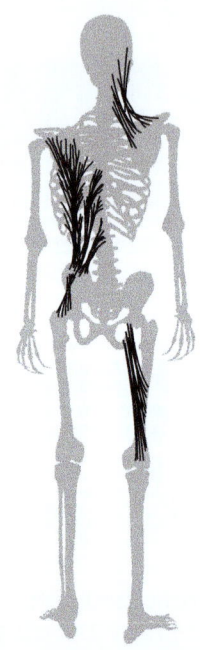

Figure A.4 Fascia adhesions in asymmetry.
(Martin 2018, p. 78, Figure 6.3)

Rotate left

Side-bend right

Neutral spine mechanics

Figure A.5 A Oppositional rotation in the transverse plane. **B** Rotation coupled with lateral flexion.
(Martin 2018; A: p. 110, Figure 4.2; B: p. 15, Figure 1.8B)

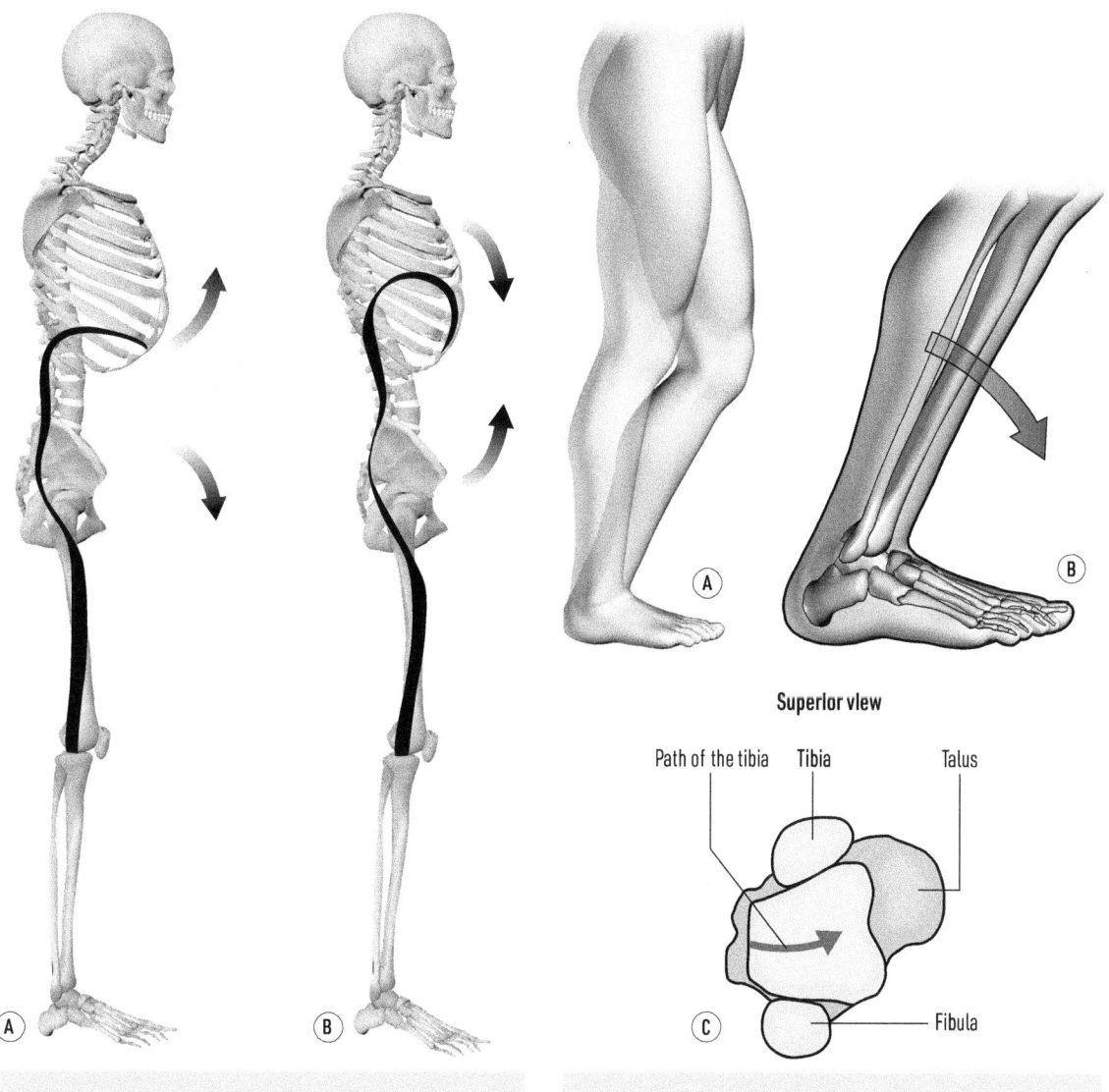

Figure A.6 Optimal relationship of feet, pelvis, thorax, cranium as relates to breathing.
(Martin 2018, p. 123, Figure 8.1 A and B)

Figure A.7 Dorsiflexion and talus glide.
(Black 2022, p. 12, Figure 1.6)

Torso and breathing

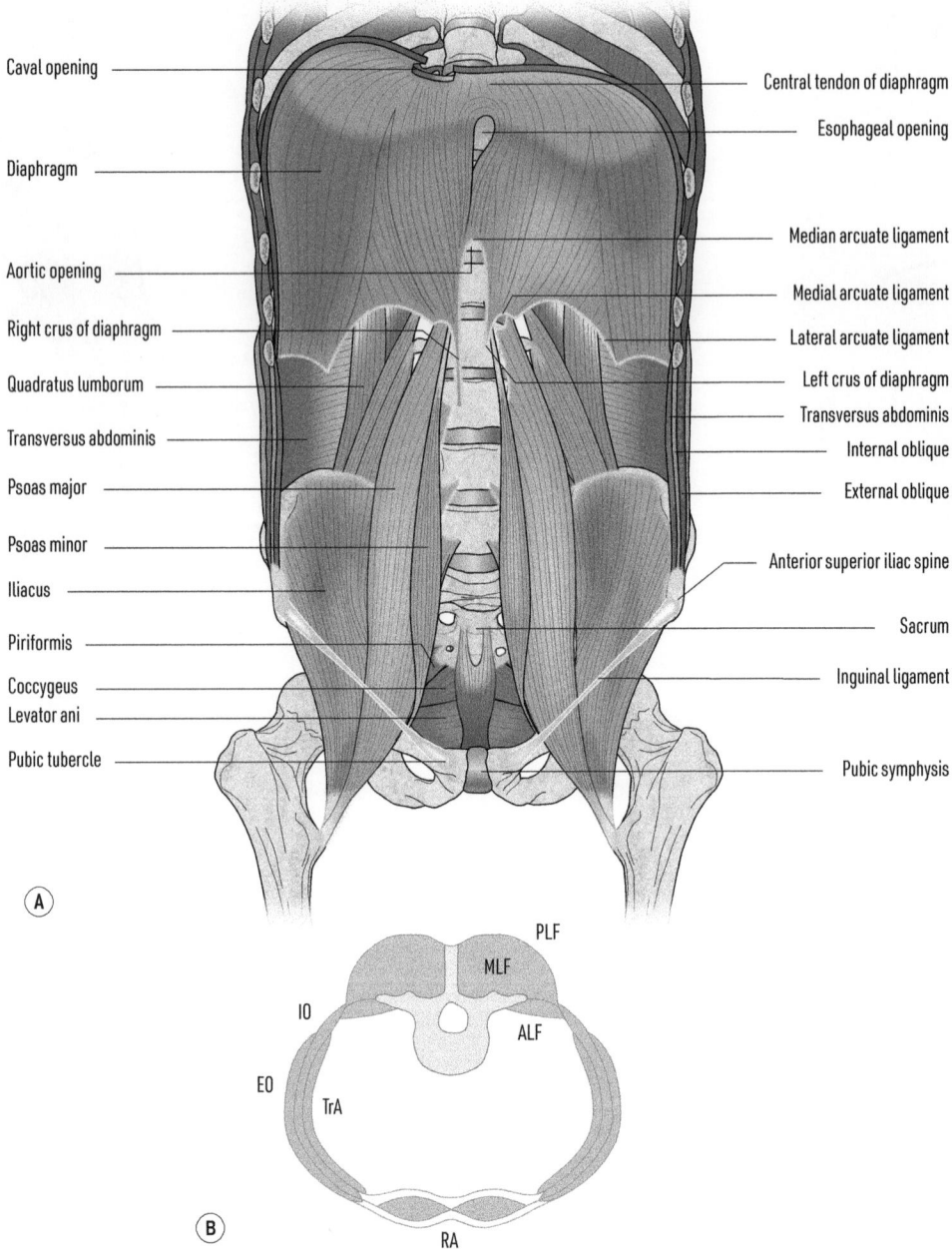

Caval opening

Diaphragm

Aortic opening

Right crus of diaphragm

Quadratus lumborum

Transversus abdominis

Psoas major

Psoas minor

Iliacus

Piriformis

Coccygeus

Levator ani

Pubic tubercle

Central tendon of diaphragm

Esophageal opening

Median arcuate ligament

Medial arcuate ligament

Lateral arcuate ligament

Left crus of diaphragm

Transversus abdominis

Internal oblique

External oblique

Anterior superior iliac spine

Sacrum

Inguinal ligament

Pubic symphysis

A

PLF

MLF

IO

ALF

EO

TrA

B

RA

Figure A.8 A Soft tissue connections between thoracic diaphragm and pelvic diaphragm. **B** Cross-section inferior to diaphragm.
(A: Martin 2018, p. 124, Figure 8.2; B: Black 2022, p. 114, Figure 4.7)

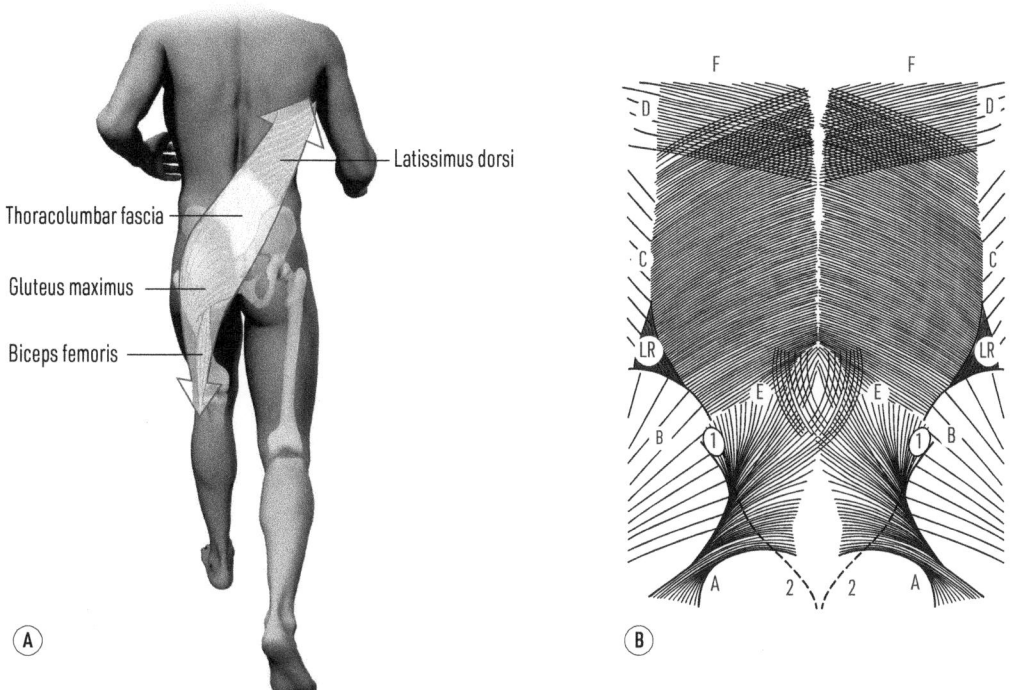

Figure A.9 A Continuum of thoracolumbar fascia with extremities. **B** The thoracolumbar fascia.
(A: Black 2022, p. 209, Figure 7.2; B: Larkam 2017, p. 40, Figure 2.5)

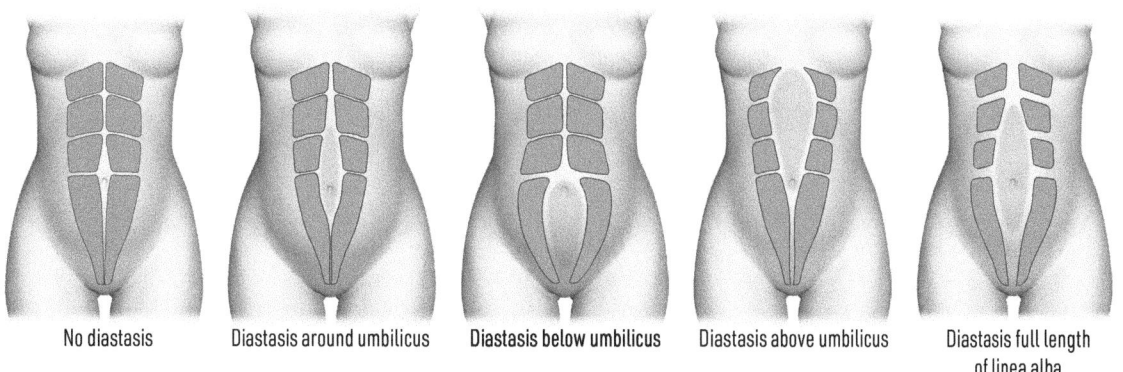

Figure A.10 Diastasis rectus.
(Mason 2023, p. 121, Figure 6.1)

363

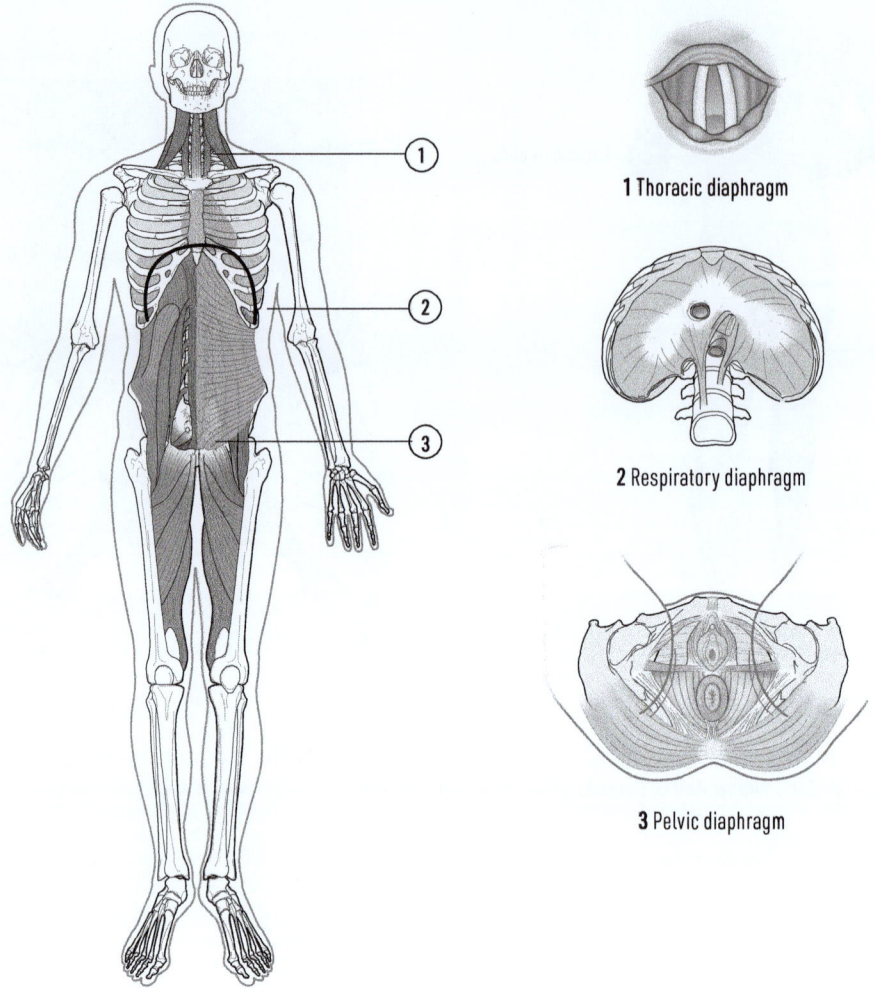

1 Thoracic diaphragm

2 Respiratory diaphragm

3 Pelvic diaphragm

Figure A.11 Diaphragms.
(Mason 2023, p. 17, Figure 1.1)

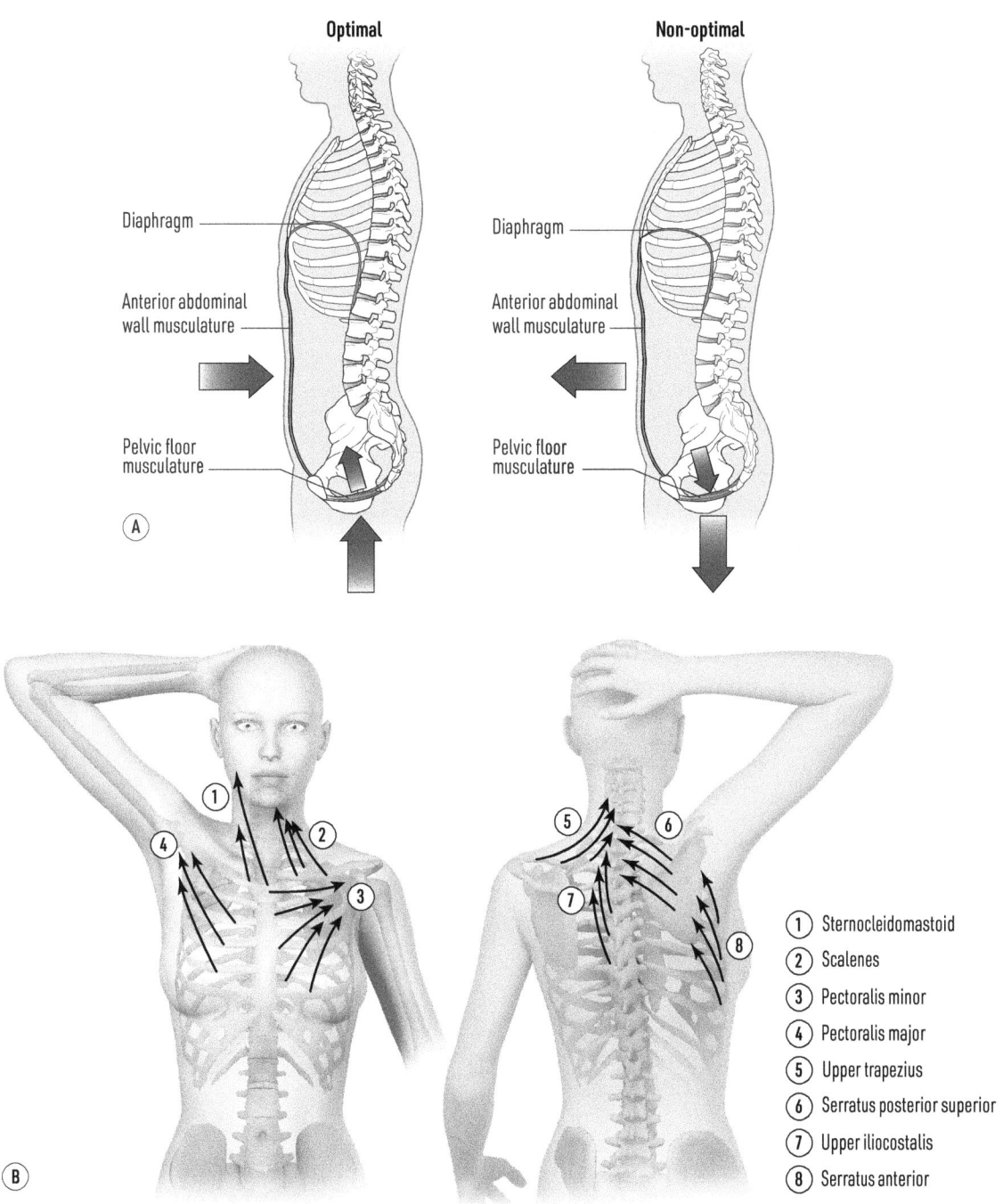

Figure A.12 A Movement relationships between the thoracic diaphragm and pelvic diaphragm. **B** Tissue response to air flow during inhalation.
(A: Martin 2018, p. 126, Figure 8.3; B: Black 2022, p. 176, Figure 6.7)

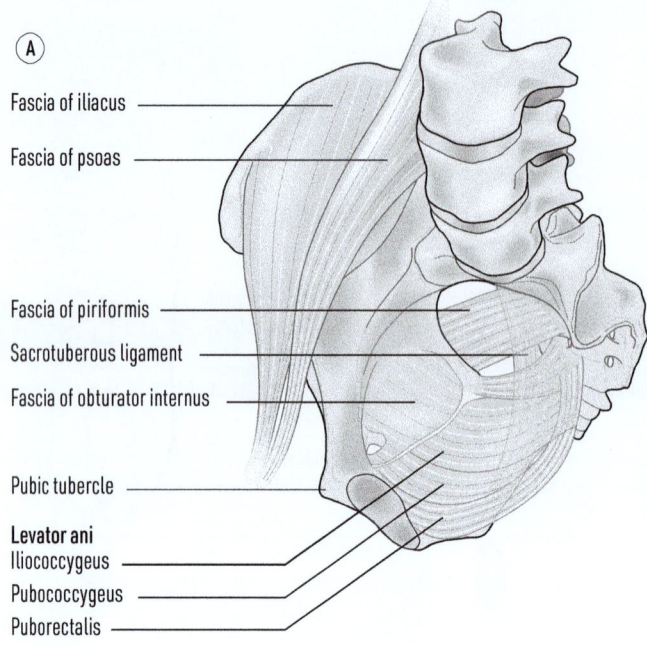

Ⓐ

Fascia of iliacus

Fascia of psoas

Fascia of piriformis

Sacrotuberous ligament

Fascia of obturator internus

Pubic tubercle

Levator ani
Iliococcygeus

Pubococcygeus

Puborectalis

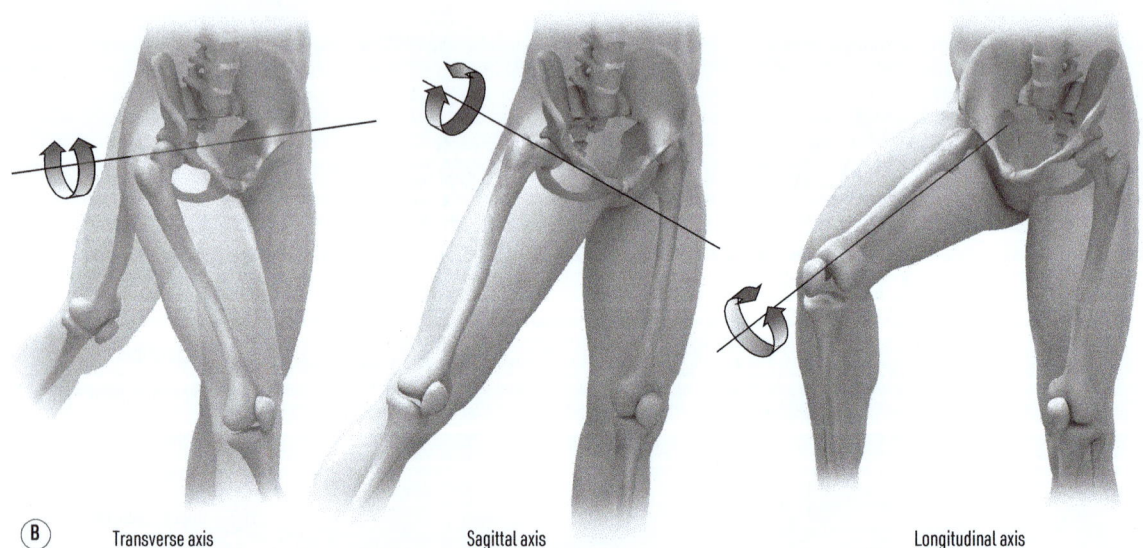

Ⓑ Transverse axis Sagittal axis Longitudinal axis

Figure A.13 Lumbopelvic-hip complex.
(Black 2022, p. 71, Figure 3.5, p. 70, Figure 3.4)

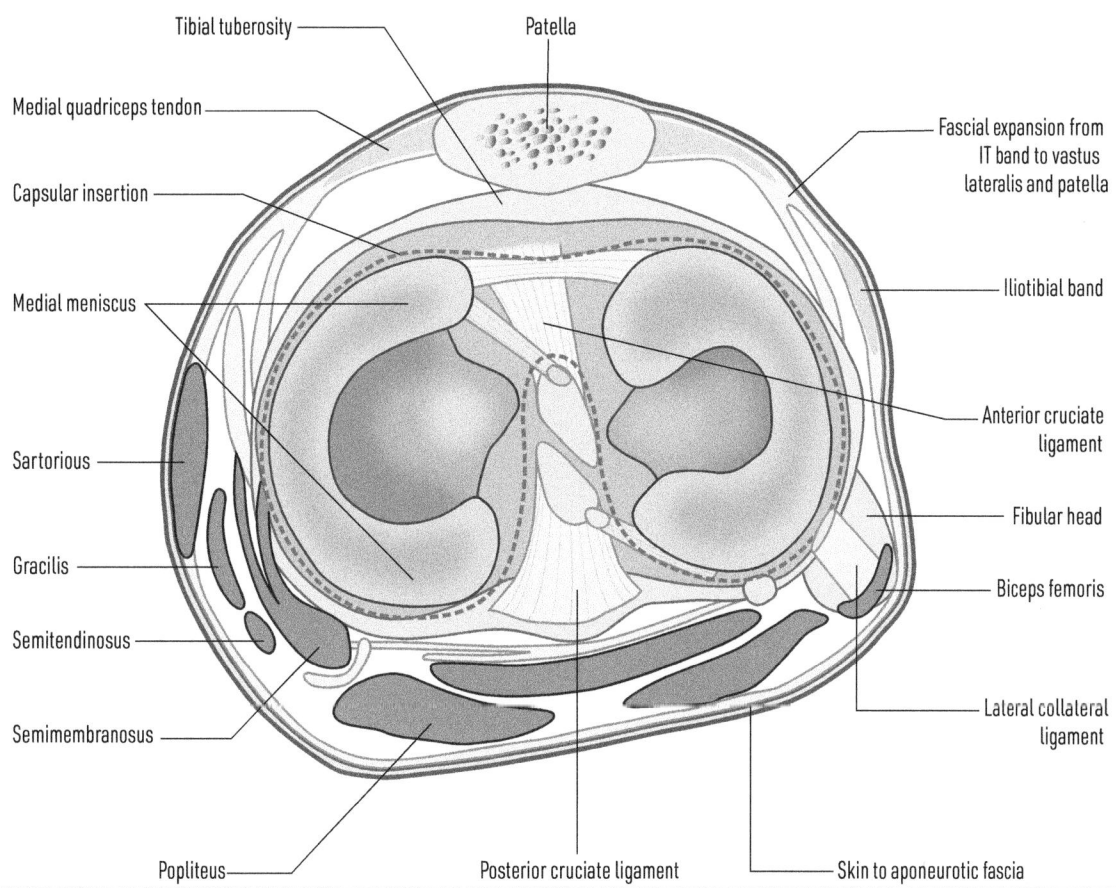

Tibial tuberosity

Patella

Medial quadriceps tendon

Capsular insertion

Medial meniscus

Sartorious

Gracilis

Semitendinosus

Semimembranosus

Popliteus

Posterior cruciate ligament

Skin to aponeurotic fascia

Fascial expansion from IT band to vastus lateralis and patella

Iliotibial band

Anterior cruciate ligament

Fibular head

Biceps femoris

Lateral collateral ligament

Figure A.14 Cross-section of knee joint.
(Black 2022, p. 38, Figure 2.4)

References

Black, M. (2022) *Centered: Organizing the Body through Kinesiology, Movement Theory and Pilates Techniques.* 2nd Ed. Edinburgh: Handspring Publishing.

Larkam, E. (2017) *Fascia in Motion: Fascia-Focused Movement for Pilates.* Edinburgh: Handspring Publishing.

Martin, S. C. (2018) *Spinal Asymmetry and Scoliosis: Movement and Function Solutions for the Spine, Ribcage and Pelvis.* Edinburgh: Handspring Publishing.

Mason, M. (2023) *Pelvic Rehabilitation: The Manual Therapy and Exercise Guide Across the Lifespan.* London: Handspring Publishing.

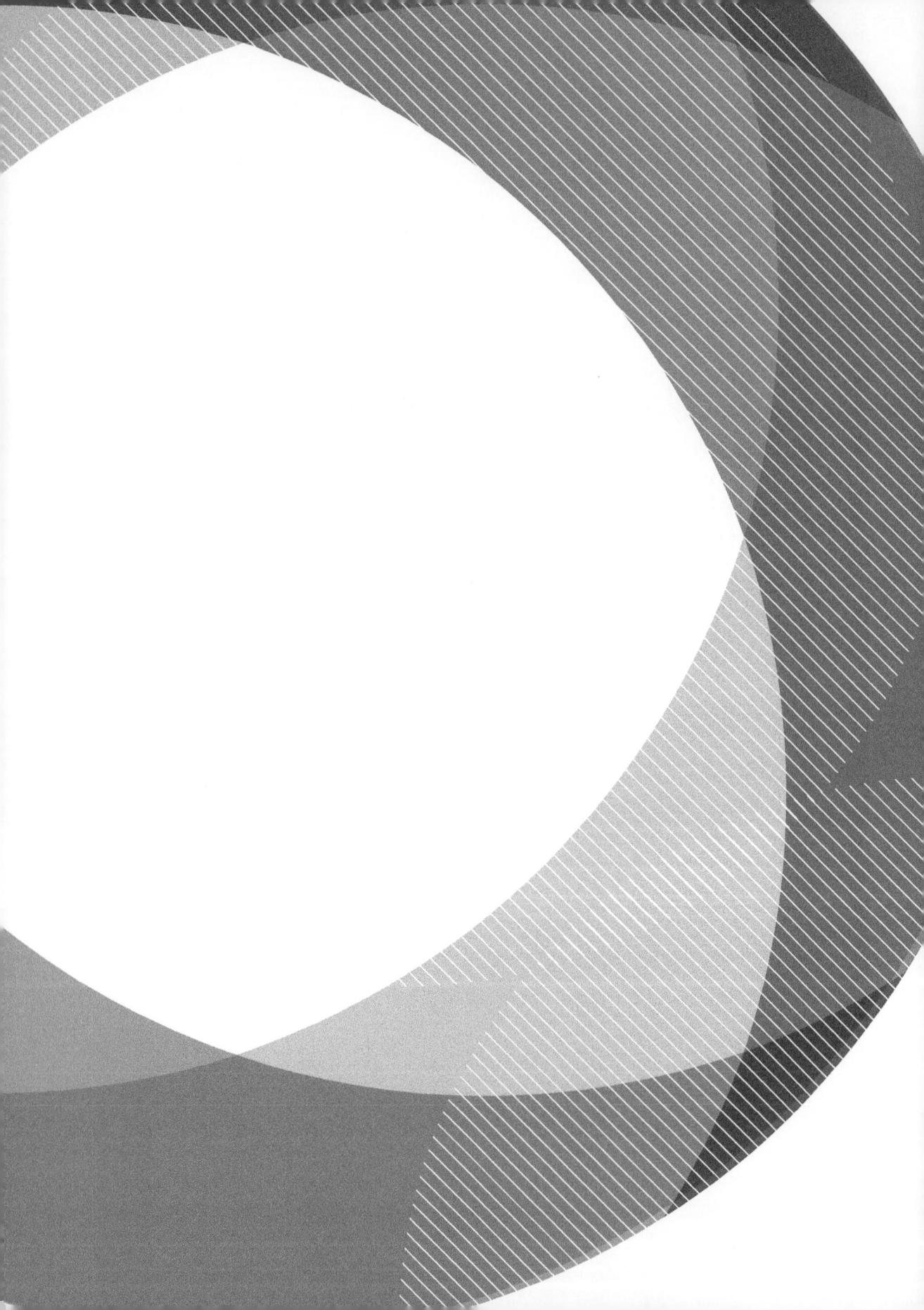

Movement Program Assessment Form

1. Walking
General overall observations of gait, with or without movement aids

Lateral view
Efficient movement

> Overall arm swing coordination with thoracic rotation

> Thorax and pelvic oppositional rotation

> Pelvifemoral motions

> Heel strike and push-off foot load transfer

> Notes on inefficient movements

2. Standing tests
Full torso rotation
Posterior and anterior views
Efficient movement

> Sequential movement from the head to feet

> Thoracic articulation from top down

> Pelvifemoral timing

> Pelvis rotates with relative femoral internal rotation

Foot and ankle articulations

> Right rotation, right foot supination and left foot pronation

> Left rotation, left foot supination and right foot pronation

> Identify and notate the efficient and inefficient movements with corresponding directions

Rotating to the right: Right side: Left side:

Rotating to the left: Right side: Left side:

Notes on inefficient movements

Hemipelvis inferior motion
Posterior view
Efficient movement

- Lumbar lateral flexion (convex side movement toward the lowering hemipelvis)

- Thorax translation opposite of lowering hemipelvis

- Hip joint internal rotation/adduction on non-dropping hemipelvis

Identify and notate the efficient and inefficient movements with corresponding directions

Right side: Left side:

Notes on inefficient movements

Hemipelvis superior motion
Posterior view
Efficient movement

- Couple movement of the superior and inferior hemipelvis

- Lumbar lateral flexion toward elevating hemipelvis

- Thoracic translation toward elevating hemipelvis thoracolumbar junction (TLJ) in midline

- Contralateral hip adduction/internal rotation

- Calcaneal inversion to plantar flex on elevating hemipelvis

Identify and notate the efficient and inefficient movements with corresponding directions

Right side: Left side:

Notes on inefficient movements

Lateral pelvic shift
Posterior and anterior views
Efficient movement

> TLJ orientated midline with S2
>
> Thoracic translation to shift direction
>
> Opposite hemipelvis 5 degrees inferior
>
> Lumbar lateral flexion toward shift direction
>
> Hip adduction/internal rotation toward shift direction (femoral glide laterally)
>
> Hip abduction/external rotation opposite of shift direction (femoral glide medially)
>
> Weight distributed on feet lateral toward shift direction, medial opposite of shift direction

Identify and notate the efficient and inefficient movements with corresponding directions

Right side: _____   Left side: _____

> Notes on inefficient movements

3. Seated tests
When seated, hip joint is 1 inch (2.5 cm) higher than knee joint

Thoracic rotation
Rotation of the thorax region in the transverse plane from cervical region to thoracolumbar junction

> Thoracic oppositional translation with rotation
>
> Weight shift on the ischial tuberosities

Hip joint and knee flexion with ankle dorsiflexion
Efficient movement

> Weight evenly distributed on ischial tuberosities
>
> Hip flexion without changes of weight on ischial tuberosities or change of torso organization

Identify and notate the efficient and inefficient movements with corresponding directions

Posterior view

Right side: _____   Left side: _____

Notes on inefficient movements

Lateral view

Right side: _____   Left side: _____

Notes on inefficient movements

Knee flexion and ankle dorsiflexion, sliding foot posteriorly, foot in contact with floor
Anterior view

Right side: _____   Left side: _____

Notes on inefficient movements

Hip flexion/abduction/external rotation
Anterior view

Right side: _____   Left side: _____

Notes on inefficient movements

Ankle dorsiflexion, lifting mid-foot and forefoot, rear foot on floor
Lateral view

Right side: Left side:

Plantar flexion, lifting rear foot and mid-foot, forefoot on floor
Lateral view

Right side: Left side:

Notes on inefficient movements

4. Sit and stand
Sit and stand from chair, three times for each view

Efficient movement

Lateral view
Hip flexion and extension

Torso angle relative to flexion and extension movements

Posterior view
TLJ orientated to midline with S2

Thorax organized to midline

Anterior view
Dorsiflexion

Hip joint centration

Torso organized to midline

Identify and notate the efficient and inefficient movements with corresponding directions

Lateral view

Right side: Left side:

Notes on inefficient movements

Posterior view

Right side: Left side:

Notes on inefficient movements

Anterior view

Right side: Left side:

Notes on inefficient movements

5. Standing balance
Time for one minute

Eyes open

Two-leg stance

One-leg stance

Cervical rotation, two-leg stance

Notes

Eyes closed

Two-leg stance

One-leg stance

Cervical rotation, two-leg stance

Notes

6. Gait

Anterior and posterior views

Each view will be a total of 5 gait cycles of 10 heel strikes

Efficient movements:

> Right step: weight transfer on to right foot
>
> Right ankle dorsiflexion and left foot push-off
>
> Pelvic rotation with oppositional thoracic rotation
>
> Arm swing amplifying thoracic rotation
>
> Left step
>
> Left ankle dorsiflexion and right foot push-off
>
> Pelvic rotation with oppositional thoracic rotation
>
> Arm swing amplifying thoracic rotation

Notes

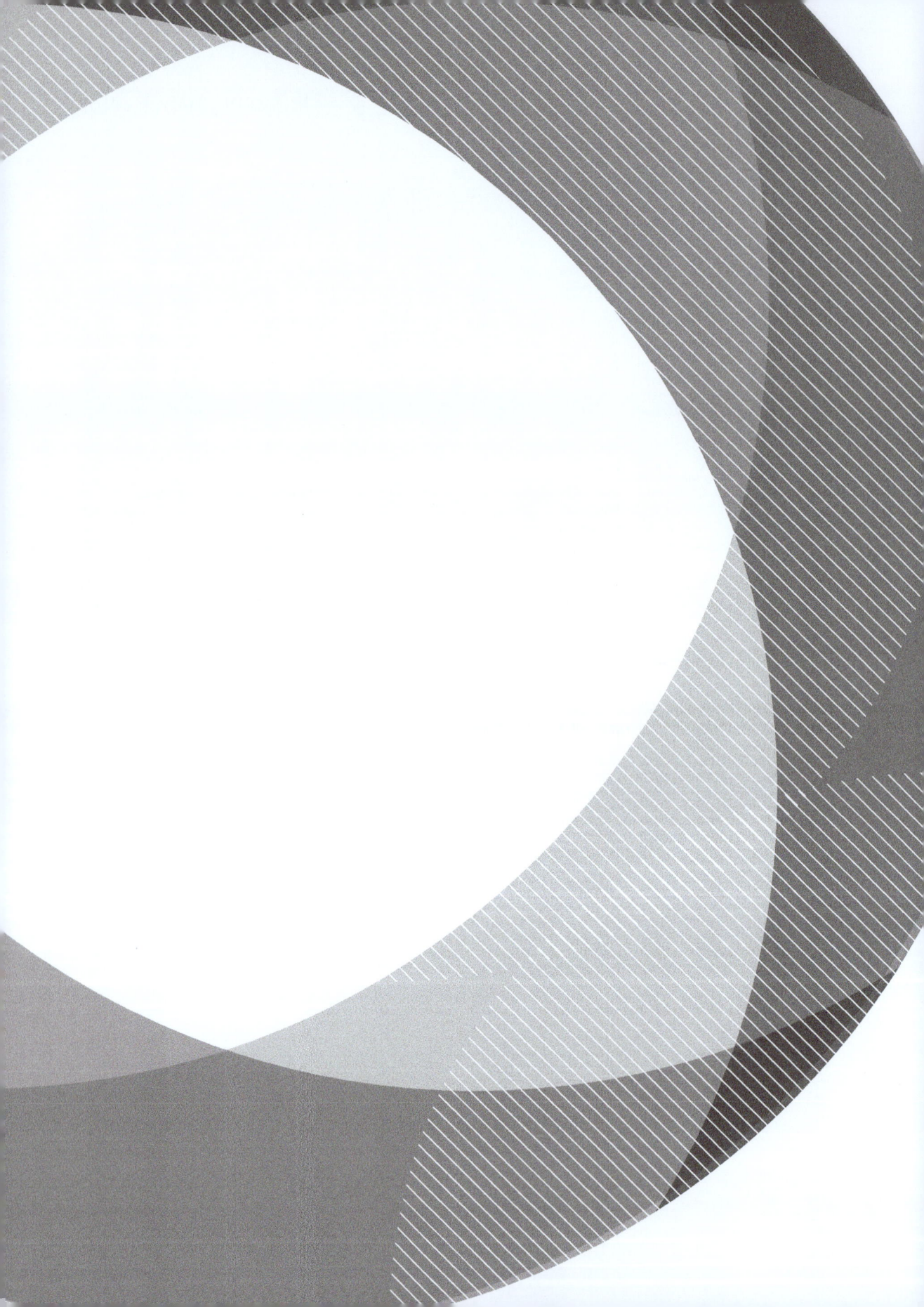

List of Equipment and Props

Equipment list via NPCE Study Guide

Universal Reformer

Trapeze Table

Wunda Chair

High Back Chair

Ladder Barrel

Spine Corrector

Magic Circle

Ped-o-Pull

Foot Corrector

Toe Corrector

Additional equipment and props

balance pad (foam pad), air cushion disc

Balansit®

balls: large, 22–26 in. (55–65 cm) in diameter; medium, 9 in. (23 cm) in diameter; small, 6 in. (15 cm) in diameter

BOSU®

carabiner

CoreAlign®

CoreAlign® resistance bands (tubing): light (peach), medium (blue), heavy (gray)

cushion/pillow, 1 in. (2.5 cm) thick

half roller

jump board

Konnector®

non-skid, rubberized pad, 7.5 x 14 x 0.5 in. (19.05 x 35.56 x 1.27 cm)

Overball

Pilates Arc®

resistance bands: light (yellow), medium (red or green), heavy (blue or black)

roller

rotator discs: no resistance, light resistance, or heavy resistance

sliders

small box

SmartSpine™

spikey balls, 4 in. (10 cm) in diameter

Stability Sling

Trapeze Table springs: very light (yellow); light (blue); medium (red); heavy (black); long springs: light (yellow); medium (purple)

Universal Reformer box, long or short orientation**

Universal Reformer springs: very light (yellow); light (blue); medium (red); heavy (green)

Universal Reformer with clinical adaption

wall ladder

wedges

Wunda Chair springs: light (white); heavy (black)

Wunda Chair with split pedal

Y-loops for feet

* The Pilates Arc® is a dense, black, foam, modular, asymmetrical version of Spine Corrector.

** The Universal Reformer box is placed in one of two directions. One is perpendicular to the long axis of the carriage and is called "short box." The other is parallel to the long axis of the carriage and is called "long box."

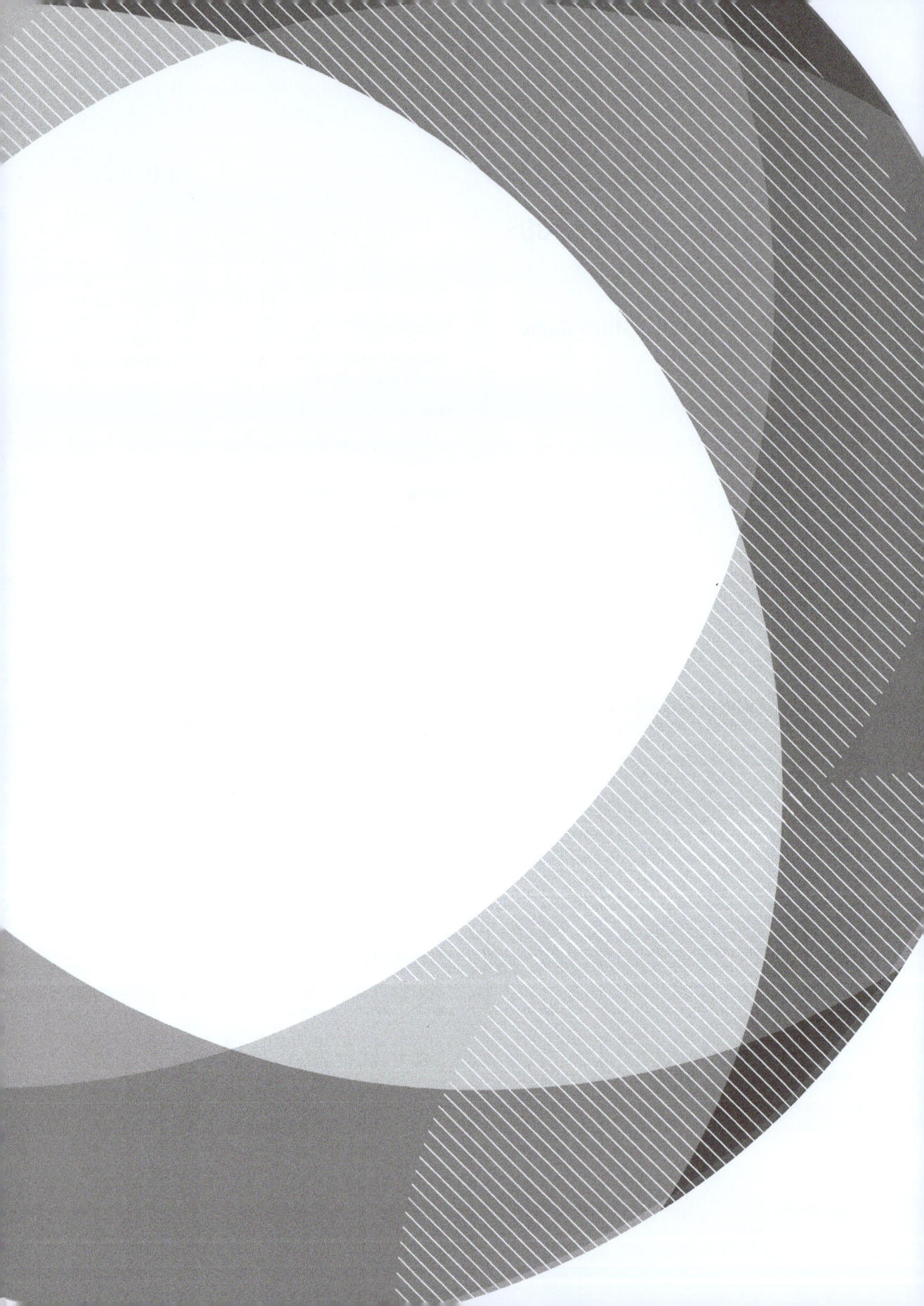

Abbreviations

ABLR	active bent leg raise		NCPT	National Certified Pilates Teacher
ADLs	activities of daily living		NPCP	National Pilates Certification Program
ASIS	anterior superior iliac spine		OA	occipitoatlantal
ASLR	active straight leg raise		PEM	post-exertional malaise
COM	center of mass		PESE	post-exertional symptom exacerbation
CT	cervicothoracic; computed tomography		PET	positron emission tomography
DIP	distal interphalangeal		PFD	pelvic floor dysfunction
DRA	diastasis recti abdominis, diastasis rectus abdominis		PIP	proximal interphalangeal
			POTS	postural orthostatic tachycardia syndrome
FABER	flexion, abduction, external rotation		PT	physical therapist; physical therapy
FAI	femoral acetabular impingement		ROM	range of motion
GHJ	glenohumeral joint		SCAN	somato (body)-cognitive (mind) action network
GT	greater trochanter		SCM	sternocleidomastoid
IAP	intra-abdominal pressure		SIJ	sacroiliac joint
ILA	inferior lateral angle		SUI	stress urinary incontinence
IRD	inter-rectus distance		TLF	thoracolumbar fascia
ISA	infrasternal angle		TLJ	thoracolumbar junction
LA	linea alba		TrA	transversus abdominis
LBP	low back pain		TRX	total resistance exercise
LE	lower extremity, lower extremities		UE	upper extremity, upper extremities
ME/CFS	myalgic encephalomyelitis/chronic fatigue syndrome		UI	urinary incontinence
			US	ultrasound
MRI	magnetic resonance imaging			
MTP	metatarsophalangeal			

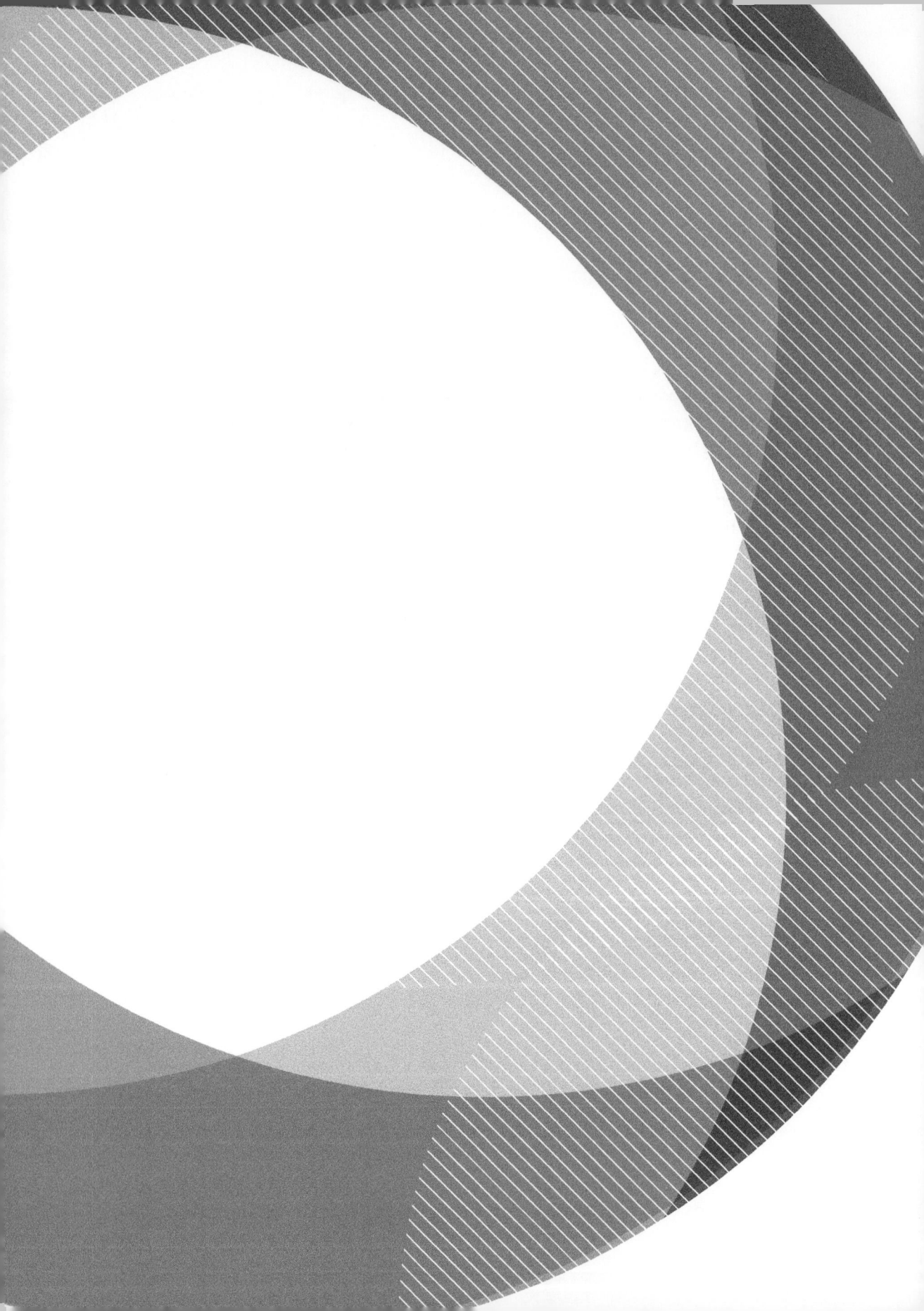

Glossary

abduction
the action of moving a limb away from the midline

activation
a stimulation of the neuromyofascial system for movement

adaptation
malleability and efficient response of the neuromyofascial system to changing conditions. Types of adaptation include fascial remodeling and reflexive responses

adduction
the action of moving a limb toward the midline

anterior
in front of or the front surface of the body

articulation
an action of creating movement through a region with anatomical congruity of the articulator surfaces and the ligaments, muscles, and fascia that support it

attenuating
refers to the reduction of magnitude of forces

auxetic
the property of a material that increases in width when "stretched." It does not narrow, become thinner and/or longer. See **stretch**

biotensegrity
a new paradigm for considering the balance of forces in a biological structure. Applied biotensegrity is an awareness of how the principles of biotensegrity are used in movement and by manual practitioners

breathe into a body area
to describe direction of the breath toward an area, stimulating activation or expansion in that region. Three-dimensional breathing is the torso's capacity to respond during inhalation in all planes of motion

clam
side lying hip joint abduction with knee flexion

closed kinematic chain
"closed kinematic chains" in biology, including human anatomy, are the coupling of multiple parts into continuous mechanical loops allowing the structure to self-regulate complex movements at all scales

compression
a force that presses or pushes together

connective tissue
provides support and framework for the body consisting of fibrous proteins and non-fibrous ground substance in varying proportions depending on their functions. This includes the tissues of muscles, fascia, fat, cartilage, bones, and blood

diaphragms
connective tissue structures at the level of the eyes (cranial diaphragm), the ring above the clavicle and shoulder girdle (thoracic outlet), the respiratory diaphragm, and the pelvic diaphragm. When these structures are activated in integrated movement they support comprehensive, whole-body movement

disassociate
a term used for intent and reasoning about treatment. To disassociate is to emphasize the articulation required for a movement task. See **articulation**

dorsiflexion
moving the dorsal surface (top) of the foot toward the shin. The articulation of the ankle occurs at the tibial talus region, the talocrural joint

elasticity
the tendency of a material to "bounce back" to its original shape after a deformation

ethmoid bone
one of the eight bones of the cranium. It is situated at the roof of the nasal cavity and between the two orbital cavities

external (lateral) rotation
the joint action of moving away from the center relative to the classical anatomical position

FABER
flexion, abduction, external rotation. These three movements combined result in a clinical pain provocation test to assist in diagnosis of pathologies at the hip, lumbar, and sacroiliac region

fascia
matrix of fibers secreted by cells that encompasses cellular structure

fascial glide
fascia facilitates movement by allowing gliding around the structures it surrounds; the ability of fascial planes and muscles to glide on each other or against other tissues

force
an effort or exertion of power

glenohumeral
the region between the scapula (shoulder blade) and the humerus (arm bone); the glenoid is the articular surface of the scapula where the head of the humerus joins forming the glenohumeral joint

ground reaction force
force exerted by the ground on a body in contact with it

hemipelvis
one half of the pelvic bone (innominate), including all the associated tissues

hip joint
the anatomical term for hip joint is "acetabulofemoral joint." The common name and most widely used term is "hip joint." The term acetabulofemoral refers to the virtual space between the head of the femur and the acetabulum of the pelvis

hip quadrant test
a physical examination test used to assess hip joint mobility and identify any restrictions in the hip joint's range of motion

idiopathic
relating to or denoting any disease or condition for which the cause is unknown

iliac crest
the superior aspect of the iliac bones that form part of the pelvis

inferior
a structure that is below another structure or directed downward

internal (medial) rotation
the joint action of moving toward the center relative to the classical anatomical position

interoception
the collection of senses signaling the internal state of the body, both conscious and unconscious; the capacity to perceive and integrate body signals generating affective states

ischial tuberosity of the ischium
one of the bilateral "sitting" bones that form part of the pelvis

kinematics
the geometry of motion

kinetics
relating to or resulting from motion

lateral
to the side of, or away from, the middle of the body

lever model
the mechanistic idea of the body as a collection of levers and pulleys operating in a uniplanar, binary, linear hierarchy

medial
toward the middle or center

menisci
Greek *meniskos*, "crescent"-shaped fibrous cartilages or "discs" that partially line a joint cavity

motor control
the process that initiates, directs, and grades purposeful movement for performing a skillful task

myofascia
"myo" refers to muscle tissue; "fascia" refers to connective tissue

parallel
a position of the legs where the second toe of each foot lines up with the mid-patella and the hip joint

pelvic list
a small degree of inferior movement of the hemipelvis

pelvifemoral
movement of the pelvis relative to the femur

plantar flexion
moving the plantar surface of the foot toward the shin. The articulation of the ankle occurs at the tibial talus region, the talocrural joint

posterior
behind or the back surface of the body

powerhouse
the cylinder of strength between the top of the pelvis and the bottom of the ribs. J. H. Pilates encouraged activation of this region to initiate all Pilates exercises (Larkam 2017)

pronation
anatomical term for rotating the distal aspects of the limbs so the plantar/palmar surface presents inferiorly; medial rotation

proprioception
the perception of the position of the body and forces acting on it

proximal
an indication of a part of a limb that is closer to the torso

reflexive stability
a motor response of the neuromyofascial system based on sensory input to a force or demand placed upon the body

sacroiliac
the region on either side of the sacrum next to the iliac bones of the pelvis

scapulohumeral rhythm
biomotion of the shoulder describing the movement of the scapula in coordination with the humerus

spiral
the spiral is a line curving continuously away from a central point

stiffness
there are distinct uses of this word with different connotations. One is a felt sense of the tissue's resistance to movement. Stiffness is a resistance to deformation. Elasticity does not just refer to the amount we can stretch. Tissue stiffness refers to the ability or capacity to restore a change in shape. In material science, stiff springs can have more elasticity than weaker springs because they store more energy and rebound more efficiently

strategies for motor control
each person has their own established motor strategies developed over a lifetime. They provide the capacity to perform a task, process sensory input, interpret dynamic activity, and respond to unpredictable, unexpected, and challenging movement

stretch
according to Jan Wilke, PhD, co-editor of *Fascia in Sport and Movement*: "The initially observed length changes during a stretch do not lead to a significant increase in strain because the collagen fibers, which are slightly wavy at rest, straighten" (Wilke 2021)

superior
a structure that is situated above another structure or directed upwards

supination
anatomical term for rotating the distal aspects of limbs so the palmar/plantar surface presents superiorly; lateral rotation

synergistic
the combining of two or more forces so that the result is more than the sum of the original two

tensegrity
tension + integrity—a term popularized by Buckminster Fuller to describe the concept of floating compression previously proposed by sculptor Kenneth Snelson

tension
a force of pulling apart

thoracolumbar
the region of the back between the thoracic (ribcage) and lumbar vertebrae

tissue
specialized regions of cellular organization between the level of the cell and the organ

translation
a term from spinal biomechanics. The ability to rotate around one axis and translate along another axis in a three-dimensional space

vector
a line that has magnitude and direction

vertical axis
the intersection of the three cardinal planes organizing around the midline of the body

vestibular
describes parts of the inner ear that control balance